MOLECULAR BASIS OF PAIN INDUCTION

MOLECULAR BASIS OF PAIN INDUCTION

Edited by

John N. Wood
Department of Biology
University College
London

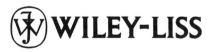
WILEY-LISS

A JOHN WILEY & SONS, INC., PUBLICATION

New York • Chichester • Weinheim • Brisbane • Singapore • Toronto

Copyright © 2000 by Wiley-Liss, Inc. All rights reserved.

Published simultaneously in Canada.

No part of this publication may be reproduced, stored in a retrieval system or transmitted in any
form or by any means, electronic, mechanical, photocopying, recording, scanning or otherwise,
except as permitted under Sections 107 or 108 of the 1976 United States Copyright Act, without
either the prior written permission of the Publisher, or authorization through payment of the
appropriate per-copy fee to the Copyright Clearance Center, 222 Rosewood Drive, Danvers, MA
01923, (978) 750-8400, fax (978) 750-4744. Requests to the Publisher for permission should be
addressed to the Permissions Department, John Wiley & Sons, Inc., 605 Third Avenue, New York,
NY 10158-0012, (212) 850-6011, fax (212) 850-6008, E-Mail: PERMREQ@WILEY.COM.

For ordering and customer service, call, 1(800)-CALLWILEY.

Library of Congress Cataloging-in-Publication Data:
Molecular basis of pain induction / edited by John N. Wood.
    p. cm.
   Includes bibliographical references and index.
   ISBN 0-471-34607-1 (alk. paper)
   1. Pain—Molecular aspects. 2. Nociceptors. I. Wood, John N.
  [DNLM: 1. Pain—physiopathology. 2. Nociceptors—physiology. WL
  704 M718 2000]
  QP451.4.M65 2000
  612.8′8—dc21
  DNLM/DLC   99-29232

Printed in the United States of America.

10 9 8 7 6 5 4 3 2 1

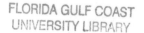

■■■■■ CONTENTS

Progress in almost every area of present-day biology is dominated by the contribution of genetics. The peripheral nervous system is no exception. Among the approaches that have revolutionized our understanding of sensory neuron development and function have been homology, expression, and difference cloning studies, which have replaced mysterious pharmacological targets with defined channels, receptors, and regulatory proteins.

In this volume we focus on recent molecular genetic studies that have given us insights into the development and function of nociceptors. New approaches to identifying transcripts present in sensory neurons are covered, as is the development of the nociceptor and its activation by a variety of chemical thermal and mechanical stimuli. There are a number of related books that complement this work. The comprehensive *Sensory Neurons* edited by Sherryl Scott focuses on much of the physiological, histochemical, and pharmacological characterization of sensory neurons, whilst the IASP volume entitled *Molecular Neurobiology of Pain* edited by David Borsook focuses on inflammation, nerve injury, and futuristic pain therapies. The present work focuses on the properties of pain-sensing sensory neurons (nociceptors) and recent advances in our understanding of their development; phenotypic variability; chemical, mechanical, and thermal activation; and mechanisms of peripheral hyperalgesia. The use of mouse null mutants is a major theme running through the book, and as problems of genetic background and behavioral studies become more widely appreciated and progress is made with tissue-specific and inducible knockouts, such animals are likely to become more and more informative. Many thanks to all the authors who participated in this work.

JOHN N. WOOD

Nicole Abson, Molecular Nociception Group, Department of Biology, University College London, London WC1E 6BT, England

Armen N. Akopian, Molecular Nociception Group, Department of Biology, University College London, London WC1E 6BT, England

David L. H. Bennett, Department of Physiology, St. Thomas' Hospital Medical School/UMDS, Lambeth Palace Road, London SE1 7EH, England

Chih-Cheng Chen, Molecular Nociception Group, Department of Biology, University College London, London WC1E 6BT, England

Michael Costigan, Neural Plasticity Research Group, Department of Anesthesia and Critical Care, Massachusetts General Hospital, Harvard Medical School, Boston, MA 02129

Alun M. Davies, School of Biomedical Sciences, Bute Medical Building, University of St. Andrews, St. Andrews, Fife KY16 9TS, Scotland

Carmen de Felipe, Instituto de Neurociencias, Universidad Miguel Hernandez, Ap. Correos 374, 03080 Alicante, Spain

Christopher A. Doyle, Faculty of Medicine, University of Manchester, G38 Stopford Building, Oxford Road, Manchester M13 9PT England

Steven England, Pfizer Central Research, Sandwich, Kent CT13 9NJ, England

Rey Garcia, Molecular Nociception Group, Department of Biology, University College London, London WC1E 6BT, England

Raymond G. Hill, Merck Sharp and Dohme Research Laboratories, Neuroscience Research Centre, Terlings Park, Harlow, Essex CM20 2QR, England

Stephen P. Hunt, Neurobiology Division, MRC Laboratory of Molecular Biology, Hills Road, Cambridge CB2 2QH, England

Iain F. James, Novartis Institute for Medical Sciences, Gower Place, London WC1E 6BN, England

Gary R. Lewin, Growth Factors and Regeneration Group, Max-Delbrück-Center for Molecular Medicine, Robert Rossle Strasse, Berlin-Buch, D-13122, Germany

Anastasia Liapi, Molecular Nociception Group, Department of Biology, University College London, London WC1E 6BT, England

Jeanette Longmore, Merck Sharp and Dohme Research Laboratories, Neuroscience Research Centre, Terlings Park, Harlow, Essex CM20 2QR, England

Richard J. Mannion, Neural Plasticity Research Group, Department of Anesthesia and Critical Care, Massachusetts General Hospital, Harvard Medical School, Boston, MA 02129

Stephen B. McMahon, Department of Physiology, St. Thomas' Hospital Medical School/UMDS, Lambeth Palace Road, London SE1 7EH, England

John A. O'Brien, Neurobiology Division, MRC Laboratory of Molecular Biology, Hills Road, Cambridge CB2 2QH, England

Kenji Okuse, Molecular Nociception Group, Department of Biology, University College London, London WC1E 6BT, England

James A. Palmer, Neurobiology Division, MRC Laboratory of Molecular Biology, Hills Road, Cambridge CB2 2QH, England

Nadia M. J. Rupniak, Merck Sharp and Dohme Research Laboratories, Neuroscience Research Centre, Terlings Park, Harlow, Essex CM20 2QR, England

Dinah W. Y. Sah, Biogen, Cambridge, MA

Inmaculada Silos-Santiago, Department of Neurobiology, Millennium Pharmaceuticals, Inc., Cambridge, MA 02139

Veronika Souslova, Molecular Nociception Group, Department of Biology, University College London, London WC1E 6BT, England

Cheryl L. Stucky, Growth Factors and Regeneration Group, Max-Delbrück-Center for Molecular Medicine, Robert Rossle Strasse, Berlin-Buch D-13122, Germany

Madhu Sukumaran, Molecular Nociception Group, Department of Biology, University College London, London WC1E 6BT, England

Ted Usdin, Section on Genetics, National Institute of Mental Health, Building 36, Room 3D06, Bethesda, MD 20892

John N. Wood, Molecular Nociception Group, Department of Biology, University College London, London WC1E 6BT, England

Clifford J. Woolf, Neural Plasticity Research Group, Department of Anesthesia and Critical Care, Massachusetts General Hospital, Harvard Medical School, Boston, MA 02129

Andreas Zimmer, Section on Genetics, National Institute of Mental Health, Building 36, Room 3D06, Bethesda, MD 20892

CHAPTER 1

Genetic Approaches to Nociceptor Development

NICOLE ABSON, MADHU SUKUMARAN, AND JOHN N. WOOD

University College
London

1.1 INTRODUCTION

A variety of cloning strategies have been used to define regulators of mammalian peripheral neuron phenotype. In this chapter we overview the embryonic origins of sensory neurons and current ideas about transcription factors that may play a role in regulating peripheral neurogenesis. The vast majority of information has come from the mapping and characterization of sensory neuron mutants in simple multicellular organisms, followed by homology cloning in rodents and the generation of mouse null mutants.

1.2 EMBRYONIC ORIGINS OF SENSORY NEURONS

Sensory neurons of the trunk originate from the neural crest, a transient population of migratory cells that emerges from the dorsal part of the neural tube. The neural crest is a pluripotent tissue that gives rise to sympathetic neurons, glia, chromaffin cells of the adrenal medulla, and melanocytes, in addition to sensory neurons. In the cephalic region, sensory neurons arise not only from the neural folds, but also from placodes, specialized areas of epithelium. Placodes give rise to ciliary and cranial sensory ganglia, glia, and to the mesectoderm, which forms much of the skeletal and connective tissues of the head.[1]

Le Douarin exploited the fact that chick-quail chimaeras allow transplanted cells and their descendants from quail embryos to be recognized un-

Molecular Basis of Pain Induction, Edited by John N. Wood
ISBN 0-471-34607-1   Copyright © 2000 by Wiley-Liss, Inc. All rights reserved.

ambiguously at later stages of development within chick hosts. Fate mapping using such chimaeras showed that neural crest of the trunk is regionalized with respect to development of the autonomic nervous system: Vagal crest (adjacent to somites 1 to 7) gives rise to enteric ganglia; trunk crest (somites 7 to 28) gives rise to sympathetic ganglia, aortic and adrenal plexuses, and the adrenal medullary paraganglia; lumbosacral crest (dorsal to somite 28) and crest derived from the region between somites 5 and 7 give rise to both enteric and sympathetic ganglia. However, crest from all these regions gives rise to the sensory nervous system.

In addition to spatial fate restriction, crest also shows temporal restriction. Weston and Butler[2] performed transplants of ^{3}H-labeled neural tube between chick embryos of differing developmental ages. They showed that the crest emerging from older neural tubes was still capable of generating all crest derivatives of that axial level if placed in a younger host environment. However, crest emerging from young neural tubes placed in older embryos formed dorsal crest derivatives, but virtually no sympathetic neurons, a ventral derivative. Hence the crest itself is still multipotent at the later age, but the older host environment restricts its endogenous potential such that it generates only dorsal derivatives. Serbedzija et al.[3,4] used fluorescent dye injection into developing chick and mouse neural tube lumen, and later into single neural tube cells[5] at various stages of development to confirm and expand these results, providing good evidence that neural crest cells populate their derivatives in a ventral-to-dorsal order.

Are neural crest cells specified before, during, or after migration; and do the cells undergo progressive restriction in fate or are individual cell types specified directly from pluripotent crest? It is important to distinguish between irreversibly committed cells, whose potential is restricted regardless of the permissiveness of the environment, and reversibly specified cells, whose fate has been selected but which can be respecified if given the appropriate environmental stimuli. Experiments analyzing the fate of individual cells during normal development show only cell specification, not their maximum potential. In vitro clonal analysis and heterotypic tissue transplants show the potential of the cell population as a whole, but usually reveal little about the commitment of individual cells since subpopulations may be being selected by the new environment.

1.2.1   In Vitro Studies

Sieber-Blum and Cohen[6] showed that single avian crest cells cultured in vitro could form adrenergic, sensory-like, and pigmented cells. More recently, multipotent crest stem cells have been isolated in vitro from both the rat and the mouse.[7] These and other studies (reviewed in Stemple and Anderson[8]) show the existence of multipotent progenitors within the early neural crest. However, the same experiments also show the concomitant existence of cells with more restricted developmental fates, despite being exposed to the same culture conditions as were the multipotent cells. Stemple and Anderson's stem cell culture goes furthest in showing that these cells are committed progenitors since the primary crest cell clones underwent a secondary round of cloning in identical culture conditions. Seventy-five percent of the originally isolated crest cells gave rise to at least one secondary clone containing neurons, glia, and other cells, demonstrating multipotency and suggesting continued stem cell potential in some of the progeny. However, many of the cells produced during the two rounds of cloning showed restricted potentials, despite being in an environment permissive to the stem cell phenotype. Some of these blast cells produced only neuronal or glial progeny, while others generated clones containing both glial cells and other cells, or both glial and neuronal cells.

1.2.2 In Vivo Studies

Such results are complemented by in vivo studies involving vital dye labeling of individual cells. Bronner-Fraser and Fraser[9] injected a fluorescent dextran into individual cells of dorsal chick neural tube or of somitic sclerotome containing migrating neural crest and observed the extent of the resulting clones 1 to 2 days later, and Serbedzija et al.[5] performed a similar set of neural tube injection experiments in mouse embryos. In both cases many of the resultant clones spanned more than one crest derivative, even when the original cell was migrating, and clones giving rise to both sensory and sympathetic neurons, in addition to putative Schwann cells were identified.

Together, these experiments demonstrate the existence of both multipotent cells and of cells with more restricted developmental fates, since in all cases some clones contained only a single derivative or a subset of derivatives. Specification of crest could therefore be due to a sequential process whereby progenitors of increasingly restricted developmental fate are generated. The variety of clones generated at any given time and position implies that specification of all progenitors for a given subset of crest derivatives does not occur simultaneously. Different clones may also show overlap in the derivatives they form, indicating that a number of different pathways can be used to generate any given postmitotic cell type.

1.2.3 External Influences on Sensory Neuron Development

Crest cells are responsive to environmental influences, since alterations in culture conditions can influence their fate. A series of heterotypic transplantation studies[1] show that alterations in the axial position, and therefore environment, of neural tube influences the fate of emerging crest. Evidence that multipotent crest is instructively influenced by the environment comes again from the work of Stemple and Anderson,[7] who found that neural crest cells cultured on fibronectin would not differentiate into neurons but that transfer to poly-D-lysine fibronectin allowed them to express their neurogenic potential. Serial subcloning showed that this was not simply selection of a subpopulation of already committed cells.

Many experiments thus support the view that premigratory crest is heterogeneous in potential. During migration, the crest becomes progressively more restricted in its potential, and this is due at least partly to environmental factors instructively influencing individual cells. At all stages, including postmigration, crest retains a greater potential than is ever expressed during normal development, which can only be revealed by experimental manipulation. We are now beginning to elucidate the methods of specification by identifying the proteins and genes involved in this process.

1.2.4   Diffusible Signaling Molecules

Among the diffusible signaling molecules implicated in cell fate specification are the neurotrophins, discussed elsewhere in this book. Other factors include:

1. *Leukemia inhibitory factor* (LIF) can promote the formation of sensory neurons (as identified by expression of substance P) from murine crest cultures and has been implicated as one of the factors promoting the initial differentiation step of the sensory neuron lineage.[10] Subsequently, a small population of sensory neurons requires LIF during development, rising to over 90% by birth.[11] In apparent contradiction to these results, mice carrying null deletions in their *LIF* genes show no overt neuronal changes, suggesting that functional redundancy may be occurring.[12]

2. *Fibroblast growth factors* (FGF) 1 and 2 have been implicated in stimulating proliferation of neural crest cells and have been shown to inhibit their differentiation, probably as a direct role of their mitogenic activity. This correlates with the expression of their genes in mouse neural tube and dorsal root ganglion (DRG) at the stage when cells are proliferating within the ganglia.[11] However, FGF1 can also promote neuronal differentiation in vitro when presented in a cell-associated context.[13]

3. *Hepatocyte growth factor* (HGF) is also involved in sensory neuron development.[14] In vitro, it cooperates with NGF to enhance axonal outgrowth from DRG neurons, and mice with mutations in the HGF receptor have a severe reduction in the number of nerves innervating the skin of the limbs and thorax.

4. *TGF-β family members,* in particular the bone morphogenic proteins (BMPs), play an important role in specifying dorsal cell fates in the neural tube, including neural crest cell fate. These dorsal cell types are induced by a contact-dependent signal from the epidermal ectoderm, which can be mimicked by BMP4 and BMP7 and which is inhibited by BMP antagonists.[15] Both BMP4 and BMP7 are expressed transiently in the dorsal ectoderm prior to neural crest specification, then subsequently in the roof-plate glia. They are therefore good candidates for a role in the induction of neural crest. At later stages there is evidence that BMPs, or related molecules such as activin A, induce at least two different dorsal interneuron cell types in the neural tube. Within peripheral nervous system (PNS) tissue, BMP2/4 can instructively promote the differentiation of clonal crest cell cultures into sympathetic neurons.[16] It can also enhance the formation of adrenergic sympathetic neurons in vitro and when expressed ectopically in the developing embryo, as can BMP7.[17]

Another TGF-β family member, glial cell line–derived neurotrophic factor (GDNF), promotes the development of neurons, including autonomic neurons, from crest cultures.[18] However, during embryogenesis, peripheral neurons do not appear to depend on GDNF for their survival. In early postnatal life, a small subset of putatively nociceptive DRG neurons develop GDNF dependency, and it has been shown that GDNF can rescue postnatal axotomized sensory neurons.[19,20]

1.2.5 Extracellular Matrix

In vitro evidence that the extracellular matrix (ECM) is also involved in directing the fate of sensory progenitors comes from the work of Stemple and Anderson[7] on fibronectin. In vitro studies have also shown that laminin, fibronectin, and type IV collagen make good substrates for crest cell migration, while others, such as tenascin, vitronectin, and various proteoglycans, are inhibitory. This correlates well with the expression of these molecules during development, with migration-permissive ECM found along crest migratory routes, and with nonpermissive ECM within surrounding areas (reviewed by Perris[21]). Mouse null mutations have shown that fibronectin, type IV collagen, and gamma 1–containing laminin isoforms might all be crucial for crest development.[21,22] In the enteric nervous system, mutations in the endothelin B receptor, a protein that binds to components of the ECM and is expressed by enteric ganglion cell progenitors, result in agangliogenesis of the colon.[23]

1.3 REGULATORY GENES INVOLVED IN PERIPHERAL NEUROGENESIS

1.3.1 Homology Cloning Strategies

A variety of genetic approaches have led to the identification of important regulators of cell fate during sensory neurogenesis. The conservation of developmental mechanisms across evolution means that lower organisms such as the fruit fly, *Drosophila melanogaster,* or nematode, *Caenorhabditis elegans,* are useful for genetic studies since their short generation times, small size, and relatively simple body plans make generation and identification of genetically mutant organisms feasible. In addition, they provide experimentally amenable systems in which to deduce the roles of new factors and to identify interacting proteins.

To date, most work has been performed with *Drosophila.* In *C. elegans,* stereotyped patterns of cell division, a small number of cells, and a transparent body have allowed[24] every neuron to be identified, and laser ablation studies have allowed the determination of interactions between these cells both during development and in adulthood.[25] More recently, the zebra fish, *Danio rerio,* has become a popular model system,[26] as it is a vertebrate with a relatively small genome and transparent embryos that develop ex utero.

Pioneering work on *Drosophila* by Nusslein-Volhard, Wieschaus, and colleagues, who performed large-scale mutagenesis, followed by isolation and breeding of mutant flies,[27] led to a detailed understanding of the gene cascades involved in laying out the *Drosophila* body plan and opened the way for analysis of other developmental processes. In *Drosophila* PNS, the thoracic and abdominal sensory neurons of the embryo form in stereotyped positions and can now all be identified using cell-specific markers.[28] Analysis of mutant PNS phenotypes has allowed regulatory genes involved in PNS development to be identified, and these genes can be divided into four major categories: proneural, neurogenic, neuronal type selector, and cell lineage.[29] Proneural genes are expressed by clusters of epidermal cells and endow them with the potential to become neuronal. Subsequent interactions between these competent cells, mediated by expression of the neurogenic genes lead to selection in most cases of a single cell from the cluster, the sensory mother cell (SMC). This cell expresses high levels of proneural genes and will give rise to the sense organ, while the remaining cells in the cluster lose proneural gene expression and differentiate into epidermal cells. Neuronal type selector genes are expressed in SMCs and control the type of sensory structure to which a precursor will give rise. Finally, cell lineage genes control the specification of the various clonally related cell types within the sensory organ (e.g., neuron, glia, or structural cell). Vertebrate homologs of a number of these *Drosophila* genes and of a few *C. elegans* genes have been identified, mainly through homology cloning. Table 1.1 summarizes many of the genes involved in *Drosophila* or *C. elegans* neural development whose mammalian homologs are known, and some of these are discussed further below.

TABLE 1.1   Invertebrate and Vertebrate Homologs as Regulators of Peripheral Neurogenesis[a]

Vertebrate Genes		Invertebrate Genes	
Genes	Comments	Genes	Comments
Proneural Genes (thought to endow cells with the potential to become neuronal precursors)			
Mash-1 (rat, mouse)	Required for development of many olfactory, enteric, and auto-nomic neurons	**Achaete–scute complex (AS-C)** Achaete, Scute, lethal of scute, asense. (*Drosophila*)	Basic HLH proteins required for external sense organ specification
CASH-1 (chick) **HASH-1** (human) **XASH1** **XASH3a, 3b** (*Xenopus*)	Xash3 converts prospective neural crest (NC) and ectodermal cells to a CNS fate		
Quox-1 (quail)	Expressed in a subpopulation of NC cells in early migration; later expressed by sensory but not sympathetic neurons	**mab-5** (*C. elegans*)	Specifies post-embryonic fates of cells in a posterior region
MATH-1, 2, 3 (mouse)	Basic HLH proteins; MATH-1 expressed in dorsal CNS during development	**Atonal** (*Drosophila*)	Basic HLH protein; specifies precursors of chordotonal organs and a class of photoreceptors
		lin-32 (*C. elegans*)	Basic HLH protein of AS-C family that acts down-stream of mab-5; necessary and in some cases sufficient for the specification of neuroblast cell fate

(continued)

TABLE 1.1 (Continued)

Vertebrate Genes		Invertebrate Genes	
Genes	Comments	Genes	Comments
Id (mouse)	HLH protein involved in neural determination and differentiation; expressed in DRG but not in sympathetic or adrenal medulla neurons	**extramacrochaetae** (*Drosophila*)	Suppressor of sensilla development; HLH protein that forms inactive heterodimers with products of the AS-C and with daughterless
snail (mouse) **sna-1** (zebra fish) **Xsna** (*Xenopus*)	Expressed in presumptive NC cells and roof plate cells; expression continues in NC cells during their migration	**snail (sna)** (*Drosophila*)	Zn finger protein required to initiate mesoderm invagination; represses genes responsible for neuroectoderm differentiation; later expressed in developing NS, first segmentally, then universally
slug (mouse)	Controls the epithelial to mesenchymal transition of premigratory NC cells		

Neuronal Genes (required during the selection of neuronal precursors from clusters of cells with the potential to become neurons; includes the neurogenic genes)

Notch-1 to 4 (rat, mouse, chick)	Transmembrane proteins involved in cell fate decisions; Notch-1 to 3 are expressed in the developing nervous system	**Notch** (*Drosophila*)	Acts as receptor in intracellular signaling events which lead to selection of cell(s) from within an equivalence group; used repeatedly in NS development
TAN-1 (human) = Notch-1			
int-3 (human) = Notch-4			
Xotch (*Xenopus*)			
		lin-12 (*C. elegans*)	Acts as receptor in intracellular signaling events that determine cell fates; see **glp-1**

(continued)

TABLE 1.1 (Continued)

Vertebrate Genes		Invertebrate Genes	
Genes	Comments	Genes	Comments
Delta-like gene 1 (mouse) **C-Delta-1** (chick) **Jagged-1** (rat) **(= Serrate-1)** (mouse) **Jagged-2** (rat) **C-Serrate-1** (chick)	Transmembrane ligands for Notch; involved in cell fate decisions	**Delta (D1)** (*Drosophila*) **Serrate** (*Drosophila*)	Transmembrane proteins which act as extracellular ligands for Notch
RBP-Jk **(= CBF1/KBF2)**	DNA-binding protein involved in nervous system differentiation; activated Notch binds to RBP-Jk, leading to trans-cription of downstream genes	**Suppressor of Hairless (Su(H))** (*Drosophila*)	First downstream target of activated Notch; found in both cytoplasm and nucleus and can bind directly to the Notch cytoplasmic domain
HES-1 to 5 (rat) **TLE family** (human)	Human homologs of E(spl) groucho; negative regu-lators of genes with E or N boxes in their promoters	**Enhancer of split complex (E(spl))** (*Drosophila*)	Seven basic HLH transcription factors required for normal sensory neuorgenesis; activated by Su(H) genes
HuD (human) **elavA,B,C,D** (mouse, *Xenopus,* zebra fish)	RNA-binding protein expressed in postmitotic CNS neurons C and D are ex-pressed only in brain	**elav** (embryonic lethal abnormal vision) (*Drosophila*)	RNA-binding protein required for correct dif-ferentiation and maintenance of neurons

Neuronal Specificity Genes (required for the generation of neuronal subtypes)

cux-1, cux-2 (mouse) **cut** (chick, human)	Homeodomain proteins; cux-1 and 2 bind to NCAM promoter; cux-1 shown to regulate NCAM promoter ex-pression; cux-2 is expressed	**cut** (*Drosophila*)	Homeodomain protein necessary and sufficient for the specification of external sen-sory (es) organ precursor cells; loss of cut activity results in conver-sion of es

(continued)

TABLE 1.1 (Continued)

Vertebrate Genes		Invertebrate Genes	
Genes	Comments	Genes	Comments
	exclusively in the nervous system		receptors to chordotonal organs
Prox-1 (mouse)	Expressed in subsets of developing neurons; thought to play a role in early development of murine CNS	**Prospero** (*Drosophila*)	Nuclear homeo-domain protein expressed in subsets of developing neurons and required for their correct speci-fication; mutation leads to delayed or arrested pio-neering of peripheral motor nerves
neurogenins ngn-1, ngn-2 (mouse, rat) **ngn-related-1 (ngnr-1)** (*Xenopus*)	Basic HLH proteins expressed by tissues imme-diately prior to their neuro-genesis; thought to be involved in neuronal determination; overexpression of ngnr-1 promotes neurogenesis	**tap** (*Drosophila*)	Basic HLH protein expressed in those neurons innervating chemosensory organs at the time of their differentiation
neuro-D (*Xenopus*)	Basic HLH protein expressed by sensory but not automatic neurons; induces neurogenesis in ectodernal tissue		
Chx10 (mouse)	Homeodomain protein expressed in neural tissues, including anterior optic vessicle; thought to be involved in	**ceh-10** (*C. elegans*)	Homeodomain protein expressed in an interneuron receiving signals from a thermosensitive

(continued)

TABLE 1.1 (Continued)

Vertebrate Genes		Invertebrate Genes	
Genes	Comments	Genes	Comments
	determination of inner nuclear layer of mature retina		photosensitive sensory neuron
Phox-2 (mouse)	Homeodomain and paired box protein expressed in autonomic but not sensory ganglia; possibly involved in expression of (nor)adrenergic phenotype; binds to and regulates NCAM promoter	**paired** (*Drosophila*)	Homeodomain and paired box transcription factor required for correct segmentation of the *Drosophila* embryo
Brn-3a (Brn-3.0) (rat, mouse, chick)	POU domain protein; required for development of subsets of sensory and CNS neurons	**unc-86** (*C. elegans*)	POU domain protein necessary for the specification of subsets of neurons, including touch receptors; required for postmitotic development of many neurons
Brn-3b (Brn-3.2) (rat, mouse, chick)	POU domain protein; essential for development of most retinal ganglion cells		
Brn-3c (Brn-3.1) (rat, mouse, chick)	POU domain protein; essential for development of hair cells of inner ear	**I-POU, tI-POU** (*Drosophila*)	POU domain proteins from alternatively spliced gene; expressed in developing neural tissue
Isl1, Isl2 (rat, mouse, chick, *Xenopus*)	LIM-homeodomain proteins expressed in developing sensory and motor neurons; Isl1 essential for generation of motor neurons	**Isl** (*Drosophila*)	LIM homeodomain protein required for axonal pathfinding by primary neurons

(continued)

TABLE 1.1 (Continued)

Vertebrate Genes		Invertebrate Genes	
Genes	Comments	Genes	Comments
DRG11 (rat)	Homeodomain and paired box protein expressed in sensory neurons and a subset of their CNS targets	**unc-4** (*C. elegans*)	Homeodomain and paired box protein required for correct synaptic input to a subset of motorneurons
PHD-1 (rat)	Expressed at lateral margins of ventricular zone in neural tube; thought to act downstream of MASH-1		

[a] NC, neural crest; AS-C, achaete-scute complex; HLH, helix–loop–helix; Zn, zinc; (C)NS, (central) nervous system; NCAM, neural cell adhesion molecule.

1.3.2 Achaete, Scute, and Mash-1

Mash-1, the mammalian homolog of two of the *Drosophila* achaete–scute complex (AS-C) genes, *achaete* and *scute,* was one of the first mammalian PNS genes identified via its homology with invertebrate genes. *Achaete* and *scute* are proneural genes and endow cells with the competence to become SMCs of either external sense (es) organs or of some types of multidendritic neuron. Their overexpression leads to many of the cells within *achaete-* or *scute*-expressing clusters generating sensory organs, while null mutations in these genes leads to loss of subsets of sensory organs. The products of the *achaete* and *scute* genes contain the basic helix–loop–helix (bHLH) motif, which allows protein dimerization and DNA binding. They act as transcriptional regulators controlling sense organ specification.

Johnson et al.[30] used PCR to identify two new rat genes, *mammalian achaete-scute homolog (Mash) 1* and *2,* which are highly conserved across the bHLH domain but diverge both from one another and from the AS-C genes outside this region. *Mash-1* is expressed exclusively in the nervous system, in the olfactory epithelium, in sympathetic and enteric precursors, and in some parasympathetic precursors, but not in sensory neurons.[31,32] Generation of mice containing a null mutation in the *Mash-1* gene showed that this gene is essential for the development of olfactory, sympathetic, parasympathetic, and some enteric neurons.[32]

Achaete and *scute* are required at the earliest stage of neuronal development, ruling over the choice between epidermal and sense organ fate, and its early expression reflects this role. *Mash-1,* however, is required only after segregation of glia and neurons has occurred. It plays no role in the formation of glia but is required to allow neuronal precursors to develop into neurons. For example, Sommer et al.[33] used primary cultures and immortalized cell lines generated from both wild-type and *Mash-1* mutant neural crest to provide evidence for the existence of a committed autonomic neuronal precursor. This cell type expresses a number of neuron-specific genes, including *NF160* and *c-ret,* but its further development, and expression of later neuronal genes such as *SCG10,* appear to require Mash-1 expression.

Many attempts have been made to try to identify further mammalian homologs of *achaete* and *scute* expressed at much earlier stages. *Xash-3* in *Xenopus* is a potential candidate,[34] but no mammalian homolog of this has yet been found. These results imply that *Mash-1* is the closest mammalian homolog to *achaete* and *scute.* It is possible that the evolutionary sequence conservation observed may reflect restrictions imposed by complex interactions with other conserved regulatory genes and the promoters of their downstream targets. Functions of the entire regulatory network may have gradually changed during evolution, but precise interactions within the network have prevented the occurrence of extensive sequence divergence. Some support for this comes from the *Drosophila* genes *daughterless, extramacrochaete, hairy, enhancer of split,* and *Notch,* all of which interact with AS-C genes in *Drosophila.* Mammalian homologs have now been identified for all these genes (Table 1.1), and evidence for their interactions with Mash-1 and one another, homologous to the interactions of their *Drosophila* homologs, is emerging. These and other results (e.g., the Notch/Delta signaling system) suggest that not only is there sequence conservation and functional conservation of individual genes, but that such conservation extends to regulatory networks of interacting genes.

1.3.3   Atonal Homologs

A number of HLH proteins related to the *Drosophila* proneural *atonal* gene have been identified in the mammalian nervous system, and a picture of the regulatory hierarchy that results in vertebrate sensory neurogenesis is now emerging.[35] In the peripheral nervous system, the atonal homologs neurogenin-1 and 2 can induce the expression of NeuroD and the formation of neuronal cells from ectodermal precursors.[36] These bHLH proteins thus appear to be neural determination genes.[37] Deletion of neurogenin 1 or 2 in transgenic mice results in the deletion of complementary subsets of proximal and distal cranial ganglia, respectively, as well as complex effects on the developing central nervous system (CNS).[38-40] Interestingly, Neurogenin-1 up-regulates a Delta-like gene and is in turn down-regulated by Notch signaling.[37,39] These genes thus appear to act at an early stage in neuronal determination, but the pathways between their appearance and the expression of later transcriptional regulators that may specify neuronal subtypes and the receptors for growth factors that finally sculpt the mature nervous system are still under investigation. Interestingly the birth of DRG nociceptive neurons is known to occur slightly later than that of other sensory neurons, and it appears that the small diameter sensory neurons expressing TrkA require the expression of Neurogenin 1, whilst larger neurons expressing TrkB and C require neurogenin-2.[61] The regulators of mature nociceptor function are of more immediate interest in the study of pain mechanisms, and POU (*Pit-Oct-Unc*) domain proteins, which may play a role in both cell-type specification and gene regulation in mature tissues, are of particular interest.

1.3.4 Unc-86 and Brn-3a, b, and c

Unc-86 encodes a *C. elegans* transcription factor identified through an uncoordinated phenotype of *unc-86* mutants.[41] It is required for the specification and differentiation of a number of sensory neurons and interneurons, including mechanosensory neurons, many of which are unrelated by lineage and do not share any obvious terminally differentiated phenotype. In *unc-86* mutants, daughter cells from several neuroblast lineages retain the phenotype of their mothers, leading to reiteration of the maternal lineage rather than the generation of phenotypically distinct daughters. A number of these cells undergo inappropriate cell death, while others differentiate into functionally incorrect neurons. During normal development of these affected lineages, *unc-86* is expressed after asymmetric division in only one of the two daughter cells. In all cases except one, *unc-86* expression is maintained in all the progeny of that daughter. Expression of *unc-86* is therefore required to allow daughter cells to differ from their mothers and from one another. In addition to its involvement in neuronal cell lineage, *unc-86* is also expressed in a large number of postmitotic neurons, where it is required, in at least some cases, for correct differentiation.[42] The role of this transcription factor is therefore strongly dependent on the context in which it is expressed.

Finney et al.[43] showed that the *unc-86* gene encodes a protein containing a homeodomain, and comparison with mammalian proteins led to the additional identification of a novel DNA-binding domain, the POU domain. POU domain proteins now constitute a large family of transcriptional regulators, expressed in distinct spatiotemporal expression patterns during development.[44,45] Sequence conservation across the POU domain has been used repeatedly in the homology cloning of new family members, including the

Brn-3 genes, which appear to be the mammalian homologs of *unc-86,* sharing extensive homology both in the POU domain and in an amino-terminal domain characteristic of class IV POU domain proteins. The three *Brn-3* genes are expressed predominantly within the nervous system, often at around the time of the last mitotic divisions in these tissues. Compared with the role of *unc-86* in the correct differentiation of a number of postmitotic neurons, these expression patterns suggest roles similar to those for the *Brn-3* genes in neuronal differentiation. However, unlike *unc-86,* expression of the *Brn-3* genes is probably restricted to postmitotic cells, ruling out roles in progenitor cell fate specification similar to those performed by the invertebrate gene.

One of the proteins shown to interact with unc-86 protein is the neural-specific mec-3, a member of the LIM-HD family of transcriptional regulators, which contain both a cysteine-rich LIM domain and a homeodomain. *Unc-86* is required in the lineage specification of a number of cells, including touch cells, which also express *mec-3*. Mutations in the *mec-3* gene do not affect the lineage of these cells but act at the differentiation stage, leading to their apparent transformation into other neuronal types.[41] It has been demonstrated that unc-86 is necessary for the activation of *mec-3* and that unc-86 and mec-3 proteins bind to the *mec-3* promoter cooperatively and are required for maintenance of *mec-3* expression.[46,47] Unc-86 and mec-3 are also both required for expression of the touch cell–specific *mec-7* gene, which encodes a β-tubulin.[41] A related LIM domain protein, Islet-1, is also expressed in developing mouse sensory neurons and is required for the formation of these and other cell types.

Brn-3a expression is detected in mouse at E9.5, appearing initially in spinal cord, then in cranial and sensory ganglia, retinal ganglion cells, and in regions of the brain, excluding the telencephalon.[45] The majority of *Brn-3a* expression is within the nervous system, although it has also been detected in the developing immune system and at low levels in the pituitary gland.[46] The expression patterns in many tissues are maintained through to adulthood.

A POU domain protein highly related to Brn-3a, named Brn-3b, is initially coexpressed in sensory ganglia, spinal cord, hindbrain, and midbrain.[47] However, *Brn-3b* expression often first appears 1 or 2 days later than *Brn-3a,* and as development progresses, the retina and PNS continue to coexpress the two genes, whereas in the CNS, the expression patterns rapidly diverge. In the adult, no *Brn-3b* expression could be detected in brain or in mature sensory neurons and only very low levels in the retina.[48]

Brn-3c shows a more restricted expression pattern than that of either of the other *Brn-3* genes.[49] In DRG and retinal ganglion cells, where high levels of *Brn-3c* are observed, there is evidence that the cells expressing *Brn-3c* constitute a subset of those expressing the other two *Brn-3* genes.[49,50] In situ hybridization patterns in other areas are not incompatible with the expression of *Brn-3c* only in subsets of *Brn-3a-* or *Brn-3b*-expressing cells, except in the cochlea, where only *Brn-3c* is found. Within the rat DRG, *Brn-3c* expression starts at around E12, when the cells are still dividing, and continues throughout development,[49] suggesting that it may be involved in the specification, development, or function of subclasses of sensory neurons.

Mice lacking *Brn-3a* exhibit a severe phenotype with defective suckling, uncoordinated limb movements, and death within 24 h of birth. Anatomical examination reveals a selective loss of subsets of those brainstem and trigeminal ganglion neurons that normally express *Brn-3a,* and correlations between the anatomical and behavioral defects can be identified.[51] The major phenotype in mice lacking *Brn-3b* is the loss of most retinal ganglion cells.[48,52] Mice heterozygous for a *Brn-3c* null allele appear normal in all respects, but *Brn-3c* homozygous null mutant mice *(Brn-3c$^{-/-}$)* exhibit complete deafness. By examining the inner ear of postnatal (P)0 and P14 mice, Erkman et al.[50] showed that the deafness was due to a failure of the sensory hair cells within the organ of Corti to differentiate. By P14 no hair cells can be identified and most spiral ganglion cells have also degenerated. Similar results were obtained by Xiang et al.[53] Disappointingly, no detailed analysis of the properties of DRG sensory neurons in Brn-3c null mutants has been carried out. However, in humans, a mutation in the human homolog of Brn-3c, named POU4F3, results in progressive hearing loss, but there are no reported abnormalities in other aspects of mechanosensation.[54,55]

A common theme in the actions of many POU domain proteins is their involvement both during the development of a given cell subtype, and subsequently in the transcriptional regulation of one or more genes expressed by that cell type. This may also hold true for the *Brn-3* genes, whose expression in a number of tissues continues into adulthood. Support for this idea comes from the in vitro findings that both Brn-3a and Brn-3c can activate the promoter of the neuronal intermediate filament gene α-internexin,[56] Brn-3a can activate the promoters of the three neurofilament genes,[57] and Brn-3b can activate the neuronal nicotinic acetylcholine receptor α2 subunit gene promoter.[58] Further work is now required to identify targets of the *Brn-3* genes farther downstream, which may be of particular interest if in the case of Brn-3c they include mechanoreceptive genes.

1.3.5   DRG11

By combining PCR with degenerate primers that hybridize with transcription factor family members, combined with differential hybridization screens, a novel paired homeobox transcription factor that is expressed exclusively in small-diameter sensory neurons and their dorsal horn spinal neuronal targets was identified.[59] This protein, named DRG11, is a homeodomain protein that is a candidate regulator of nociceptor phenotype, as it is found in TrkA-positive neurons but not in glia or sympathetic neurons.

1.4 CONCLUSIONS

Many of the genetic mechanisms involved in sensory neuron specification are conserved to a greater or lesser extent across evolution. A better understanding of the regulation of these programs of gene expression may eventually have practical significance in terms of pain therapies, not only in understanding the genetic repertoires that define the limits of sensory neuron plasticity, but also in providing new targets for analgesic drugs that modulate the production of sensory neuron receptors and channels involved in nociception.[60]

ACKNOWLEDGMENTS

We thank the Wellcome Trust, the Medical Research Council, and the Royal Society for their support.

REFERENCES

1. Le Douarin, N. M. (1982). The neural crest, Cambridge University Press, Cambridge.
2. Weston, J. A., and Butler, S. L. (1966). Temporal factors affecting localisation of neural crest cells in the chicken embryo. Dev. Biol. 14:246–266.
3. Serbedzija, G. N., Fraser, S. E., and Bronner-Fraser, M. (1990). Pathways of trunk neural crest migration in the mouse embryo as revealed by vital dye labelling. Development 108:605–612.
4. Serbedzija, G. N., Bronner-Fraser, M., and Fraser, S. E. (1989). A vital dye analysis of the timing and pathways of avian neural crest cell migration. Development 106:809–819.
5. Serbedzija, G. N., Bronner-Fraser, M., and Fraser, S. E. (1994). Developmental potential of trunk neural crest cells in the mouse. Development 120:1709–1718.
6. Sieber-Blum, M., and Cohen, A. M. (1980). Clonal analysis of quail neural crest cells: they are pluripotent and differentiate in vitro in the absence of non-crest cells. Dev. Biol. 80:96–106.
7. Stemple, D. L., and Anderson, D. J. (1992). Isolation of a stem cell for neurons and glia from the mammalian neural crest. Cell 71:973–985.

8. Stemple, D. L., and Anderson, D. J. (1993). Lineage diversification of the neural crest: in vitro investigations. Dev. Biol. 159:12–23.

9. Bronner-Fraser, M., and Fraser, S. E. (1991). Cell lineage analysis of the avian neural crest. Dev. Suppl. 2:17–22.

10. Murphy, M., Reid, K., Brown, M. A., and Bartlett, P. F. (1993). Involvement of leukemia inhibitory factor and nerve growth factor in the development of dorsal root ganglion neurons. Development 117:1173–1182.

11. Murphy, M., Reid, K., Ford, M., Furness, J. B., and Bartlett, P. F. (1994). FGF2 regulates proliferation of neural crest cells, with subsequent neuronal differentiation regulated by LIF or related factors. Development 120:3519–3528.

12. Stewart, C. L., Kaspar, P., Brunet, L. J., Bhatt, H., Gadi, I., Kontgen, F., and Abbondanzo, S. J. (1992). Blastocyst implantation depends on maternal expression of leukaemia inhibitory factor. Nature Sept. 3; 359(6390):76–79.

13. Brill, G., Vaisman, N., Neufeld, G., and Kalcheim, C. (1992). BHK-21-derived cell lines that produce basic fibroblast growth factor, but not parental BHK-21 cells, initiate neuronal differentiation of neural crest progenitors. Development 115(4):1059–1069.

14. Maina, F., Hilton, M. C., Ponzetto, C., Davies, A. M., and Klein, R. (1997). Met receptor signaling is required for sensory nerve development and HGF promotes axonal growth and survival of sensory neurons. Genes Dev. 11:3341–3350.

15. Liem, K. F., Jr., Tremml, G., Roelink, H., and Jessell, T. M. (1995). Dorsal differentiation of neural plate cells induced by BMP-mediated signals from ectoderm. Cell 82(6):969–979.

16. Shah, N. M., Groves, A. K., and Anderson, D. J. (1996). alternative neural crest cell fates are instructively promoted by TGFβ superfamily members. Cell 85:331–343.

17. Reissmann, E., Ernsberger, U., Francis-West, P. H., Rueger, D., Brickell, P. M., and Rohrer, H. (1996). Involvement of bone morphogenetic protein-4 and bone morphogenetic protein-7 in the differentiation of the adrenergic phenotype in developing sympathetic neurons. Development 122:2079–2088.

18. Maxwell, G. D., Reid, K., Elefanty, A., Bartlett, P. F., and Murphy, M. (1996). Glial cell line–derived neurotrophic factor promotes the development of adrenergic neurons in mouse neural crest cultures. Proc. Natl. Acad. Sci. USA 93:13274–13279.

19. Molliver, D. C., Wright, D. E., Leitner, M. L., Parsadanian, A. S., Doster, K., Wen, D., Yan, Q., and Snider, W. D. (1997). IB4-binding DRG neurones switch from NGF to GDNF dependence in early postnatal life. Neuron 19:849–861.

20. Matheson, C. R., Carnahan, J., Urich, J. L., Bocangel, D., Zhang, T. J., and Yan, Q. (1997). Glial cell line–derived neurotrophic factor (GDNF) is a neurotrophic factor for sensory neurons: comparison with the effects of the neurotrophins. J. Neurobiol. 32:22–32.

21. Perris, R. (1997). The extracellular matrix in neural crest-cell migration. TINS 20:23–31.

22. George, E. L., Georges-Labouesse, E. N., Patel-King, R. S., Rayburn, H., and Hynes, R. O. (1993). Defects in mesoderm, neural tube and vascular development in mouse embryos lacking fibronectin. Development 119:1079–1091.

23. Hosoda, K., Hammer, R. E., Richardson, J. A., Baynash, A. G., Cheung, J. C., Giaid, A., and Yanagisawa, M. (1994). Targeted and natural (piebald-lethal) mutations of endothelin-B receptor gene produce megacolon associated with spotted coat color in mice. Cell 79:1267–1276.

24. Brenner, S. (1974). The genetics of *Caenorhabditis elegans.* Genetics 77:71–94.

25. Chalfie, M., Sulston, J. E., White, J. G., Southgate, E., Thomson, J. N., and Brenner, S. (1985). The neural circuit for touch sensitivity in *Caenorhabditis elegans.* J. Neurosci. 5:956–964.

26. Mullins, M. C., Hammerschmidt, M., Haffter, P., and Nusslein-Volhard, C. (1994). Large-scale mutagenesis in the zebrafish: in search of genes controlling development in a vertebrate. Curr. Biol. 4:189–202.

27. Nusslein-Volhard, C., and Wieschaus, E. (1980). Mutations affecting segment number and polarity in *Drosophila.* Nature 287(5785):795–801.

28. Campos-Ortega, J. A., and Hartenstein, V. (1985). In: The embryogenic development of *Drosophila melanogaster,* Springer-Verlag, New York, pp. 1–227.

29. Ghysen, A., Dambly-Chaudiere, C., Jan, L. Y., and Jan, Y.-N. (1993). Cell interactions and gene interactions in peripheral neurogenesis. Genes Dev. 7:723–733.

30. Johnson, J. E., Birren, S. J., and Anderson, D. J. (1990). Two rat homologues of *Drosophila achaete-scute* specifically expressed in neuronal precursors. Nature 346:858–861.

31. Guillemot, F., Lo, L.-C., Johnson, J. E., Auerbach, A., Anderson, D. J., and Joyner, A. L. (1993). Mammalian *achaete-scute* homologue 1 is required for the early development of olfactory and autonomic neurons. Cell 75:463–476.

32. Guillemot, F., and Joyner, A. L. (1993). Dynamic expression of the murine *achaete-scute* homologue *Mash-1* in the developing nervous system. Mech. Dev. 42:171–185.

33. Sommer, L., Shah, N., Rao, M., and Anderson, D. J. (1995). The cellular function of MASH1 in autonomic neurogenesis. Neuron 15:1245–1258.

34. Zimmerman, K., Shih, J., Bars, J., Collazo, A., and Anderson, D. J. (1993). XASH-3, a novel *Xenopus achaete-scute* homolog, provides an early marker of planar neural induction and position along the mediolateral axis of the neural plate. Development 119:221–232.

35. Ma, Q., Kintner, C., and Anderson, D. J. (1996). Identification of neurogenin, a vertebrate neuronal determination gene. Cell Oct. 4; 87(1):43–52.

36. Lee, J. E., Hollenberg, S. M., Snider, L., Turner, D. L., Lipnick, N., and Weintraub, H. (1995). Conversion of *Xenopus* ectoderm into neurons by neuroD, a basic helix–loop–helix protein. Science 268:836–844.

37. Ma, Q., Sommer, L., Cserjesi, P., and Anderson, D. J. (1997). Mash1 and neurogenin1 expression patterns define complementary domains of neuroepithelium

in the developing CNS and are correlated with regions expressing notch ligands. J. Neurosci. May 15; 17(10):3644–3652.

38. Schwab, M. H., Druffel-Augustin, S., Gass, P., Jung, M., Klugmann, M., Batholomae, A., Rossner, M. J., and Nave, K. A. (1998). Neuronal basic helix–loop–helix proteins (NEX, neuroD, NDRF): spatiotemporal expression and targeted disruption of the NEX gene in transgenic mice. J. Neurosci. 18(4):1408–1418.

39. Ma, Q., Chen, Z., del Barco Barrantes, I., Luis de la Pompa, J., and Anderson, D. J. (1998). Neurogenin 1 is essential for the determination of neuronal precursors for proximal cranial sensory ganglia. Neuron 20:469–482.

40. Fode, C., Gradwohl, G., Morin, X., Dierich, A., Lemeur, M., Goridis, C., and Guillemot, F. (1998). Neurogenin 2 is a determination factor for epibranchial placode derived sensory neurons. Neuron 20:483–494.

41. Chalfie, M., and Sulston, J. E. (1981). Developmental genetics of the mechanosensory neurons of *C. elegans*. Dev. Biol. 82:358–370.

42. Finney, M., and Ruvkun, G. (1990). The *unc-86* gene product couples cell lineage and cell identity in *C. elegans*. Cell 63:895–905.

43. Finney, M., Ruvkun, G., and Horvitz, H. R. (1988). The *C. elegans* cell lineage and differentiation gene *unc-86* encodes a protein containing a homeodomain and extended sequence similarity to mammalian transcription factors. Cell 55:757–769.

44. Wegner, M., Drolet, D. W., and Rosenfeld, M. G. (1993). POU-domain proteins: structure and function of developmental regulators. Curr. Opin. Cell Biol. June; 5(3):488–498.

45. He, X., Treacy, M. N., Simmons, D. M., Ingraham, H. A., Swanson, L. W., and Rosenfeld, M. G. (1989). Expression of a large family of POU-domain regulatory genes in mammalian brain development. Nature 340(6228):35–41.

46. Xue, D., Finney, M., Ruvkun, G., and Chalfie, M. (1992). Regulation of the *mec-3* gene by the *C. elegans* homeoproteins unc-86 and mec-3. EMBO J. 11:4969–4979.

47. Xue, D., Tu, Y., and Chalfie, M. (1993). Cooperative interactions between the *Caenorhabditis elegans* homeoproteins unc-86 and mec-3. Science 261: 1324–1328.

48. Gerrero, M. R., McEvilly, R. J., Turner, E., Lin, C. R., O'Connell, S., Jenne, K. J., Hobbs, M. V., and Rosenfeld, M. G. (1993). Brn-3.0: a POU-domain protein expressed in the sensory, immune, and endocrine systems that functions on elements distinct from known octamer motifs. Proc. Natl. Acad. Sci. USA 90: 10841–10845.

49. Turner, E. E., Jenne, K. J., and Rosenfeld, M. G. (1994). Brn-3.2: a Brn-3-related transcription factor with distinctive central nervous system expression and regulation by retinoic acid. Neuron 1:205–218.

50. Erkman, L., McEvilly, R. J., Luo, L., Ryan, A. K., Hooshmand, F., O'Connell, S. M., Keithley, E. M., Rapaport, D. H., Ryan, A. F., and Rosenfeld, M. G. (1996). Role of transcription factors Brn-3.1 and Brn-3.2 in auditory and visual system development. Nature 381:603–606.

51. Ninkina, N. N., Stevens, G. E. M., Wood, J. N., and Richardson, W. D. (1993). A novel *Brn-3*-like POU transcription factor expressed in subsets of rat sensory and spinal cord neurones. Nucleic Acids Res. 21:3175–3182.

52. Xiang, M., Zhou, L., Make, J. P., Yoshioka, T., Hendry, S. H., Eddy, R. L., Shows, T. B., and Nathans, J. (1995). The Brn-3 family of POU-domain factors: primary structure, binding specificity, and expression in subsets of retinal ganglion cells and somatosensory neurons. J. Neurosci. 15:4762–4785.

53. Xiang, M., Gan, L., Zhou, L., Klein, W. H., and Nathans, J. (1996). Targeted deletion of the mouse POU domain gene *Brn-3a* causes a selective loss of neurons in the brainstem and trigeminal ganglion, uncoordinated limb movement, and impaired suckling. Proc. Natl. Acad. Sci. USA 93:11950–11955.

54. Xiang, M., Gan, L., Li, D., Chen, Z. Y., Zhou, L., O'Malley, B. W., Jr., Klein, W., and Nathans, J. (1997). Essential role of POU-domain factor Brn-3c in auditory and vestibular hair cell development. Proc. Natl. Acad. Sci. USA 94:9445–9450.

55. Vahava, O., Morell, R., Lynch, E. D., Weiss, S., Kagan, M. E., Ahituv, N., Morrow, J. E., Lee, M. K., Skvorak, A. B., Morton, C. C., Blumenfeld, A., Frydman, M., Friedman, T. B., King, M. C., and Avraham, K. B. (1998). Mutation in transcription factor POU4F3 associated with inherited progressive hearing loss in humans. Science Mar. 20; 279(5358):1950–1954.

56. Budhram-Mahadeo, V., Morris, P. J., Lakin, N. D., Theil, T., Ching, G. Y., Lillycrop, K. A., Moroy, T., Liem, R. K., and Latchman, D. S. (1995). Activation of the alpha-internexin promoter by the Brn-3a transcription factor is dependent on the N-terminal region of the protein. J. Biol. Chem. 270:2853–2858.

57. Smith, M. D., Morris, P. J., Dawson, S. J., Schwartz, M. L., Schlaepfer, W. W., and Latchman, D. S. (1997). Coordinate induction of the three neurofilament genes by the Brn-3a transcription factor. J. Biol. Chem. 272:21325–21333.

58. Milton, N. G., Bessis, A., Changeux, J.-P., and Latchman, D. S. (1995). The neuronal nicotinic acetylcholine receptor a2 subunit gene promoter is activated by the Brn-3b POU family transcription factor and not by Brn-3a or Brn-3c. J. Biol. Chem. 270:15143–15147.

59. Saito, T., Greenwood, A., Sun, Q., and Anderson, D. J. (1995). Identification by differential RT-PCR of a novel paired homeodomain protein specifically expressed in sensory neurons and a subset of their CNS targets. Mol. Cell Neurosci. 3:280–292.

60. Akopian, A. N., Abson, N. C., and Wood, J. N. (1996). Molecular genetic approaches to nociceptor development and function. TINS 19:240–245.

61. Ma, Q., Fode, C., Guillemot, F., and Anderson, D. J. (1999). Neurogenin 1 and 2 control two distinct waves of neurogenesis in developing DRG. Genes Dev 13:1717–1728.

CHAPTER 2

Neurotrophic Factor Requirements of Developing Sensory Neurons

ALUN M. DAVIES

University of St. Andrews
St. Andrews, Scotland

2.1 INTRODUCTION

Neurons are generated in excess in the developing vertebrate nervous system, superfluous neurons being eliminated during a phase of cell death that occurs shortly after their axons reach their targets. The relative ease with which different populations of sensory neurons can be studied in culture from the earliest stages of their development together with in vivo studies of sensory neurons in normal and mutant mice has generated a great wealth of information about the factors that regulate their survival. A very complex picture is emerging of multiple neurotrophic factors acting on different kinds of sensory neurons at various stages of their development. Neurotrophic factors are not only synthesized by the peripheral and central targets of sensory neurons but also by cells lying en route to these targets and by some sensory neurons themselves. Despite this complexity, some general principles have emerged. Most sensory neurons survive initially independent of neurotrophic factors. For some populations of sensory neurons the duration of neurotrophic factor independence is related to the distance and time it takes their axons to reach their targets, suggesting that these neurons may not require trophic support until they start innervating their targets. Other populations of sensory neurons have only a brief period or neurotrophic factor independence and may require trophic support from the cells that lie en route to their targets. These neurons switch their neurotrophic factor requirements from one set of neurotrophins to another early in their development. During

Molecular Basis of Pain Induction, Edited by John N. Wood

the stage of development when the number of neurons is matched to the requirements of their target fields by a phase of cell death, the neurotrophin survival requirements of sensory neurons are related to their sensory modality. In addition to regulating neuronal survival, neurotrophic factors influence several other aspects of sensory neuron development, including the growth and branching of sensory axons and the regulation of neuropeptide expression. The latter aspects of sensory neuronal development are beyond the scope of the present review, which is focused exclusively on regulation of neuronal survival by neurotrophic factors.

2.2   NEUROTROPHIC FACTOR INDEPENDENCE

The observation that neurites grow from trigeminal ganglion explants independent of added neurotrophins at the stage when axons normally emerge from this ganglion in vivo led to the suggestion that neurons initially survive and grow independent of such factors.[1] This assumption has been strengthened by studies involving (1) dissociated cultures of early sympathetic and sensory neurons,[2,3] which eliminate the possibility of direct trophic support from contiguous cells in explant cultures; (2) single neuron cultures,[4] which eliminate the possibility of trophic support from other cells in mixed dissociated cultures; and (3) cultures of early neurons grown in completely defined medium,[5] which eliminate the possibility that the complex mixtures of factors present in the serum supplements used in previous studies could have promoted neuronal survival.

Although early neurons are able to survive in culture medium that has not been supplemented with neurotrophins, it is possible that they are dependent on neurotrophins for survival but obtain these by an autocrine route. Although there is direct experimental evidence for the operation of a brain-derived neurotrophic factor (BDNF) autocrine loop in a subset of early dorsal root ganglion neurons, this appears to play a role in enhancing an early maturational change in these neurons but has no effect on survival.[4] A BDNF autocrine loop may, however, be important in sustaining the survival of a subset of adult dorsal root ganglion (DRG) neurons.[6]

Evidence that the duration of neurotrophin independence is correlated with target distance for certain populations of developing sensory neurons has come from comparative studies of the survival of placode-derived cranial sensory neurons of the chicken embryo. The neurons of the vestibular, geniculate, petrosal, and nodose ganglia are derived from neurogenic placodes that are born over the same period of development and start extending axons to their targets at approximately the same time, but the distances the axons have to grow to reach their peripheral and central targets differ greatly. Vestibular neurons have the closest targets, geniculate and petrosal neurons have more distant targets, and nodose neurons have the most distant targets. Although the rate at which these neurons extend axons to their targets is correlated with target distance,[7] it nonetheless takes longer for the axons of neurons with more distant targets to reach these targets.[8] When grown in low-density dissociated cultures early in their development, these neurons die at different rates in the absence of neurotrophins: vestibular neurons die rapidly, nodose neurons die very slowly, and geniculate and petrosal neurons die at intermediate rates,[8] suggesting that the duration of neurotrophin independence is correlated with the distance and time it takes the axons of these neurons to reach their targets where BDNF is synthesized.[9]

The majority of vestibular, geniculate, petrosal, and nodose neurons become dependent on BDNF for survival with time in culture. As with the duration of neurotrophin independence, the timing of these survival responses and the expression of the BDNF tyrosine kinase receptor (TrkB) are correlated with target distance.[8,9] Studies of the survival of neurons that differentiate from the corresponding placodal cells in culture suggest that progenitor cells present in neurogenic placodes are specified to differentiate into neurons with the appropriate survival characteristics.[8] Heterotopic grafting of the regions of head ectoderm from which vestibular and nodose neurons derive suggest that the ectodermal cells becomes so specified only after the placodes have formed.[10]

Unlike populations of placode-derived sensory neurons, which have a regulated period of neurotrophin-independent survival related to target distance, other populations of sensory neurons survive only briefly in culture without neurotrophins during the earliest stages of their development. Many of these neurons switch their survival requirements from one set of neurotrophins to another during an early stage in their development, as outlined below.

2.3 NEUROTROPHIN SWITCHING IN EARLY DEVELOPMENTAL STAGES

The most comprehensive evidence that neurons switch their neurotrophin survival requirements during an early stage of their development has come from detailed in vitro and in vivo studies of the trigeminal ganglion neurons of the mouse embryo. When these neurons are grown at very low density in defined medium at E10, the stage when the earliest trigeminal axons are starting to grow to their targets, they initially survive independently of neurotrophins. Between 24 and 48 h in vitro, corresponding to the time when the earliest trigeminal axons approach their peripheral targets in vivo, the neurons die unless BDNF or neurotrophin-3 (NT3) is present in the culture medium.[5,11]

Although nerve growth factor (NGF) has a negligible effect on the survival of E10 trigeminal neurons, in cultures established at later stages, NGF supports an increasing proportion of the neurons. Concomitant with the acquisition of NGF dependence, responsiveness to BDNF and NT3 is rapidly lost in all neurons except a small subset. During the switchover period there is negligible additional neuronal survival in cultures containing NGF plus BDNF or NT3, indicating that the neurons pass through a phase when they are capable of responding to each of these neurotrophins.[5] Moreover, lack of an additive effect between NGF and BDNF or NGF and NT3 on neuronal survival in E11 and E12 cultures suggests that there are not completely separate subsets of NGF-, BDNF-, and NT3-responsive neurons in the ganglion during this stage of development but that many neurons coexpress functionally significant levels of different Trk receptors. Single-cell PCR has indeed shown that individual neurons in the developing rat trigeminal ganglion do coexpress mRNAs encoding different trk receptors.[12] Because neurons are generated in the trigeminal ganglion up to at least E13[13] and the majority of neurons respond to NGF by E12, it is likely that only neurons born in the early stages of ganglion formation switch neurotrophin responsiveness from BDNF and NT3 to NGF and that late-born neurons do not pass through a transient period of responsiveness to BDNF and NT3 before becoming NGF responsive, but respond to NGF from the outset. Indeed, direct evidence that this is the case has recently been obtained using bromo-deoxyuridine (BrdU) incorporation in vivo to identify late-born neurons which respond predominantly to NGF in culture, not BDNF or NT3 (Y. Enokido and A.M. Davies, unpublished results).

The acquisition and loss of responsiveness to different neurotrophins is not, however, a simple on–off phenomenon occurring at a defined stage in development. As neurons mature in vivo, the length of time they are able to survive with BDNF or NT3 in vitro decreases with age, whereas the length of time they are able to survive with NGF increases with age.[11] The dose responses of the neurons to BDNF and NT3 also shift by several orders of magnitude to higher concentrations with age.[14]

The physiological relevance of in vitro studies of neurotrophin switching in developing trigeminal neurons has been confirmed by studying the timing of neuronal death in the trigeminal ganglia of embryos that have null mutations in the neurotrophin genes and in the *trkA, trkB,* and *trkC* genes, which encode receptor tyrosine kinases for NGF, BDNF, and NT3, respectively. In *trkB*[-/-] embryos, the number of trigeminal neurons undergoing apoptosis is increased markedly during the early developmental stages when neurons are responsive to BDNF in vitro. In *trkA*[-/-] embryos, neuronal apoptosis is markedly elevated later in development when neurons are responsive to NGF in vitro.[15] Thus many neurons depend on trkB signaling for survival in the early trigeminal ganglion before becoming dependent on trkA signaling. Although early trigeminal neurons survive in culture equally well with either of the two preferred trkB ligands, BDNF and NT4,[16] BDNF appears to be the physiologically relevant trkB ligand for these neurons in vivo because there is a significant reduction in the neuronal complement of the neonatal trigeminal ganglia of $BDNF^{-/-}$ mice[17,18] but not $NT4^{-/-}$ mice.[19,20] Furthermore, excess loss of trigeminal neurons takes place in $BDNF^{-/-}$ embryos early in development (P. Ernfors, personal communication).

There is also a large decrease in the neuronal complement of the trigeminal ganglion of $NT3^{-/-}$ embryos before the peak of naturally occurring neuronal death,[21,22] implying that like BDNF, endogenous NT3 is also required at an early stage in trigeminal ganglion development. There are, however, conflicting views on the precise role of NT3 in the ganglion during this stage. It has been reported that the majority of the dying cells in the early trigeminal ganglia of $NT3^{-/-}$ embryos had incorporated BrdU administered 5 h earlier and expressed nestin, a marker for precursor cells. This, together with finding that there is a reduction in the number of proliferating cells in early trigeminal ganglia of $NT3^{-/-}$ embryos led to the conclusion that NT3 promotes the survival of proliferating precursor cells.[21] In contrast, the complement of neurons and nonneuronal cells (mostly precursor cells) is unchanged in the trigeminal ganglia of $NT3^{-/-}$ embryos during the earliest stages of gangliogenesis at E10.5, and subsequent rapid depletion of neurons occurs initially without significant change in the number of nonneuronal cells and proliferating cells in the ganglion, suggesting that NT3 acts as a survival factor for at least a proportion of early neurons.[22]

It is unlikely that the response of early trigeminal neurons to NT3 is mediated by its preferred receptor, trkC, because there is not a marked loss of neurons in the early trigeminal ganglia of $trkC^{-/-}$ embryos.[15] However, because the survival of early trigeminal neurons depends on trkB and not trkA signaling[15] and because NT3 is able to promote the survival of embryonic sensory neurons by signaling via trkB,[23] it is likely that NT3 acts on early trigeminal neurons predominantly via trkB.

Corresponding changes in the expression of neurotrophins and their receptors accompany the changing survival requirements of developing trigeminal neurons. BDNF and NT3 mRNAs are expressed in the peripheral trigeminal territory prior to arrival of the earliest sensory axons,[5,24] and NGF mRNA and protein are expressed later with the arrival of sensory axons.[25] The levels of BDNF and NT3 mRNAs are initially highest in the mesenchyme through which the axons grow to the periphery,[5,22,24] whereas NGF mRNA is expressed predominantly in the target field epithelium.[25]

TrkB mRNA is expressed at very low levels in the trigeminal ganglion during the period of neurotrophin independence when the earliest sensory axons are growing toward their targets.[26] The onset of BDNF dependence is correlated with increased expression of trkB mRNA, whereas loss of BDNF responsiveness is associated with increasing expression of trkB transcripts coding for variants that lack the catalytic tyrosine kinase domain and function as negative modulators of BDNF signaling in neurons.[26] Although trkA and p75 (a neurotrophin receptor that enhances the survival response of embryonic trigeminal neurons to NGF[27]) are expressed at very low levels in the trigeminal ganglion before the axons reach their targets,[28,29] the acquisition of a sustained NGF survival response is associated with a marked increased expression of these receptors in trigeminal neurons.[28] Similar temporal patterns of trk transcripts have been described in the developing chicken embryo trigeminal ganglion.[30]

Contrary to the demonstration that NGF treatment increases trkA and p75 expression in neurons and cell lines, the finding that the increase in trkA and p75 mRNA expression that accompanies the onset of a sustained NGF survival in developing trigeminal neurons is unaffected in *NGF*[−/−] embryos suggests that target-derived NGF is not involved in regulating NGF receptor expression and dependence during this period of development.[31] In vitro studies suggest that other signals are required for the acquisition of NGF dependence and the loss of BDNF and NT3 dependence. When trigeminal neurons are cultured before they respond to NGF, they survive with BDNF well beyond the switchover period from BDNF to NGF dependence, and when these early neurons are switched from BDNF to NGF after various times in culture, they die as rapidly as neurotrophin-deprived neurons. However, neurons switched from BDNF or NT3 to NGF in cultures set up at stages throughout the switchover period exhibit an NGF survival response that improves with age.[11] These results suggest that the switch from BDNF/NT3 to NGF dependence is due to signals that act on the neurons during the switchover period.

In addition to mouse trigeminal neurons, evidence for an early developmental change in neurotrophin survival responses has been obtained for other populations of neural crest-derived sensory neurons, including those of the jugular ganglion and a subset of dorsal root ganglion neurons. At an early stage of development, embryonic chicken jugular neurons are supported by BDNF, NT3, and NGF in culture. With increasing age, the neurons lose responsiveness to BDNF and NT3 but retain responsiveness to NGF.[14] In vitro studies of the survival requirements of embryonic chicken dorsal root ganglia (DRG) neurons from an early stage of their development have shown that after a brief phase of neurotrophin independence, the survival of the great majority of neurons is promoted by either NGF or BDNF, whereas later in development DRG contains two distinct subpopulations of neurons that are dependent on either NGF or BDNF for survival.[3,32] Similarly, NGF, BDNF, NT3, and neurotrophin-4 (NT4) increase the number of surviving neurons in cultures of early DRG cells from rat and chicken embryos,[33,34] whereas only NGF among the neurotrophins has a major survival-promoting effect on neonatal DRG neurons in culture.[33] These findings suggest that many DRG neurons are responsive to multiple neurotrophins early in development before becoming more restricted

in survival requirements later. Accordingly, the loss of DRG neurons in
$trkA^{-/-};trkB^{-/-}$ double knockout mice is not significantly greater than that occurring in $trkA^{-/-}$ mice,[35] suggesting that at least some DRG neurons are dependent on both trkA and trkB signaling pathways for survival.

There is a marked increase in the number of cells undergoing apoptosis
and a large reduction in the number of neurons in the DRG of $NT3^{-/-}$ and
$trkC^{-/-}$ embryos during the early stages of ganglion formation.[36–39] This is due
at least in part to the death of postmitotic neurons because in the DRG of E11
$NT3^{-/-}$ embryos there is a significant reduction in the number of neurofilament positive cells in the absence of any change in the precursor population,[39]
suggesting that endogenous NT3 is required for the survival of a proportion
of newly differentiated neurons.

There is growing evidence, however, that NT3 also acts on sensory neuron
precursor cells. $TrkC$ mRNA[40–42] and TrkC protein[34] are expressed by the majority of cells in DRG during the early stages of gangliogenesis and become
restricted to a subset of large neurons later in development. Function-block-
ing anti-NT3[43] and anti-trkC[34] antibodies cause a substantial reduction in the
number of neurons in DRG when administered to avian embryos during gangliogenesis. A transient elevation in neurogenesis between E11 and E12 in the
DRG of $NT3^{-/-}$ embryos concomitant with a reduction in precursor cell numbers that is not apparently due to the death of these cells or a reduction in their
rate of proliferation[39] suggests that in the absence of NT3 precursor, cells differentiate into neurons prematurely. The consequent depletion of the precursor cell pool results in the failure of neurons to accumulate in the DRG of
NT3-deficient embryos between E12 and E13 when more than half of the
neurons are normally generated.[39] This suggests that endogenous NT3 plays a
role in keeping precursor cells in the proliferative state and prevents their differentiation. Paradoxically, however, the administration of NT3 to quail embryos during gangliogenesis causes a substantial reduction in the neuronal
complement of DRG.[44] This is associated with a reduction in cell division in
early DRG, suggesting that exogenous NT3 inhibits precursor cell proliferation in this experimental paradigm. However, the levels of exogenous NT3
may have been high enough to activate nonpreferred trk receptors, which may
not be physiologically relevant at this stage of development. In addition to
regulating precursor cell proliferation, it has been suggested that endogenous
NT3 is required for precursor cell survival because the majority of cells undergoing apoptosis in the early DRG of $NT3^{-/-}$ embryos [recognized by the
terminal transferase UTP nick end labeling (TUNEL) technique for DNA
fragmentation] had also incorporated BrdU administered 5 h earlier.[38]
However, in another study, no BrdU-positive/TUNEL-positive cells were observed in the early DRG of $NT3^{-/-}$ embryos, although BrdU-positive/neuro-
filament-positive cells were observed.[39]

The expression of *NT3* mRNA in tissues adjacent to DRG[37,39] suggests that NT3 is available to precursor cells and newly differentiated DRG neurons when their axons are starting to grow to their targets. Because the majority of early DRG neurons survive in single-cell cultures in defined medium in the absence of neurotrophins for 24 h,[4] it is possible that DRG neurons may not require NT3 for survival during the earliest stages of axonal outgrowth in vivo. NT3 does, however, promote a maturational change in cultured DRG neurons during this early stage of their development; the cell bodies change from being small and spindle shaped to being larger and spherical, with long bipolar axonal processes.[4] BDNF has a similar effect on neuronal morphology at this stage, and experiments with antisense oligonucleotides suggest that endogenous BDNF acts by an autocrine loop on the neurons at this stage.[4] It is likely, however, that many DRG neurons are dependent for their survival on a supply of NT3 from the tissues en route to their peripheral targets since the duration of neurotrophin independence observed in culture is not long enough to permit the axons to reach distant peripheral targets without intermediate support.

It is not clear why some populations of sensory neurons undergo a switch in neurotrophin dependence during an early stage in their development. It is interesting, however, that sensory neurons that switch dependence from BDNF/NT3 to NGF survive only briefly without neurotrophins in culture during the earliest stages of their development,[3–5] whereas sensory neurons that do not switch have a regulated period of neurotrophin independence that is correlated with target distance.[8] Because the peripheral axons of sensory neurons that undergo a switch in neurotrophin dependence appear to be exposed to BDNF and NT3 en route to their peripheral targets,[5,24,37,39] it is possible that these neurotrophins play a role in sustaining neurons before their axons reach the peripheral tissues where NGF is produced.[25,45] Sensory neurons that do not exhibit a switch in neurotrophin dependence survive in vitro for different lengths of time without neurotrophins for as long as it would take their axons to reach their targets in vivo; neurons with more distant targets survive longer than neurons with nearby targets.[8] Thus it is possible that these populations of neurons are not dependent on intermediate support before encountering their targets.

2.4   LATE DEVELOPMENTAL CHANGES IN NEUROTROPHIC FACTOR RESPONSIVENESS

Additional changes in neurotrophic factor responses are observed in some sensory neurons well after their axons have reached and innervated their targets. A clear example is provided by the neurons of the embryonic mouse trigeminal ganglion, which acquire a late survival response to the neu-rotrophic cytokines ciliary neurotrophic factor (CNTF), leukemia inhibitory factor (LIF), oncostatin-M (OSM), and cardiotrophin-1 (CT-1) several days after they have become dependent on NGF for survival.[46] Similarly, in vitro studies of mouse DRG neurons have shown that a small percentage of these neurons respond to LIF with enhanced survival in the late fetal period and that the majority are LIF-responsive postnatally.[47] Embryonic chicken trigem-inal neurons also acquire a late survival response to glia cell–derived neu-rotrophic factor (GDNF) several days after they start responding to neurotrophins.[48] Similarly, a subset of DRG neurons that are dependent on NGF for survival during embryonic development become responsive to GDNF in the postnatal period.[49] It should be pointed out, however, that not all sensory neurons have a late survival requirement for neurotrophic cytokines and GDNF. Nodose ganglion neurons, for example, can be supported in cul-ture by CNTF, LIF, OSM, CT-1, and GDNF throughout the same period of embryonic development as they respond to BDNF. However, whereas the physiological relevance of the in vitro responses of developing sensory neu-rons to neurotrophins has been substantiated by detailed developmental stud-ies of the timing of sensory neuron loss in mouse embryos with mutated neurotrophin and trk genes, similar detailed studies have yet to be carried out of the timing of sensory neuron death in embryos with null mutations in genes encoding other neurotrophic factors and their receptors.

2.5 RELATIONSHIP BETWEEN NEUROTROPHIN DEPENDENCE AND SENSORY MODALITY

Although several populations or subsets of sensory neurons switch their sur-vival requirements from one neurotrophin to another during an early stage of their development, there is considerable evidence that during and beyond the peak period of naturally occurring neuronal death, the neurotrophin depen-dence of many sensory neurons is related to sensory modality.[50,51] The first clear evidence that the neurotrophin requirements of sensory neurons are re-lated to modality during this period of development came from detailed in vitro studies of the neurotrophin responses of cranial sensory neurons which are segregated into groups that serve different sensory modalities (reviewed in Refs. 48 and 49). This idea has been confirmed and extended by elegant and detailed studies of the trk receptors expressed by different kinds of sensory neurons[52–55] and by studies of the types of sensory neurons eliminated in mice with null mutations in genes encoding neurotrophins and their recep-tors.[17–20,36,55–63] However, it should be pointed out that the interpretation of these studies is not always straightforward, for several reasons. First, because of the switches in neurotrophin dependence that occur in some subsets of sensory neurons during development,[5,11,14] the loss or reduction of a subset of neurons in mice with null mutations in a particular neurotrophin, for example, may result from dependence on this neurotrophin at a very early stage in development before characteristic sensory receptors have differentiated in the periphery. Second, the interpretation of the significance of trk receptor expression and the loss of neurons in mice with mutations in trk genes is complicated by the multiple ligand specificities of the trk's. Whereas expression studies in cell lines have shown that trkA is the receptor for NGF,[64-66] trkB is the receptor for BDNF and NT4,[67-73] and trkC is the receptor for NT3,[74] studies of trk receptor tyrosine kinases expressed in cell lines have shown that NT3 is also able to signal through trkA and trkB.[71,72,74,75] Although such receptor crosstalk has not been observed in all neuronal cell lines,[76-79] the demonstration that NT3 can promote the in vitro survival of NGF- and BDNF-dependent sensory neurons from embryos that have a null mutation in the *trk*C gene and that NT3 responsiveness is abolished by additional null mutations in the *trk*A and *trk*B genes show that NT3 also signals through trkA and trkB in developing neurons.[23] Such signaling may explain why the phenotype of NT3$^{-/-}$ mice[57,58] is more severe than that of *trk*C$^{-/-}$ mice.[61-80] Finally, the loss of a particular class of sensory receptor organs or failure of their innervation to develop does not necessarily reflect the death of the neurons that normally innervate these structures. With these caveats in mind, the following is a brief account of the neurotrophin dependencies of several functionally distinct kinds of sensory neurons during development.

2.5.1 Proprioceptive Neurons

Proprioceptive neurons convey sensory information about joint position and movement. The elucidation of the neurotrophin requirements of these neurons was facilitated by the development of methods to isolate, purify, and culture trigeminal mesencephalic nucleus (TMN) neurons,[81] a population of cranial sensory neurons that innervate muscle spindles and tendon organs in the masticatory muscles. The survival of these neurons is unaffected by NGF[82] and is promoted by BDNF[83] and a muscle-derived factor[81] that has turned out to be NT3.[84] Because DRG that innervates limbs contains more proprioceptive neurons than that innervating nonlimb regions, the finding that NT3 promotes the survival of more neurons in cultures of limb DRG compared with cultures of nonlimb DRG[85] provided some indirect evidence that NT3 promotes the survival of proprioceptive neurons. Direct evidence that proprioceptive neurons in DRG are dependent on NT3 has come from the demonstration that these neurons are eliminated by treating chicken embryos with anti-NT3 antiserum[86] and the finding that these neurons are absent in *NT3*$^{-/-}$ neonatal mice[36,57,58] and *trkC*[-/-] neonatal mice.[61] Interestingly, the number of muscle spindles is reduced by half in *NT3*[+/-] mice, suggesting that the concentration of NT3 is limiting during development. The demonstration that introduction of an NT3 transgene into muscle selectively rescues proprioceptive neurons in mice lacking endogenous NT3 suggests that these neurons require NT3 from muscle for their survival.[87] The conclusions of in vitro studies of the survival requirements of TMN neurons have been confirmed by the finding that there is an approximate 50% reduction in the number of these neurons in both *BDNF*[-/-] mice,[17,18] and *NT3*[-/-] mice.[57] The generality of the lack of effect of NGF on proprioceptive neuron survival observed in cultured TMN neurons has been confirmed in studies of *trkA*[-/-] and *NGF*[-/-] mice in which small-diameter but not large-diameter DRG neurons are lost.[56,59]

2.5.2 Thermoceptive and Nociceptive Neurons

Thermoceptive and nociceptive neurons have small cell bodies and unmyelinated (group C) or thinly myelinated (group Aδ) nerve fibers. Evidence that these sensory neurons are dependent on NGF for survival first came from studying the effects of anti-NGF antibodies on fetal rodents. Pups that were exposed to anti-NGF antibodies in utero were unresponsive to a variety of painful stimuli and had selective loss of small-diameter DRG neurons, substantially reduced numbers of unmyelinated and thinly myelinated axons in spinal nerve dorsal roots, and almost no sensory axons projecting to laminas I and II in the dorsal horn.[88-91] Similarly, among populations of cranial sensory neurons, only those comprised of small-diameter cutaneous sensory neurons are supported by NGF in vitro.[92] TrkA mRNA is expressed mainly by small-diameter DRG neurons,[52-54] and the phenotype of *trkA*[-/-] and NGF[-/-] mice is consistent with the loss of nociceptive and thermoceptive neurons.[56,59] Additional evidence for an association between NGF and nociception comes from the finding that chronic administration of anti-NGF to rats at birth and later ages results in the virtual absence of Aδ cutaneous nociceptors.[93] This loss is due partly to sensory neuron death in the early postnatal period and partly to Aδ fibers switching from their predominant innervation of cutaneous nociceptors to innervating hair follicles,[94] suggesting that NGF is required for the development of Aδ cutaneous nociceptors.

2.5.3 Cutaneous Mechanoreceptive Neurons

Cutaneous afferents innervating D-hair receptors and low-threshold slowly adapting mechanoreceptors and their end organs, the Merkel cells, are lost during the first postnatal week in *NT3*[-/-] mice.[62] Merkel cell innervation is also lost in *trkC*[-/-] mice, although this occurs later in development than in

$NT3^{-/-}$ mice.[55] A subset of Merkel cell afferents in whisker follicles are also eliminated in $NGF^{-/-}$ and $trkA^{-/-}$ mice, suggesting that the innervation of some Merkel cells may also depend on NGF.[55] Studies of the innervation of whisker follicles in $BDNF^{-/-}$ and $trkB^{-/-}$ mice has shown that the development of Ruffini endings and longitudinal lanceolate endings is dependent on BDNF.[55] Reticular endings in whisker follicles and some longitudinal lanceolate endings are also deficient in $NGF^{-/-}$ and $trkA^{-/-}$ mice.

2.5.4   Visceral Sensory Neurons

Visceral sensory neurons convey a variety of sensations from the viscera. The nodose ganglion neurons which convey sensory information from the viscera have provided an opportunity to study the neurotrophin requirements of visceral neurons. In vitro studies have shown that the nodose ganglion is comprised of two subsets of neurons: a major subset that is supported by BDNF and NT4[16,32,95] and a minor subset supported by NT3.[27,84] Consistent with the results of these in vitro studies is the demonstration that in ovo administration of BDNF to quail embryos during the period of naturally occurring neuronal death in the nodose ganglion rescues a large number of the neurons that would otherwise die.[96] Not surprisingly, there are major reductions in the number of neurons in the nodose ganglia of $BDNF^{-/-}$, NT4–/–, $trkB^{-/-}$, and $NT3^{-/-}$ mice.[17–20,57,97,98] Although the neurotrophin requirements of the sacral DRG neurons that innervate the lower gastrointestinal and pelvic viscera have not been studied directly, the finding that these neurons express both trkB mRNA and trkA mRNA in adult rats[53] suggests that they respond to both BDNF and NGF. Whether the potential response of these neurons to NGF is a feature of adult visceral sensory neurons or reflects a difference between visceral neurons of spinal and cranial nerves is unclear.

2.5.5   Vestibulocochlear Neurons

These sensory neurons, located in the ganglia of the eighth cranial nerve, innervate the hair cells of the organs of hearing and balance. In vitro studies have demonstrated that the survival of vestibular neurons is promoted by BDNF[8,95] but not by NGF.[92] Accordingly, BDNF mRNA and NT3 mRNA are expressed in the inner ear targets of these neurons during development.[99–103] The number of vestibular neurons is reduced markedly in $BDNF^{-/-}$ or $trkB^{-/-}$ mice and reduced to a lesser extent in $NT3^{-/-}$ or $trkC^{-/-}$ mice. The number of cochlear neurons is reduced markedly in $NT3^{-/-}$ or $trkC^{-/-}$ mice and reduced to a lesser extent in $BDNF^{-/-}$ or $trkB^{-/-}$ mice.[35,80,104] These observations suggest that the majority of vestibular neurons are dependent on BDNF for survival in vivo, whereas the majority of cochlear neurons are dependent on NT3.

REFERENCES

1. Davies, A. M., Lumsden, A. G. S., Slavkin, H. C., and Burnstock, G. (1981). Influence of nerve growth factor on the embryonic mouse trigeminal ganglion in culture. Dev. Neurosci. 4:150–156.

2. Ernsberger, U., Edgar, D., and Rohrer, H. (1989). The survival of early chick sympathetic neurons in vitro is dependent on a suitable substrate but independent of NGF. Dev. Biol. 135:250–262.

3. Ernsberger, U., and Rohrer, H. (1988). Neuronal precursor cells in chick dorsal root ganglia: differentiation and survival in vitro. Dev. Biol. 126:420–432.

4. Wright, E. M., Vogel, K. S., and Davies, A. M. (1992). Neurotrophic factors promote the maturation of developing sensory neurons before they become dependent on these factors for survival. Neuron 9:139–150.

5. Buchman, V. L., and Davies, A. M. (1993). Different neurotrophins are expressed and act in a developmental sequence to promote the survival of embryonic sensory neurons. Development 118:989–1001.

6. Acheson, A., Conover, J. C., Fandl, J. P., DeChlara, T. M., Russell, M., Thadani, A., Squinto, S. P., Yancopoulos, G. D., and Lindsay, R. M. (1995). A BDNF autocrine loop in adult sensory neurons prevents cell death. Nature 374:450–453.

7. Davies, A. M. (1989). Intrinsic differences in the growth rate of early nerve fibres related to target distance. Nature 337:553–555.

8. Vogel, K. S., and Davies, A. M. (1991). The duration of neurotrophic factor independence in early sensory neurons is matched to the time course of target field innervation. Neuron 7:819–830.

9. Robinson, M., Adu, J., and Davies, A. M. (1996). Timing and regulation of *trkB* and *BDNF* mRNA expression in placode-derived sensory neurons and their targets. Eur. J. Neurosci. 8:2399–2406.

10. Vogel, K. S., and Davies, A. M. (1993). Heterotopic transplantation of presumptive placodal ectoderm influences the fate of sensory neuron precursors. Development 119:263–277.

11. Paul, G., and Davies, A. M. (1995). Trigeminal sensory neurons require extrinsic signals to switch neurotrophin dependence during the early stages of target field innervation. Dev. Biol. 171:590–605.

12. Moshnyakov, M., Arumae, U., and Saarma, M. (1996). mRNAs for one, two or three members of trk receptor family are expressed in single rat trigeminal ganglion neurons. Mol. Brain Res. 43:141–148.

13. Davies, A. M., and Lumsden, A. (1984). Relation of target encounter and neuronal death to nerve growth factor responsiveness in the developing mouse trigeminal ganglion. J. Comp. Neurol. 223:124–137.

14. Buj-Bello, A., Piñón, L. G., and Davies, A. M. (1994). The survival of NGF-dependent but not BDNF-dependent cranial sensory neurons is promoted by several different neurotrophins early in their development. Development 120:1573–1580.

15. Piñón, L. G. P., Minichiello, L., Klein, R., and Davies, A. M. (1996). Timing of neuronal death in *trkA*, *trkB* and *trkC* mutant embryos reveals developmental changes in sensory neuron dependence on Trk signalling. Development 122:3255–3261.

16. Davies, A. M., Horton, A., Burton, L. E., Schmelzer, C., Vandlen, R., and Rosenthal, A. (1993). Neurotrophin-4/5 is a mammalian-specific survival factor for distinct populations of sensory neurons. J. Neurosci. 13:4961–4967.

17. Ernfors, P., Lee, K. F., and Jaenisch, R. (1994). Mice lacking brain-derived neurotrophic factor develop with sensory deficits. Nature 368:147–150.

18. Jones, K. R., Farinas, I., Backus, C., and Reichardt, L. F. (1994). Targeted disruption of the BDNF gene perturbs brain and sensory neuron development but not motor neuron development. Cell 76:989–999.

19. Conover, J. C., Erickson, J. T., Katz, D. M., Bianchi, L. M., Poueymirou, W. T., McClain, J., Pan, L., Helgren, M., Ip, N. Y., Boland, P., Friedman, B., Wiegand, S., Vejsada, R., Kato, A. C., DeClara, T. M., and Yancopoulas, G. D. (1995). Neuronal deficits, not involving motor neurons, in mice lacking BDNF and NT4. Nature 375:235–238.

20. Liu, X., Ernfors, P., Wu, H., and Jaenisch, R. (1995). Sensory but not motor neuron deficits in mice lacking NT4 and BDNF. Nature 375:238–241.

21. El Shamy, W. M., and Ernfors, P. (1996). Requirement of neurotrophin-3 for the survival of proliferating trigeminal ganglion progenitor cells. Development 122:2405–2414.

22. Wilkinson, G. A., Fariñas, I., Backus, C., Yoshida, C. K., and Reichardt, L. F. (1996). Neurotrophin-3 is a survival factor in vivo for early mouse trigeminal neurons. J. Neurosci. 16:7661–7669.

23. Davies, A. M., Minichiello, L., and Klein, R. (1995). Developmental changes in NT3 signalling via TrkA and TrkB in embryonic neurons. EMBO J. 14:4482–4489.

24. Arumae, U., Pirvola, U., Palgi, J., Kiema, T. R., Palm, K., Moshnyakov, M., Ylikoski, J., and Saarma, M. (1993). Neurotrophins and their receptors in rat peripheral trigeminal system during maxillary nerve growth. J. Cell Biol. 122:1053–1065.

25. Davies, A. M., Bandtlow, C., Heumann, R., Korsching, S., Rohrer, H., and Thoenen, H. (1987). Timing and site of nerve growth factor synthesis in developing skin in relation to innervation and expression of the receptor. Nature 326:353–358.

26. Ninkina, N., Adu, J., Fischer, A., Piñón, L. G., Buchman, V. L., and Davies, A. M. (1996). Expression and function of TrkB variants in developing sensory neurons. EMBO J. 15:6385–6393.

27. Davies, A. M., Lee, K. F., and Jaenisch, R. (1993). p75-deficient trigeminal sensory neurons have an altered response to NGF but not to other neurotrophins. Neuron 11:565–574.

28. Wyatt, S., and Davies, A. M. (1993). Regulation of expression of mRNAs encoding the nerve growth factor receptors p75 and trkA in developing sensory neurons. Development 119:635–648.

29. Schropel, A., von Shack, D., Dechant, G., and Barde, Y. A. (1995). Early expression of the nerve growth factor receptor trkA in chick sympathetic and sensory ganglia. Mol. Cell. Neurosci. 6:544–556.

30. Williams, R., Backstrom, A., Kullander, K., Hallbook, F., and Ebendal, T. (1995). Developmentally regulated expression of mRNA for neurotrophin high-affinity (*trk*) receptors within chick trigeminal neurons. Eur. J. Neurosci. 7:116–128.

31. Davies, A. M., Wyatt, S., Nishimura, M., and Phillips, H. (1995). NGF receptor expression in sensory neurons develops normally in embryos lacking NGF. Dev. Biol. 171:434–438.

32. Lindsay, R. M., Thoenen, H., and Barde, Y. A. (1985). Placode and neural crest–derived sensory neurons are responsive at early developmental stages to brain-derived neurotrophic factor. Dev. Biol. 112:319–328.

33. Memberg, S. P., and Hall, A. K. (1996). Proliferation, differentiation, and survival of rat sensory neuron precursors in vitro require specific trophic factors. Mol. Cell. Neurosci. 6:323–335.

34. Lefcort, F., Clary, D. O., Rusoff, A. C., and Reichardt, L. F. (1996). Inhibition of the NT3 receptor TrkC, early in chick embryogenesis, results in severe reductions in multiple neuronal subpopulations in the dorsal root ganglia. J. Neurosci. 16:3704–3713.

35. Minichiello, L., Piehl, F., Vazquez, E., Schimmang, T., Hokfelt, T., Represa, J., and Klein, R. (1995). Differential effects of combined trk receptor mutations on dorsal root ganglion and inner ear sensory neurons. Development 121:4067–4075.

36. Tessarollo, L., Vogel, K. S., Palko, M. E., Reid, S. W., and Parada, L. F. (1994). Targeted mutation in the neurotrophin-3 gene results in loss of muscle sensory neurons. Proc. Natl. Acad. Sci. USA 91:11844–11848.

37. White, F. A., Silos-Santiago, I., Molliver, D. C., Nishimura, M., Phillips, H., Barbacid, M., and Snider, W. D. (1996). Synchronous onset of NGF and TrkA survival dependence in developing dorsal root ganglia. J. Neurosci. 16:4662–4672.

38. ElShamy, W. M., and Ernfors, P. (1996). A local action of neurotrophin-3 prevents the death of proliferating sensory neuron precursor cells. Neuron 16:963–972.

39. Farinas, I., Yoshida, C. K., Backus, C., and Reichardt, L. F. (1996). Lack of neurotrophin-3 results in death of spinal sensory neurons and premature differentiation of their precursors. Neuron 17:1065–1078.

40. Lamballe, F., Smeyne, R. J., and Barbacid, M. (1994). Developmental expression of trkC, the neurotrophin-3 receptor, in the mammalian nervous system. J. Neurosci. 14:14–28.

41. Kahane, N., and Kalcheim, C. (1994). Expression of trkC receptor mRNA during development of the avian nervous system. J. Neurobiol. 25:571–584.

42. Zhang, D., Yao, L., and Bernd, P. (1994). Expression of *trk* and neurotrophin mRNA in dorsal root and sympathetic ganglia of the quail during development. J. Neurobiol. 25:1517–1532.

43. Gaese, F., Kolbeck, R., and Barde, Y. A. (1994). Sensory ganglia require neurotrophin-3 early in development. Development 120:1613–1619.

44. Ockel, M., Lewin, G. R., and Barde, Y. A. (1996). In vivo effects of neurotrophin-3 during sensory neurogenesis. Development 122:301–307.

45. Harper, S., and Davies, A. M. (1990). NGF mRNA expression in developing cutaneous epithelium related to innervation density. Development 110:515–519.

46. Horton, A. R., Bartlett, P. F., Pennica, D., and Davies, A. M. (in press). Cytokines promote the survival of cranial sensory neurons at different developmental stages. Eur. J. Neurosci.

47. Murphy, M., Reid, K., Brown, M. A., and Bartlett, P. F. (1993). Involvement of leukemia inhibitory factor and nerve growth factor in the development of dorsal root ganglion neurons. Development 117:1173–1182.

48. Buj-Bello, A., Buchman, V. L., Horton, A., Rosenthal, A., and Davies, A. M. (1995). GDNF is an age-specific survival factor for sensory and autonomic neurons. Neuron 15:821–828.

49. Molliver, D. C., Wright, D. E., Leitner, M. L., Parsadanian, A. S., Doster, K., Wen, D., Yan, Q., and Snider, W. D. (1997). IB4-binding DRG neurons switch from NGF to GDNF dependence in early postnatal life. Neuron 19:849–861.

50. Davies, A. M. (1987). Molecular and cellular aspects of patterning sensory neuron connections in the vertebrate nervous system. Development 101:185–208.

51. Davies, A. M. (1994). The role of neurotrophins during successive stages of sensory neuron development. Prog. Growth Factor Res. 5:263–289.

52. Mu, X., Silos-Santiago, I., Carroll, S. L., and Snider, W. D. (1993). Neurotrophin receptor genes are expressed in distinct patterns in developing dorsal root ganglia. J. Neurosci. 13:4029–4041.

53. McMahon, S. B., Armanini, M. P., Ling, L. H., and Phillips, H. S. (1994). Expression and coexpression of Trk receptors in subpopulations of adult primary sensory neurons projecting to identified peripheral targets. Neuron 12:1161–1171.

54. Wright, D. E., and Snider, W. D. (1995). Neurotrophin receptor mRNA expression defines distinct populations of neurons in rat dorsal root ganglia. J. Comp. Neurol. 351:329–338.

55. Fundin, B. T., Silos-Santiago, I., Ernfors, P., Fagan, A. M., Aldskogius, H., DeChiara, T. M., Phillips, H. S., Barbacid, M., Yancopoulos, G. D., and Rice, F. L. (1997). Differential dependency of cutaneous mechanoreceptors on neurotrophins, trk receptors, and p75 LNGFR. Dev. Biol. 190:94–116.

56. Crowley, C., Spencer, S. D., Nishimura, M. C., Chen, K. S., Pitts-Meek, S., Armanini, M. P., Ling, L. H., McMahon, S. B., Shelton, D. L., Levinson, A. D., and Phillips, H. S. (1994). Mice lacking nerve growth factor display perinatal

loss of sensory and sympathetic neurons yet develop basal forebrain cholinergic neurons. Cell 76:1001–1011.

57. Ernfors, P., Lee, K. F., Kucera, J., and Jaenisch, R. (1994). Lack of neurotrophin-3 leads to deficiencies in the peripheral nervous system and loss of limb proprioceptive afferents. Cell 77:503–512.

58. Farinas, I., Jones, K. R., Backus, C., Wang, X. Y., and Reichardt, L. F. (1994). Severe sensory and sympathetic deficits in mice lacking neurotrophin-3. Nature 369:658–661.

59. Smeyne, R. J., Klein, R., Schnapp, A., Long, L. K., Bryant, S., Lewin, A., Lira, SA., and Barbacid, M. (1994). Severe sensory and sympathetic neuropathies in mice carrying a disrupted Trk/NGF receptor gene. Nature 368:246–249.

60. Klein, R., Smeyne, R. J., Wurst, W., Long, L. K., Auerbach, B. A., Joyner, A. L., and Barbacid, M. (1993). Targeted disruption of the trkB neurotrophin receptor gene results in nervous system lesions and neonatal death. Cell 75:113–122.

61. Klein, R., Silos, S. I., Smeyne, R. J., Lira, S. A., Brambilla, R., Bryant, S., Zhang, L., Snider, W. D., and Barbacid, M. (1994). Disruption of the neurotrophin-3 receptor gene trkC eliminates Ia muscle afferents and results in abnormal movements. Nature 368:249–251.

62. Airaksinen, M. S., Koltzenburg, M., Lewin, G. R., Masu, Y., Helbig, C., Wolf, E., Brem, G., Toyka, K. V., Thoenen, H., and Meyer, M. (1996). Specific subsets of cutaneous mechanoreceptors require neurotrophin-3 following peripheral target innervation. Neuron 16:287–295.

63. Silos-Santiago, I., Molliver, D. C., Ozaki, S., Smeyne, R. J., Fagan, A. M., Barbacid, M., and Snider, W. D. (1995). Non-TrkA-expressing small DRG neurons are lost in TrkA deficient mice. J. Neurosci. 15:5929–5942.

64. Hempstead, B. L., Martin, Z. D., Kaplan, D. R., Parada, L. F., and Chao, M. V. (1991). High-affinity NGF binding requires coexpression of the trk proto-oncogene and the low-affinity NGF receptor. Nature 350:678–683.

65. Kaplan, D. R., Martin, Z. D., and Parada, L. F. (1991). Tyrosine phosphorylation and tyrosine kinase activity of the trk proto-oncogene product induced by NGF. Nature 350:158–160.

66. Klein, R., Jing, S. Q., Nanduri, V., O'Rourke, E., and Barbacid, M. (1991). The trk proto-oncogene encodes a receptor for nerve growth factor. Cell 65:189–197.

67. Berkemeier, L. R., Winslow, J. W., Kaplan, D. R., Nikolics, K., Goeddel, D. V., and Rosenthal, A. (1991). Neurotrophin-5: a novel neurotrophic factor that activates trk and trkB. Neuron 7:857–866.

68. Glass, D. J., Nye, S. H., Hantzopoulos, P., Macchi, M. J., Squinto, S. P., Goldfarb, M., and Yancopoulos, G. D. (1991). TrkB mediates BDNF/NT-3-dependent survival and proliferation in fibroblasts lacking the low affinity NGF receptor. Cell 66:405–413.

69. Klein, R., Nanduri, V., Jing, S. A., Lamballe, F., Tapley, P., Bryant, S., Cordon, C. C., Jones, K. R., Reichardt, L. F., and Barbacid, M. (1991). The trkB tyrosine

protein kinase is a receptor for brain-derived neurotrophic factor and neurotrophin-3. Cell 66:395–403.

70. Klein, R., Lamballe, F., Bryant, S., and Barbacid, M. (1992). The trkB tyrosine protein kinase is a receptor for neurotrophin-4. Neuron 8:947–956.

71. Soppet, D., Escandon, E., Maragos, J., Middlemas, D. S., Reid, S. W., Blair, J., Burton, L. E., Stanton, B. R., Kaplan, D. R., Hunter, T., Nikolics, K., and Parada, L. F. (1991). The neurotrophic factors, brain-derived neurotrophic factor and neurotrophin-3 are ligands for the trkB tyrosine kinase receptor. Cell 65:895–903.

72. Squinto, S. P., Aldrich, T. H., Lindsay, R. M., Morrissey, D. M., Panayotatos, N., Bianco, S. M., Furth, M. E., and Yancopoulos, G. D. (1990). Identification of functional receptors for ciliary neurotrophic factor on neuronal cell lines and primary neurons. Neuron 5:757–766.

73. Ip, N. Y., Ibanez, C. F., Nye, S. H., McClain, J., Jones, P. F., Gies, D. R., Belluscio, L., Le, B. M., Espinosa, R., 3d, Squinto, S. P., Persson, H., and Yancopoulas, G. D. (1992). Mammalian neurotrophin-4: structure, chromosomal localization, tissue distribution, and receptor specificity. Proc. Natl. Acad. Sci. USA 89:3060–3064.

74. Lamballe, F., Klein, R., and Barbacid, M. (1991). trkC, a new member of the trk family of tyrosine protein kinases, is a receptor for neurotrophin-3. Cell 66:967–979.

75. Ip, N. Y., Stitt, T. N., Tapley, P., Klein, R., Glass, D. J., Fandl, J., Greene, L. A., Barbacid, M., and Yancopoulos, G. D. (1993). Similarities and differences in the way neurotrophins interact with the Trk receptors in neuronal and nonneuronal cells. Neuron 10:137–149.

76. Lamballe, F., Tapley, P., and Barbacid, M. (1993). trkC encodes multiple neurotrophin-3 receptors with distinct biological properties and substrate specificities. EMBO J. 12:3083–3094.

77. Valenzuela, D. M., Maisonpierre, P. C., Glass, D. J., Rojas, E., Nunez, L., Kong, Y., Gies, D. R., Stitt, T. N., Ip, N. Y., and Yancopoulos, G. D. (1993). Alternative forms of rat TrkC with different functional capabilities. Neuron 10:963–974.

78. Tsoulfas, P., Soppet, D., Escandon, E., Tessarollo, L., Mendoza, R. J., Rosenthal, A., Nikolics, K., and Parada, L. F. (1993). The rat trkC locus encodes multiple neurogenic receptors that exhibit differential response to neurotrophin-3 in PC12 cells. Neuron 10:975–990.

79. Garner, A. S., and Large, T. H. (1994). Isoforms of the avian TrkC receptor: a novel kinase insertion dissociates transformation and process outgrowth from survival. Neuron 13:457–472.

80. Schimmang, T., Minichiello, L., Vazquez, E., Joac, I. S., Giraldez, F., Klein, R., and Represa, J. (1995). Developing inner ear sensory neurons require TrkB and TrkC receptors for innervation of their peripheral targets. Development 121:3381–3391.

81. Davies, A. M. (1986). The survival and growth of embryonic proprioceptive neurons is promoted by a factor present in skeletal muscle. Dev. Biol. 115:56–67.

82. Davies, A. M., Lumsden, A. G., and Rohrer, H. (1987). Neural crest-derived proprioceptive neurons express nerve growth factor receptors but are not supported by nerve growth factor in culture. Neuroscience 20:37–46.

83. Davies, A. M., Thoenen, H., and Barde, Y. A. (1986). Different factors from the central nervous system and periphery regulate the survival of sensory neurones. Nature 319:497–499.

84. Hohn, A., Leibrock, J., Bailey, K., and Barde, Y. A. (1990). Identification and characterization of a novel member of the nerve growth factor/brain-derived neurotrophic factor family. Nature 344:339–341.

85. Hory-Lee, F., Russell, M., Lindsay, R. M., and Frank, E. (1993). Neurotrophin 3 supports the survival of developing muscle sensory neurons in culture. Proc. Natl. Acad. Sci. USA 90:2613–2617.

86. Oakley, R. A., Garner, A. S., Large, T. H., and Frank, E. (1995). Muscle sensory neurons require neurotrophin-3 from peripheral tissues during the period of normal cell death. Development 121:1341–1350.

87. Wright, D. E., Zhou, L., Kucera, J., and Snider, W. D. (1997). Introduction of a neurotrophin-3 transgene into muscle selectively rescues proprioceptive neurons in mice lacking endogenous neurotrophin-3. Neuron 19:503–517.

88. Johnson, E. M., Gorin, P. D., Brandeis, L. D., and Pearson, J. (1980). Dorsal root ganglion neurons are destroyed by in utero exposure to maternal antibody to nerve growth factor. Science 210:916–918.

89. Johnson, E. M., Osborne, P. A., Rydel, R. E., Schmidt, R. E., and Pearson, J. (1983). Characterisation of the effects of autoimmune nerve growth factor deprivation in the developing guinea pig. Neuroscience 8:631–642.

90. Goedert, M., Otten, U., Hunt, S. P., Bond, A., Chapman, D., Schlumpf, M., and Lichtensteiger, W. (1984). Biochemical and anatomical effects of antibodies against nerve growth factor on developing rat sensory ganglia. Proc. Natl. Acad. Sci. USA 81:1580–1584.

91. Ruit, K. G., Elliott, J. L., Osborne, P. A., Yan, Q., and Snider, W. D. (1992). Selective dependence of mammalian dorsal root ganglion neurons on nerve growth factor during embryonic development. Neuron 8:573–587.

92. Davies, A. M., and Lindsay, R. M. (1985). The cranial sensory ganglia in culture: differences in the response of placode-derived and neural crest-derived neurons to nerve growth factor. Dev. Biol. 111:62–72.

93. Ritter, A. M., Lewin, G. R., Kremer, N. E., and Mendell, L. M. (1991). Requirement for nerve growth factor in the development of myelinated nociceptors in vivo. Nature 350:500–502.

94. Lewin, G. R., Ritter, A. M., and Mendell, L. M. (1992). On the role of nerve growth factor in the development of myelinated nociceptors. J. Neurosci. 12:1896–1905.

95. Davies, A. M., Thoenen, H., and Barde, Y. A. (1986). The response of chick sensory neurons to brain-derived neurotrophic factor. J. Neurosci. 6:1897–1904.

96. Hofer, M. M., and Barde, Y. A. (1988). Brain-derived neurotrophic factor prevents neuronal death in vivo. Nature 331:261–262.

97. Erickson, J. T., Conover, J. C., Borday, V., Champagnat, J., Barbacid, M., Yancopoulos G, and Katz, D. M. (1996). Mice lacking brain-derived neurotrophic factor exhibit visceral sensory neuron losses distinct from mice lacking NT4 and display a severe developmental deficit in control of breathing. J. Neurosci. 16:5361–5371.

98. ElShamy, W. M., and Ernfors, P. (1997). Brain-derived neurotrophic factor, neurotrophin-3, and neurotrophin-4 complement and cooperate with each other sequentially during visceral neuron development. J. Neurosci. 17:8667–8675.

99. Pirvola, U., Ylikoski, J., Palgi, J., Lehtonen, E., Arumae, U., and Saarma, M. (1992). Brain-derived neurotrophic factor and neurotrophin 3 mRNAs in the peripheral target fields of developing inner ear ganglia. Proc. Natl. Acad. Sci. USA 89:9915–9919.

100. Pirvola, U., Arumae, U., Moshnyakov, M., Palgi, J., Saarma, M., and Ylikoski, J. (1994). Coordinated expression and function of neurotrophins and their receptors in the rat inner ear during target innervation. Hear. Res. 75:131–144.

101. Ylikoski, J., Pirvola, U., Moshnyakov, M., Palgi, J., Arumae, U., and Saarma, M. (1993). Expression patterns of neurotrophin and their receptor mRNAs in the rat inner ear. Hear. Res. 65:69–78.

102. Vazquez, E., Van D. W. T., Del, V. M., Vega, J. A., Staecker, H., Giraldez, F., and Represa, J. (1994). Pattern of trkB protein-like immunoreactivity in vivo and the in vitro effects of brain-derived neurotrophic factor (BDNF) on developing cochlear and vestibular neurons. Anat. Embryol. (Berl.) 189:157–167.

103. Schecterson, L. C., and Bothwell, M. (1994). Neurotrophin and neurotrophin receptor mRNA expression in developing inner ear. Hear. Res. 73:92–100.

104. Ernfors, P., Van Der Water, T., Loring, J., and Jaenisch, R. (1995). Complementary roles of BDNF and NT3 in vestibular and auditory development. Neuron 14:1153–1164.

CHAPTER 3

Neurotrophic Signaling and Sensory Neuron Survival and Function

INMACULADA SILOS-SANTIAGO

Millennium Pharmaceuticals Inc.
Cambridge, Massachusetts

3.1 INTRODUCTION

Neurotrophic factors are a family of secreted soluble proteins that exert their biological actions upon high-affinity binding to their respective tyrosine kinase (trk) receptors. Genetically engineered mice in which different members of the neurotrophin family or their receptors have been inactivated by homologous recombination have revealed new aspects in the development of sensory neurons. For example, the specificity of neurotrophin signaling in promoting survival of subpopulations of neurons involved in a particular sensory modality is now clear. In general, it appears that a specific neurotrophin, signaling through a specific trk receptor, is required for the survival of a particular population of sensory neurons. Furthermore, neurotrophin/trk signaling dependency for survival occurs very early in embryonic development, before the newly postmitotic neuron reaches its target field. Interestingly, this temporal frame in neurotrophin/trk signaling requirement is the same for most of the sensory neuronal populations independent of their embryonic origin.

More recently, in vitro and in vivo experiments are suggesting novel roles for neurotrophin/trk signaling in neural development and maintenance of the adult nervous system. For instance, these growth factors may be involved in the regulation of the terminal arborization of nerve cells in their target fields.[1,2] Detailed analysis of different neurotrophin- and neurotrophin-receptor-deficient mice, as well as of transgenic mice that overexpress neurotrophins and

Molecular Basis of Pain Induction, Edited by John N. Wood
ISBN 0-471-34607-1   Copyright © 2000 by Wiley-Liss, Inc. All rights reserved.

conditional deficient mice, are now under way and in the near future they will reveal another important biological effect of neurotrophin/trk signaling in other aspects of the development of sensory neurons.

3.2   NEUROTROPHIN SIGNALING AND NEURONAL SURVIVAL DURING DEVELOPMENT

Neurotrophins bind trk receptors in the membrane of the responsive cells to elicit their biological effects. Upon ligand binding, the trk receptors dimerize, and this dimerization induces the autophosphorylation of the kinase domain in tyrosine residues.[3,4] The phosphorylation of the receptor recruits and phosphorylates cytoplasmic proteins that initiate different signal transduction pathways.[5] The end result of this kinase activity is the regulation of neuronal survival as well as other developmental processes.

The role of neurotrophin signaling in promoting survival of neurons during embryonic and early postnatal life has clearly been established with the use of genetically engineered mice. Some of these mice lack different members of the neurotrophin family (neurotrophin knockout mice). Other mice are carrying germ-line mutations in the catalytic domains of each of the trk kinase receptors (trk kinase-deficient mice) (reviewed in Refs. 6 to 8). The phenotypes of mice defective for each trk receptor have turned out to be strikingly similar to mice lacking their cognate neurotrophins (see below). These observations represent the most compelling evidence that the trk receptors mediate most, if not all, neurotrophin activities in vivo. Furthermore, these mice have revealed the specificity of neurotrophin signaling in promoting survival of subpopulations of neurons involved in specific sensory modalities. This fact raised great hopes for the potential use of specific neurotrophins in the treatment of a specific peripheral neuropathy.

3.2.1   NGF/TrkA Signaling and Survival of Nociceptive Neurons During Embryonic Development

Nerve growth factor (NGF), the first characterized member of the neurotrophin family, was discovered in the 1950s as a molecule that appeared to be required for survival and maturation of sensory and sympathetic neurons. In the 1960s and 1970s in vivo and in vitro experiments using an antiserum against NGF or exogenous NGF confirmed that the major effect of NGF is to promote neuronal survival[9] of sympathetic neurons and certain populations of sensory neurons. Since NGF deprivation enhances the death of these neuronal populations, it seems plausible that regulation of the neuronal number during embryonic and early postnatal development depends on the availability of NGF.

In the 1980s the receptors for NGF were discovered,[10,11] and in 1990 it was established that NGF binds the trkA tyrosine kinase receptor with high affinity. Mice in which the NGF gene or the trkA kinase domain have been eliminated display very similar phenotypes, characterized by the total absence of response to painful stimuli and their death in early postnatal life.[12-14] This indicates that the biological effects of NGF are mediated by its high-affinity receptor, trkA.

Studies in which NGF antibodies were injected or generated by pregnant rats led to the suggestion that among other biological functions, NGF promotes the survival of small DRG neurons.[15] Analysis of the trkA kinase-deficient mice has confirmed all these previous studies and has established the role of NGF/trkA signaling in promoting the survival of nociceptive neurons as well as BSI-positive neurons in vivo.[6,12-14] Mice defective in trkA catalytic receptors or NGF display severe sensory deficits characterized by a complete loss of response to noxious mechanical and thermal stimuli. Histological analysis revealed profound neuronal loss (70 to 80%) in sensory ganglia including dorsal root ganglia (DRG) and trigeminal ganglia (TRG)[12-14,16-18] (Fig. 3.1). Within the DRG the vast majority of missing neurons correspond to those of small size as well as some of medium size.[14] Immunohistochemical and in situ hybridization analysis using calcitonin gene–related peptide

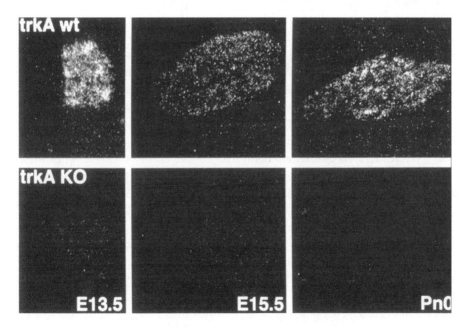

Figure 3.1 TrkA expression in the trigeminal ganglia of trkA kinase-deficient mice (trkA KO) and their wild-type littermates (trkA wt) at different stages of development. Note the absence of trkA transcripts in all mutant mice.

(CGRP), substance P, and trkA, markers expressed in small to medium-sized DRG neurons[19,20] have shown that most of these neurons are absent in DRGs from NGF-deficient and trkA kinase-deficient mice.[12,14,16] Furthermore, axonal processes from these neurons were completely absent in both the dorsal horn of the spinal cord and in the skin of NGF-deficient and trkA kinase-deficient mice.[12,14] Consistent with these results, virtually all unmyelinated and approximately 50% of myelinated (those in the range 2 to 5 μm) fibers are absent in the dorsal roots (DRs) of these mice.[14] These observations confirmed the dependence of peptidergic DRG neurons on NGF for survival.[12,14,16] Interestingly, however, trkA kinase-deficient mice also lack small nonpeptidergic neurons that bind the lectin BSI-B4 and do not express trkA postnatally. These neurons project to the inner part of lamina II in the dorsal horn of the spinal cord. As a consequence, the entire DR projection to the superficial dorsal horn appears to be lost in these mice.[14] These results indicate that virtually all DRG neurons with a nociceptive phenotype as well as small neurons that bind BSI-B4 are lost in trkA kinase-deficient mice.

Similarly to the DRG system, in the TRG system Rice et al.[21] have recently shown that innervation of the epidermis and upper dermis in the mystacial pad is drastically affected in NGF- and trkA-deficient mice. Interestingly, peptidergic and nonpeptidergic innervations appear to be equally compromised. For instance, unmyelinated nonpeptidergic axons that innervate the epidermis as well as the mouth of hair follicles are absent throughout the postnatal period in NGF- and trkA-kinase deficient mice. Unmyelinated peptidergic, small myelinated, and sympathetic axons are also absent in these mice. In fact, only one set of unmyelinated innervation survived in NGF- and trkA kinase-deficient mice. This innervation may be parasympathetic in nature.[21]

More recently it has been suggested that all functional subclasses of nociceptive neurons may be not affected equally in these mice. Analysis of the cornea in trkA kinase-deficient mice has shown that corneal innervation, although drastically reduced, is not eliminated completely.[22] The cornea receives innervation from various subclasses of nociceptive neurons, including mechanonociceptive neurons, polymodal nociceptive neurons, and cold nociceptive neurons. As mentioned above, trkA and NGF deficient mice do not respond to noxious or thermal stimuli on their skin. However, residual sensitivity to noxious stimuli remains in the cornea of the trkA kinase-deficient mice. These mice do not respond to cold stimulus or to capsaicin application. Furthermore, the response to mechanical and heat stimulation is minimal. However, acid stimulation was most effective in inducing a response in these mice. These observations suggest that polymodal nociceptors are surviving in trkA kinase-deficient mice and indicate that the remaining corneal innervation is sensory in nature.[22] Consistent with these data is the residual presence of substance P and CGRP-positive neurons in the TRG of trkA kinase-deficient mice (I. Silos-Santiago, unpublished observations).

These genetically engineered mice have also shown that NGF/trkA signaling is not necessary for neurogenesis, expression of neuronal markers, or initial axon growth in sensory neurons. Studies during embryonic development of these neuronal populations have demonstrated that NGF-dependent neurons are born in NGF- and trkA kinase-deficient mice and extend axons toward their peripheral targets. Although some of these neurons are able to reach their proximal targets, most NGF-dependent neurons die prior to final target innervation[18,23] (Fig. 3.2).

3.2.2   NT-3/trkC Signaling and Embryonic Survival of Proprioceptive Neurons

Disruption of the *trk*C or neurotrophin-3 (NT3) genes also result in severe sensory deficits but distinct in nature from those observed in trkA- or NGF-defective mice. Mice lacking NT3 or trkC receptors develop abnormal, athetotic movements when walking, and at rest they display abnormal

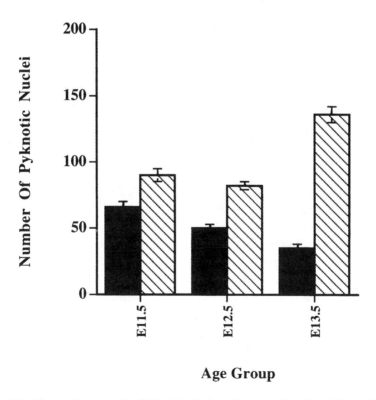

Figure 3.2   Temporal pattern of cell death in the dorsal root ganglia of trkA kinase-deficient mice. At all stages analyzed the number of pyknotic nuclei is significantly higher in the trkA kinase-deficient mice (hatched bars) than in their wild-type littermates (shaded bars).

postures.[24–29] This sensory defect is due to complete absence of Ia muscle afferents, the projections derived from large proprioceptive DRG neurons that connect primary endings of muscle spindles in the periphery to motor pools in the ventral region of the spinal cord. The trkC kinase-deficient mice survive for 2 to 3 weeks. Examination of the DRGs histologically reveals a modest reduction in DRG neuronal numbers of approximately 20 to 30%, roughly the percentage of neurons that express trkC in the adult mouse DRG.[16,26,28,29] The dorsal roots are substantially depleted of large-caliber axons, losing approximately 50% of myelinated axons. A clue to the nature of DRG neuronal loss was provided by application of the lipid-soluble tracer DiI to the DRG, allowing visualization of the central axonal projections of the DRG neurons.[26,30] Remarkably, these mutant mice have no axons that extend into the ventral horn or into the region of Clarke's column in the intermediate zone. The results show that the collateral branches of Ia afferents are eliminated completely. These are the afferents thought to be involved in the sense of proprioception. Consistent with these results, parvalbumin (PV)-positive neurons are drastically reduced in the DRG of trkC kinase-deficient mice.[30] Analysis of these mice during embryonic development have shown that these afferents never enter the spinal cord, consistent with the fact that the parent neurons are lost at an early stage of development[18] (Fig. 3.3). As a consequence of the early loss of proprioceptive neurons, these mice never develop muscle spindles.

Interestingly, the sensory phenotype of trkC and NT3 null mutant mice,[24,25,27–29] although it parallels many aspects of that of trkC kinase-deficient mice, is far more severe. These animals rarely survive more than 1 day postnatal, and most sensory and sympathetic ganglia analyzed display an important neuronal loss.[24,25,27,31–35] Although the onset of cell death is similar in trkC kinase-deficient mice and in NT3 or trkC null mutant mice,[17,29,31,34,36] the percentage of cell death in NT3 null mutant mice is higher than that observed in trkC kinase-deficient or trkC null mutant mice,[26,28,29] suggesting that NT3 may act through other trk receptors. In NT3 null mutant mice, consistent with abnormal limb movements and body postures, the Ia dorsal root (DR) projection to the motor pools is absent as well as PV-immunoreactive and carbonic anhydrase–positive neurons.[24,25,27,29,36] Similarly to the trkC kinase-deficient mice, NT3 null mutant mice do not develop muscle spindles.[24,25,36]

Consistent with the role of NT3/trkC signaling in promoting the survival of proprioceptive neurons is the approximately 50% reduction in the number of neurons in the trigeminal mesencephalic nucleus in these mutant mice (I. Silos-Santiago and E. Peña, unpublished observations; see also Refs. 24 and 25). Proprioceptive neurons innervating muscles in the neck and face reside in this brain stem nucleus.

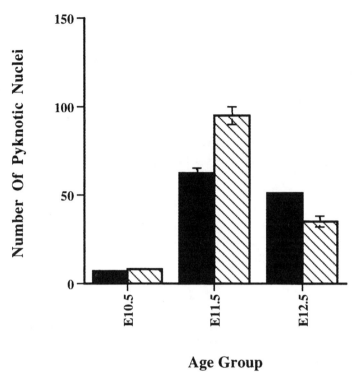

Figure 3.3 Temporal pattern of cell death in the dorsal root ganglia of trkC kinase-deficient mice. Massive cell death occurs at embryonic day 11.5 in trkC kinase-deficient mice (hatched bars) and wild-type littermates (shaded bars).

3.2.3 Neurotrophins and Survival of Different Subsets of Mechanoreceptors

Cutaneous mechanoreceptive neurons are a very heterogeneous group that supply a variety of distinct endings to various components of the skin and adjacent subcutaneous connective tissue. Corresponding to this heterogeneity is the complex trophic dependence of this group of neurons. Very recently it has been shown that in the mystacial pad, neurotrophin/trk signaling plays an important role in the development of all cutaneous mechanoreceptors that are supplied by medium to large-caliber myelinated afferents (Fig. 3.4). This work has shown that neurotrophins acting through trk receptors are involved in the survival of mechanoreceptive neurons and/or in the formation of their sensory endings. For example, the absence of NGF/trkA signaling results in the absence of transverse lanceolate and reticular endings as well as their source axons. Interestingly, the reticular endings were also decreased in NT3 homozygous mutant mice but were

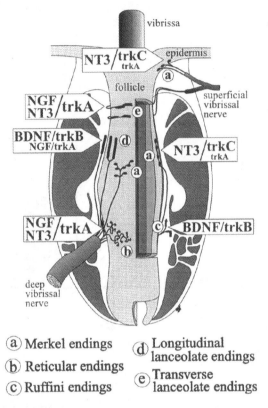

ⓐ Merkel endings   ⓓ Longitudinal lanceolate endings

ⓑ Reticular endings   ⓔ Transverse lanceolate endings

ⓒ Ruffini endings

Figure 3.4   Schematic representation of the neurotrophin/trk signaling dependence of vibrissal mechanoreceptors for survival. (Modified from Ref. 37.)

increased dramatically in the trkC kinase-deficient mice. This fact suggested to the authors that the effect of NT3 may be mediated through the trkA receptor. Merkel cell–neurite complexes seem to require NT3/trkC signaling for their development.[37] However, the loss of Merkel innervation occurs earlier in NT3 null mutant mice than in trkC kinase-deficient mice, possibly due to a reduced dependence on NT3/trkA signaling. Other sets of cutaneous mechanoreceptors appear to be dependent on BDNF/trkB signaling. Ruffini endings and their axons are eliminated entirely in homozygous BDNF or trkB knockouts. Longitudinal lanceolate endings were reduced but never totally eliminated in the absence of BDNF or trkB as well as NGF or trkA. Thus the longitudinal lanceolate afferents may have a simultaneous co-dependency on two signaling mechanisms. Interestingly, although neurotrophin-4 (NT4) also binds with high affinity to the trkB receptor, the absence of NT4 had no obvious detrimental effect among the mechanoreceptors assessed to date in the mystacial pad.

The role of all neurotrophins and their receptors in the survival and maintenance of the mystacial pad innervation is consistent with the loss of trigeminal ganglion neurons in the neurotrophin null mutant mice as well as in the trk kinase-deficient mice[13,17,24,25,29,35,38,39] (Fig. 3.5).

Electrophysiological studies have also shown that NT3 is essential for maintenance of the innervation of two subsets of cutaneous mechanoreceptors in skin: D-hair receptors and the slowly adapting mechanoreceptors (SA1), Merkel cells.[40] Interestingly, both studies suggest that the NT3/trkC signaling dependence of some cutaneous afferents occurs postnatally after target innervation, since at birth NT3 mutant mice have a normal complement of Merkel cells and innervating sensory axons. This differs from the muscle afferents that innervate muscle spindles, which require NT3/trkC signaling for survival before final target innervation.[6,27,36,41,42]

The fact that some mechanoreceptors do not become dependent on NT3 until the postnatal period suggests that these sensory neurons may require another growth factor for embryonic survival and then change their dependence on NT3 postnatally. This switch in growth factor dependence for survival also seems to occur in a subset of sensory neurons that express trkA during embryonic development and down-regulate the trkA expression postnatally. Whether this population responds to NT3 later remains to be determined.

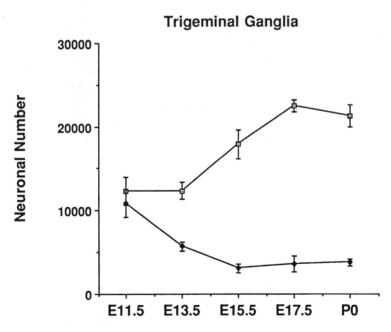

Figure 3.5   Neuronal numbers in the trigeminal ganglia of trkA kinase-deficient mice at different stages of development: trkA kinase-deficient mice (diamonds); wild-type mice (squares).

The trophic dependence of the remainder of the cutaneous mechano-receptors present in the skin remains to be determined. The role of BDNF/trkB signaling in the development of skin mechanoreceptors has been very elusive. Although previous studies have reported as many as 30% fewer neurons in newborn trkB kinase-deficient or BDNF null mutant mice compared to their wild-type littermates,[16,29,43] other studies have found no DRG neuronal loss at this stage. In newborn BDNF null mutant mice as well as in newborn trkB kinase-deficient mice, DRG neuronal numbers are similar to those of their wild-type littermates (I. Fariñas and G. Yancopoulos, personal communications; see also Ref. 30). Consistent with these results the dorsal root projection to the spinal cord appears normal at this stage of development.[30] In addition, it has been reported that there is about 30% reduction in the number of DRG neurons in 2-week-old BDNF null mutant mice[38,44] or trkB kinase-deficient mice (I. Silos-Santiago, unpublished observations). The identity of these neurons is unknown. However, immunohistochemical and electron microscopy analysis by Vega and collaborators have shown that Meissner corpuscles are absent in 2-week-old trkB kinase-deficient mice (J.A. Vega and I. Silos-Santiago, unpublished observations) and in the BDNF null mutant mice (J.A. Vega and I. Fariñas, unpublished observations). These results suggest that neurons that give rise to these sensory receptors may be absent in these mutant mice. This is the first indication that BDNF/trkB signaling is required for the survival of a subpopulation of cutaneous mechanoreceptors in glabrous skin. Other cutaneous mechanoreceptors, such as Pacinian corpuscles, are still present in these mice. To date no survival factor has been described for this subtype of cutaneous mechanoreceptors.

Interestingly, newborn mice that lack both trkB and trkC kinase domains display a higher percentage of neuronal cell loss (40%) than do single kinase-deficient mice.[30] These data suggest that the loss of additional neurons observed in the trkB/trkC doubly deficient mice is due to the elimination of compensatory signaling between trkB and trkC. The identity of those neurons remains to be established.

3.2.4   NT3/trkC and BDNF/trkB Signaling in Normal Development of the Inner Ear

In situ hybridization studies have revealed that trkB and trkC are expressed in the sensory neurons of vestibular and spiral ganglia. The ligands for these receptors, BDNF and NT3, are expressed in the sensory epithelia of the inner ear. Interestingly, expression of the ligands shows no clear pattern in terms of sensory hair cell types. However, there is a clear spatial expression pattern in different regions of the inner ear. For example, BDNF is heavily expressed in the semicircular canals, whereas NT3 is not expressed in these structures. Both BDNF and NT3 are expressed in the saccule and utricule as well as in the cochlea.[45,46] In the latter region, however, a gradient of neurotrophin expression appears to exist, with NT3 present mainly in the basal turn and BDNF in the apical turn (as judged from mutant mouse innervation). Analysis of trkB, trkC, NT3, BDNF, trkB/C double, and NT3/BDNF double knockout mice have demonstrated the role of BDNF/trkB and NT3/trkC signaling in development of the inner ear.[16,24,25,29,30,38,39,44,47–52]

The *trk*B targeted mice carry a deletion in their tyrosine kinase sequences that prevents expression of the trkB receptor but not of the noncatalytic isoforms.[43] Similar to the BDNF null mutant mice, these mice develop to birth; however, most of them die between 2 and 3 weeks of age, and their phenotype is characterized by severe deficiencies in coordination and balance.[38,43,44,47]

The lack of balance in these mice, apparent on the day of birth, is due to an important neuronal loss in the vestibular ganglion where only a small percentage of its neuronal population remains by postnatal day 0[16,30,47,51,52] (Fig. 3.6). The neurogenesis of this ganglion appears normal as early as E12.5, when the

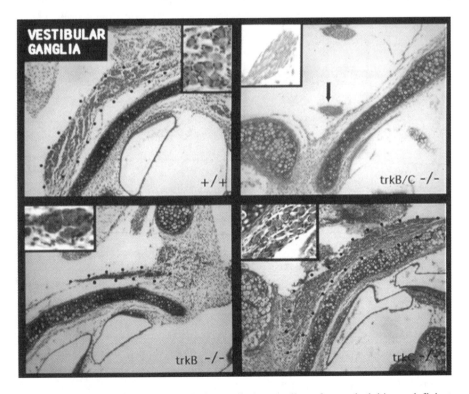

Figure 3.6 Paraffin sections through the vestibular ganglion of several trk kinase-deficient mice showing neuronal loss in newborn mice. Dotted line delineates the vestibular ganglion.

axons of some vestibular neurons are able to reach some of the sensory epithelia.[47,48] However, in newborn mice, all innervation to the semicircular canals is absent, and innervation to the utricle and saccule is very reduced.[16,47,48,50–52] Elimination of the innervation of these structures appears to occur very early during embryonic development.[47,48] In the cochlear ganglion of these mice a small reduction in the number of neurons has also been observed by postnatal day 0.[16,30,47,51,52] This is consistent with a small reduction in the cochlea innervation (apical turn) that has been described in trkB kinase-deficient mice.[48,50]

In contrast, trkC kinase-deficient mice as well as NT3 null mutant mice display severe neuronal loss in the cochlear ganglion and a small reduction in the number of vestibular neurons.[16,24,25,30,47,49–51] The 85% loss of cochlear neurons is not equally distributed throughout the cochlea. This results in an apparent reduction of all innervation in the basal turn of the cochlea in both NT3 and trkC kinase-deficient mice.[48–50]

The most dramatic effect in the development of the inner ear has been observed in newborn trkB/trkC kinase-deficient and NT3/BDNF null mutant mice. In these animals, the vestibular and cochlear ganglia are completely absent.[29,30,47,48,50] This cell loss led to complete loss of all afferent ear innervation at birth, indicating that the two neurotrophins (NT3 and BDNF) and their two

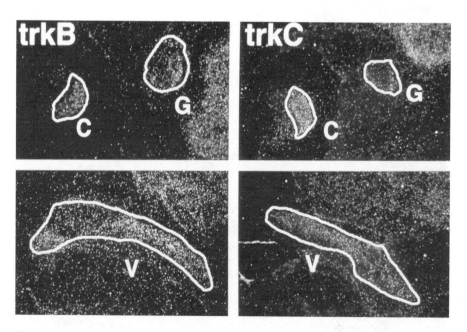

Figure 3.7   TrkB (left panels) and trkC (right panels) expression in the cochlear (C, upper panels), geniculate (G, upper panels), and vestibular (V, lower panels) ganglia in wild-type mice.

receptors (trkB and trkC) are all that is required to maintain the survival of these neuronal populations as well as innervation of the inner ear. Interestingly, the sensory epithelia of the inner ear that are innervated by these ganglia did develop in these mice and are still present at birth. These data indicate that the initial development of sensory epithelia as well as the early structural maturation of hair cells is not dependent on nerve fiber innervation.

Also interesting is the fact that mice heterozygous for the NT3 or BDNF mutation lack about half of the vestibular and cochlear neuronal complement.[47,52] This gene dosage dependence for neuronal survival confirms two facts: the necessity of minimal levels of growth factors to support survival of these neurons, and the fact that NT3 and BDNF are produced in limited amounts in the inner ear. In addition, it has been shown that trkB/C double-mutant mice, in which one allele is homozygous for the mutation (trkB$^{-/-}$ or trkC$^{-/-}$) and the other allele is heterozygous (trkC$^{+/-}$ or trkB$^{+/-}$) display a more dramatic reduction in sensory neurons than do single homozygous mutants.[16,48,50] Similarly, the innervation pattern of the inner ear is affected more severely in these mice.[48,50] These data suggest a certain degree of cooperation of the trkB and trkC receptors in inner ear sensory neurons, consistent with the known overlap in gene expression (Fig. 3.7).

3.2.5   TrkB Signaling and Survival of Geniculate and Nodose–Petrosal Neurons

In vitro it has been shown that different populations of cranial sensory neurons also require neurotrophins for survival.[53] As expected, the survival of neurons in specific cranial ganglia is affected by the absence of different trk/neurotrophin signaling pathways. For instance, there is a severe neuronal loss in the geniculate ganglia of trkB kinase-deficient mice[30,54] (Fig. 3.8). Only about 5% of geniculate neurons are present in these mice the day of birth. Consistent with these data is the fact that in both BDNF and NT4 null mutant mice only about 50% of the sensory neurons are detected in the geniculate ganglion.[29,44,55] In double BDNF/NT4 null mutant mice only 6% of geniculate neurons survive.[55] These data indicate that both BDNF and NT4 acting through trkB are essential for survival of these sensory neurons. Furthermore, this additive effect suggests that at least two different neuronal populations that require different neurotrophic factors for survival may exist within the geniculate ganglia, and that BDNF or NT4 may not compensate for each other in promoting survival of these neuronal populations. The identity of these sensory neurons remain to be determined. Interestingly, however, a percentage of geniculate neurons are also eliminated in trkC (Fig. 3.8) and in NT3 null mutant mice.[25,29,30] The fact that in trkB kinase-deficient mice the majority of geniculate neurons are eliminated and that there is no additive

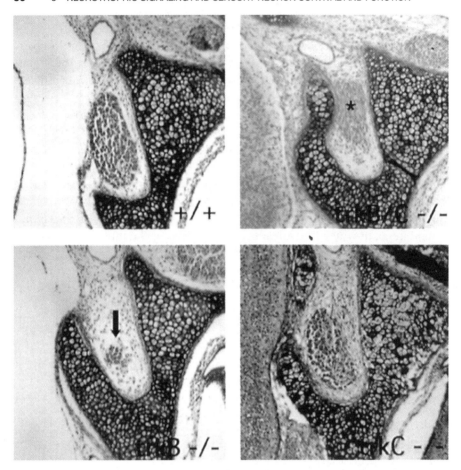

Figure 3.8 Paraffin sections through the geniculate ganglion of several trk kinase-deficient mice showing neuronal loss in newborn mice.

effect in double trkB/C kinase-deficient mice (Fig. 3.8) or in double BDNF/NT3 null mutant mice[29,30] suggests that NT3/trkC-dependent neurons are a subpopulation of the geniculate neurons that require trkB signaling for survival at some stage of development. Whether NT3/trkC-dependent neurons also require BDNF, NT4, or both at different stages of development remains unknown.

Consistent with these results, lingual deficits have been described in trkB kinase-deficient mice and in BDNF and NT3 null mutant mice.[54,56,57] Although some taste buds can be identified in these mutant mice, in BDNF and trkB mice taste buds are reduced in number and malformed. Furthermore, intragemmal innervation cannot be observed in the remaining taste buds, although some extragemmal fibers are present between taste buds cells.

In contrast, in NT3 null mutant mice there is a massive loss of somatosensory innervation of lingual structures with no effect on taste buds.

A very similar situation has been described in placode-derived visceral neurons of nodose–petrosal ganglia. Neurons in this complex relay visceral sensory information from the cardiovascular, respiratory, and gastrointestinal systems to the central nervous system (CNS). Therefore, it is possible that significant loss of these neurons accounts for the death of the trkB kinase-defective mice. Neurons in the nodose–petrosal ganglia are affected by the lack of all neurotrophins[24,25,29,38,39,44,45,58,59] but NGF.[12] In agreement with these results, analysis of trk kinase-deficient mice have shown that these neurons depend on trkB and trkC signaling for survival during development[30,58] (Fig. 3.9). Recent studies have shown that some populations of nodose–petrosal sensory neurons depend exclusively on BDNF for survival, whereas others depend on NT4. In

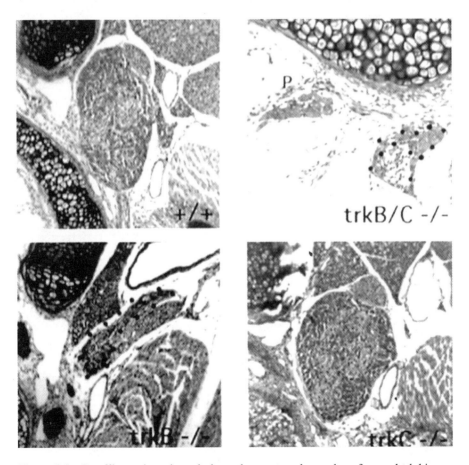

Figure 3.9 Paraffin sections through the nodose–petrosal complex of several trk kinase-deficient mice showing neuronal loss in newborn mice. Dots delineate the nodose ganglion.

addition it appears that there may be another group of these neurons that require either BDNF or NT4.[58] The latter group corresponds to a subset of dopaminergic neurons. Erikson et al.[58] have shown that BDNF and NT4 can compensate for each other to support some dopaminergic neurons in the nodose–petrosal ganglia. Erikson et al. have also demonstrated that dopaminergic neurons that innervate the carotid body are severely depleted in trkB kinase-deficient mice as well as in BDNF null mutant mice. Loss of these neurons is responsible for the abnormal breathing reflexes in these mice, which may contribute to their early postnatal death. The majority of these neurons are not affected in NT4 null mutant mice that survive until adulthood.

Another interesting aspect of this work is the fact that similar to the inner ear system, mice heterozygous for BDNF deletions display half of the neuronal loss described in BDNF null mutant mice. However, NT4 heterozygous mice have the same neuronal complement in the nodose/petrosal complex as that of wild-type mice. These data suggest that BDNF is produced in limited quantities, whereas similar to NGF, NT4 is not produced in limited amounts.

As mentioned above, a small percentage of nodose–petrosal neurons are lost in the absence of NT3/trkC signaling[24,25,29,30] (Fig. 3.9). However, there is not an additive effect in trkB/C kinase-deficient or BDNF/NT3 null mutant mice, suggesting that neurons that depend on NT3/trkC signaling for survival are a subset of those that require trkB signaling, which may require NT3 at different stages of development. In this sense, ElShamy and Ernfors[59] have recently shown that NT3 and NT4 are survival factors for these visceral neurons very early during embryonic development and that BDNF appears to be required for survival at later stages.

3.3   P75-DEFICIENT MICE

The role of p75, the low-affinity receptor for all the neurotrophins, remains elusive. Mice that lack this low-affinity neurotrophin receptor are viable and fertile, although they develop skin ulcers in the distal extremities.[60] Analysis of the DRG have shown that there is a 50% neuronal loss in mice homozygous for the mutation. However, using electrophysiological and immunohistochemical techniques, it appears that p75 is not required for the survival of one specific subpopulation of sensory neurons.[61,62] In vitro analysis of different populations of peripheral neurons have shown that p75 can modulate neurotrophin sensitivity in those neurons.[63] Whether this mechanism is involved in the neuronal loss observed in mice that lack p75 receptor remains to be elucidated.

3.4 FUTURE DIRECTIONS

The generation of genetically engineered mice in which neurotrophins and their receptors have been eliminated by homologous recombination has clearly defined its role during embryonic and early postnatal development. Analysis of these mice has established the survival requirements for various populations of neurons in the PNS as well as in the CNS. However, due to the short life span of these mice, whether neurotrophin/trk signaling is important for the maintenance and function of the nervous system in adult life remains to be determined. Generation of conditional knockout or knock-in mice, now well under way, will help to identify the role of neurotrophin/trk signaling in adulthood and therefore to establish the potential of these molecules in the treatment of human diseases.

REFERENCES

1. Katz, L. C., and Shatz, C. J. (1996). Synaptic activity and the construction of cortical circuits. Science 274:1133–1138.
2. Thoenen, H. (1995). Neurotrophins and neuronal plasticity. Science 270:593–598.
3. Kaplan, D. R., and Stephens, R. M. (1994). Neurotrophin signal transduction by the Trk receptor J. Neurobiol. 25:1404–1417.
4. Barbacid, M. (1995). Neurotrophic factors and their receptors. Curr. Opin. Cell Biol. 7:148–155.
5. Segal, R., and Greenberg, M. E. (1996). Intracellular signaling pathways activated by neurotrophic factors. Annu. Rev. Neurosci. 19:463–489.
6. Snider, W. D. (1994). Functions of the neurotrophins during nervous system development: what the knockouts are teaching us. Cell 77:627–638.
7. Fariñas, I., and Reichardt, L. F. (1996). Neurotrophic factors and their receptors: implications of genetic studies. Semin. Neurosci. 8:133–143.
8. Snider, W. D., and Silos-Santiago, I. (1996). Dorsal root ganglion neurons require functional neurotrophin receptors for survival during development. Philos. Trans. R. Soc. Lond. B 351:395–403.
9. Levi-Montalcini, R. (1987). The nerve growth factor 35 years later. Science 237:1154–1162.
10. Chao, M. V., Bothwell, M. A., Ross, A. H., Koprowski, H., Lanahan, A. A., Buck, C. R., and Sehgal, A. (1986). Gene transfer and molecular cloning of the human NGF receptor. Science 232:518–521.
11. Martín-Zanca, D., Hughes, S. H., and Barbacid, M. (1986). A human oncogene formed by the fusion of truncated tropomyosin and protein tyrosine kinase sequences. Nature 319: 743–749.

12. Crowley, C., Spencer, S. D., Nishimura, M., Chen, K. S., Pitts-Meek, S., Armanini, M. P., Ling, L. H., McMahon, S. B., Shelton, L., Levinson, A. D., and Philips, H. S. (1994). Mice lacking nerve growth factor display perinatal loss of sensory and sympathetic neurons yet develop basal forebrain cholinergic neurons. Cell 76:1001–1011.

13. Smeyne, R. J., Klein, R., Schnapp, A., Long, L. K., Bryant, S., Lewin, A., Lira, S. A., and Barbacid, M. (1994). Severe sensory and sympathetic neuropathies in mice carrying a disrupted Trk/NGF receptor gene. Nature 368:246–249.

14. Silos-Santiago, I., Molliver, D. C., Ozaki, S., Smeyne, R. J., Fagan, A. M., Barbacid, M., and Snider, W. D. (1995). Non-trkA-expressing small DRG neurons are lost in *trk*A deficient mice, J. Neurosci. 15:5929–5942.

15. Johnson, E. M., Gorin, P. D., Brandeis, L. D., and Pearson, J. (1980). Dorsal root ganglion neurons are destroyed by exposure in utero to maternal antibody to nerve growth factor. Science 219:916–918.

16. Minichiello, L., Piehl, F., Vazquez, E., Schimmang, T., Hokfelt, T., Represa, J., and Klein, R. (1995). Differential effects of combined *trk* receptor mutations on dorsal root ganglion and inner ear sensory neurons. Development 121:4067–4075.

17. Piñón, L. G. P., Minichiello, L., Klein, R., and Davies A. M. (1996). Timing of neuronal death in *trk*A, *trk*B and *trk*C mutant embryos reveals developmental changes in sensory neuron dependence on Trk signalling. Development 122:3255–3261.

18. White, F. A., Silos-Santiago, I., Molliver, D. C., Nishimura, M., Philips, H. S., Barbacid, M., and Snider, W. D. (1996). Synchronous onset of NGF and trkA survival dependence in developing dorsal root ganglia. J. Neurosci. 16:4662–4672.

19. Lawson, S. N. (1992). Morphological and biochemical cell types of sensory neurons. In: Sensory neurons, ed. Scott, S. A., Oxford University Press, New York, pp. 27–59.

20. Molliver, D. C., Radeke, M. J., Feinstein, S. C., and Snider, W. D. (1995). Presence or absence of TrkA protein distinguishes subsets of small sensory neurons with unique cytochemical characteristics and dorsal horn projections. J. Comp. Neurol. 361:404–416.

21. Rice, F. L., Albers, K. M., Davies, B. M., Silos-Santiago, I., Wilkinson, G. A., LaMaster, A. M., Ernfors, P., Smeyne, R. J., Aldskogius, H., DeChiara, T. M., Philips, H. S., Reichardt, L. F., Barbacid, M., Yancopoulos, G. D., and Fundin, B. T. (1998). Differential dependency of unmyelinated and aδ epidermal and upper dermal innervation on neurotrophins, trk receptors and p75 LNGFR. Dev. Biol. 198:57–81.

22. de Castro, F., Silos-Santiago, I., Lopez de Armentia, M., Barbacid, M., and Belmonte, C. (1998). Corneal innervation and sensitivity to noxious stimuli in trkA knockout mice. Eur. J. Neurosci.

23. Fagan, A. M., Zhang, H., Landis, S., Smeyne, R. J., Silos-Santiago, I., and Barbacid, M. (1996). TrkA, but not TrkC, receptors are essential for survival of sympathetic neurons in vivo. J. Neurosci. 16:6208–6218.

24. Ernfors, P., Lee, K. F., Kucera, J., and Jaenisch, R. (1994). Lack of neurotrophin-3 leads to deficiencies in the peripheral nervous system and loss of limb proprioceptive afferents. Cell 77:503–512.

25. Fariñas, I., Jones, K. R., Backus, C., Wang, X. Y., and Reichardt, L. F. (1994). Severe sensory and sympathetic deficits in mice lacking neurotrophin-3. Nature 369:658–661.

26. Klein, R., Silos-Santiago, I., Smeyne, R. J., Lira, S. A., Brambilla, R., Bryant, S., Zhang, L., Snider, W. D., and Barbacid, M. (1994). Disruption of the neurotrophin-3 receptor gene *trk*C eliminates Ia muscle afferents and results in abnormal movements. Nature 368:249–251.

27. Tessarollo, L., Vogel, K. S., Palko, M. E., Reid, S. W., and Parada, L. F. (1994). Targeted mutation in the neurotrophin-3 gene results in loss of muscle sensory neurons. Proc. Natl. Acad. Sci. USA 91:11844–11848.

28. Tessarollo, L., Tsoulfas, P., Donovan, M. J., Palko, M. E., Blair-Flynn, J., Hemstead, B. L., and Parada, L. F. (1997). Targeted deletion of all isoforms of the trkC gene suggest the use of alternate receptors by its ligand neurotrophin-3 in neuronal development and implicates trkC in normal cardiogenesis. Proc. Natl. Acad. Sci. USA 94:14776–14778.

29. Liebl, D. J., Tessarrollo, L., Palko, M. E., and Parada, L. F. (1997). Absence of sensory neurons before target innervation in brain-derived neurotrophic factor–, neurotrophin 3–, and trkC-deficient embryonic mice. J. Neurosci. 17:9113–9121.

30. Silos-Santiago, I., Fagan, A. M., Garber, M., Fritzsch, B., and Barbacid, M. (1997). Severe sensory deficits but normal CNS development in newborn mice lacking trkB and trkC tyrosine protein kinase receptors. Eur. J. Neurosci. 9:2045–2056.

31. ElShamy, W. M., and Ernfors, P. (1996). A local action of neurotrophin-3 prevents the death of proliferating sensory neuron precursor cells. Neuron 16:963–972.

32. ElShamy, W. M., and Ernfors, P. (1996). Requirement of neurotrophin-3 for the survival of proliferating trigeminal ganglion progenitor cells. Development 122:2405–2414.

33. ElShamy, W. M., Linnarsson, S., Lee, K.-F., Jaenisch, R., and Ernfors, P. (1996). Prenatal and postnatal requirements of NT-3 for sympathetic neuroblast survival and innervation of specific targets. Development 122:491–500.

34. Fariñas, I., Yoshida, C. K., Backus, C., and Reichardt, L. F. (1996). Lack of neurotrophin-3 results in death of spinal sensory neurons and premature differentiation of their precursors. Neuron 17:1065–1078.

35. Wilkinson, G. A., Fariñas, I., Backus, C., Yoshida, C. K., and Reichardt, L. F. (1996). Neurotrophin-3 is a survival factor in vivo for early mouse trigeminal neurons. J. Neurosci. 16:7661–7669.

36. Kucera, J., Fan, G., Jaenisch, R., Linnarsson, S., and Ernfors, P. (1995). Dependence of developing group Ia afferents on neurotrophin-3. J. Comp. Neurol. 363:307–320.

37. Fundin, B. T., Silos-Santiago, I., Ernfors, P., Fagan, A. M., Aldskogius, H., DeChiara, T. M., Philips, H. S., Barbacid, M., Yancopoulos, G. D., and Rice, F. L. (1997). Differential dependency of mechanoreceptors on neurotrophins, trk receptors and p75 LNGFR. Dev. Biol. 190:94–116.

38. Ernfors, P., Lee, K. F., and Jaenisch, R. (1994). Mice lacking brain-derived neurotrophic factor develop with sensory deficits. Nature 368:147–150.

39. Conover, J. C., Erickson, J. T., Katz, D. M., Bianchi, L. M., Poueymirou, W. T., McClain, J., J. R., Pan, L., Helgren, M., Ip, N. Y., Boland, P., Friedman, B., Wiegand, S., Vejsada, Kato, A. C., DeChiara, T. M., and Yancopoulos, G. D. (1995). Neuronal deficits, not involving motor neurons, in mice lacking BDNF and/or NT-4. Nature 375:235–238.

40. Airaksinen, M. S., Koltzenburg, M., Lewin, G. R., Masu, Y., Helbig, C., Wolf, E., Brem, G., Toyka, K. V., Thoenen, H., and Meyer, M. (1996). Specific subtypes of cutaneous mechanoreceptors require neurotrophin-3 following peripheral target innervation. Neuron 16:287–295.

41. Gaese, F., Kolbeck, R., and Barde, Y.-A. (1994). Sensory ganglia require neurotrophin-3 early in development. Development 120: 1613–1619.

42. Lefcort, F., Clary, D. O., Rusoff, A. C., and Reichardt, L. F. (1996). Inhibition of the NT-3 receptor trkC, early in chick embryogenesis, results in severe reductions in multiple neuronal subpopulations in the dorsal root ganglia. J. Neurosci. 16:3704–3713.

43. Klein, R., Smeyne, R. J., Wurst, W., Long, L. K., Auerbach, B, A,, Joyner, A. L., and Barbacid, M. (1993). Targeted disruption of the trkB neurotrophin receptor gene results in nervous system lesions and neonatal death. Cell 75:113–122.

44. Jones, K. R., Fariñas, I., Backus, C., and Reichardt, L. F. (1994). Targeted disruption of the BDNF gene perturbs brain and sensory neuron development but not motor neuron development. Cell 76:989–999.

45. Pirvola, U., Ylikoski, J., Palgi, J., Lehtonen, E., and Arumae, U. (1992). Brain-derived neurotrophic factor and neurotrophin-3 mRNA in the peripheral target fields of developing inner ear ganglia. Proc. Natl. Acad. Sci. USA 89:9915–9919.

46. Pirvola, U., Arumae, U., Moshnyakov, M., Palgi, J., Saarma, M., and Ylikoski, J. (1994). Coordinated expression and function of neurotrophins and their receptors in the inner ear during target innervation. Hear. Res. 75:131–144.

47. Ernfors, P., Van Der Water, T., Loring, J., and Jaenisch, R. (1995). Complementary roles of BDNF and NT-3 in vestibular and auditory development. Neuron 14:1153–1164.

48. Fritzsch, B., Silos-Santiago, I., Smeyne, R. J., Fagan, A. M., and Barbacid, M. (1995). Reduction and loss of inner ear innervation in trkB and trkC receptor knock out mice: a whole mount DiI and SEM analysis. Auditory Neurosci. 1: 401–417.

49. Fritzsch, B., Fariñas, I., and Reichardt, L. F. (1997). Lack of neurotrophin 3 causes losses of both classes of spiral ganglion neurons in the cochlea in a region-specific fashion. J. Neurosci. 17:6213–6225.

50. Fritzsch, B., Silos-Santiago, I., Bianchi, L. M., and Fariñas, I. (1997). The role of neurotrophic factors in regulating the development of the inner ear innervation. TINS 20:159–164.

51. Schimmang, T., Minichiello, L., Vázquez, E., San José, I., Giráldez, F., Klein, R., and Represa, J. (1995). Developing inner ear sensory neurons require trkB and TrkC receptors for innervation of their peripheral targets. Development 121:3381–3391.

52. Bianchi, L. M., Conover, J. C., Fritzsch, B., DeChiara, T., Lindsay, R. M., and Yancopoulos, G. D. (1996). Degeneration of vestibular neurons in late embryogenesis of both heterozygous and homozygous BDNF null mutant mice. Development 122:1965–1973.

53. Davies, A. M. (1994). The role of neurotrophins in the developing nervous system. J. Neurobiol. 25: 1334–1348.

54. Fritzsch, B., Sarai, P. A., Barbacid, M., and Silos-Santiago, I. (1997). Mice with a targeted disruption of the neurotrophin receptor trkB lose their gustatory ganglion cells early but do develop taste buds. Int. J. Dev. Neurosci. 15: 563–576.

55. Liu, X., Ernfors, P., Wu, H., and Jaenisch, R. (1995). Sensory but not motor neuron deficits in mice lacking NT4 and BDNF. Nature 375:238–241.

56. Nosrat, C. A., Blomlof, J., ElShamy, W. M., Ernfors, P., and Olson, L. (1997). Lingual deficits in BDNF and NT-3 mutant mice leading to gustatory and somatosensory disturbances, respectively. Development 124:1333–1342.

57. Oakley, B., Brandemihl, A., Cooper, D., Lau, D., Lawton, A., and Zhang, C. (1998). The morphogenesis of mouse vallate gustatory epithelium and taste buds requires BDNF- dependent taste neurons. Dev. Brain Res. 105:85–96.

58. Erickson, J. T., Conover, J. C., Borday, V., Champagnat, J., Barbacid, M., Yancopoulos, G. D., and Katz, D. M. (1996). Mice lacking brain-derived neurotrophic factor exhibit visceral sensory neuron losses distinct from mice lacking NT-4 and display a severe developmental deficit in control of breathing. J. Neurosci. 16: 5361–5371.

59. ElShamy, W. M., and Ernfors, P. (1997). Brain-derived neurotrophic factor, neurotrophin-3, and neurotrophin-4 complement and cooperate with each other sequentially during visceral neuron development. J. Neurosci. 17:8667–8675.

60. Lee, K.-L., Davies, A. M., and Jaenisch, R. (1994). p75-deficient embryonic dorsal root sensory and neonatal sympathetic neurons display a decreased sensitivity to NGF. Development 120:1027–1033.

61. Bergmann, I., Priestley, J. V., McMahon, S. B., Brocker, E. B., Toyka, K. V., and Koltzenburg, M. (1997). Analysis of cutaneous sensory neurons in transgenic mice lacking the low affinity neurotrophin receptor p75. Eur. J. Neurosci. 9:18–28.

62. Stucky, C. L., and Koltzenburg, M. (1997). The low-affinity neurotrophin receptor p75 regulates the function but not the selective survival of specific subpopulations of sensory neurons. J. Neurosci. 17:4398–4405.

63. Lee, K.-L., Li, E., Huber, J., Landis, S. C., Sharpe, A. H., Chao, M. V., and Jaenisch, R. (1992). Targeted mutation of the gene encoding the low affinity NGF receptor p75 leads to deficits in the peripheral sensory nervous system. Cell 69:737–749.

CHAPTER 4

Glial Cell Line–Derived Neurotrophic Factor and Nociceptive Neurons

STEPHEN B. MCMAHON AND DAVID L. H. BENNETT

Neuroscience Research Centre, King's College
London

4.1 INTRODUCTION

The neurotrophins nerve growth factor (NGF), brain-derived neurotrophic factor (BDNF), neurotrophin-3 (NT3), and neurotrophin-4 and 5 (NT4/5) are critical in development and maintenance of the nervous system. Sensory neurons have provided a model system for investigating the actions of these molecules. During development, neurotrophins regulate the survival of specific populations of sensory neurons during the period of naturally occurring cell death.[1] Neurotrophins also exert more subtle effects on sensory neuron differentiation and in adulthood are important for phenotypic maintenance of sensory neurons. Of particular interest has been the demonstration that NGF powerfully regulates the sensitivity of many nociceptive afferents to noxious stimuli and has a critical role in the generation of inflammatory pain.[2–4] Another area of interest has been the possible therapeutic use of neurotrophins in the treatment of peripheral neuropathy[5] and indeed, clinical trials are in progress to test the efficacy of NGF in the treatment of diabetic neuropathy.

It has been shown that there is a family of neurotrophic factors that belong to the TGFβ superfamily which are structurally distinct from the neurotrophins. This family includes glial cell line–derived neurotrophic factor (GDNF), neuturin (NTN), and persephin (PSP). We and others have begun to investigate whether members of this novel family of trophic factors have an important role in sensory neuron development and in the regulation of sensory neuron properties during adulthood. In this chapter we focus on the actions of GDNF, as

Molecular Basis of Pain Induction, Edited by John N. Wood

most recent work has concentrated on this factor. An important concept to arise from this work is the idea that adult small-diameter nociceptive afferents can be divided into two roughly equal-sized groups. The first group expresses tyrosine kinase A (trkA), the high-affinity NGF receptor, and is responsive to this factor, while the second group expresses GDNF receptor components (but not trkA) and is GDNF sensitive. These findings suggest an important role for GDNF family members in the maintenance of adult nociceptive properties and suggest further that these trophic factors or their antagonists might find therapeutic applications in the treatment of chronic pain states.

4.2   GDNF: A NEUROTROPHIC FACTOR DISTINCT FROM THE NEUROTROPHINS

GDNF, the first member of this family to be characterized, was purified as a consequence of its ability to support embryonic midbrain dopaminergic neurons in vitro.[6] GDNF exists as a homodimer of two 134-amino acid subunits. GDNF has potent survival-promoting effects on a variety of neuronal populations within both the peripheral nervous system (PNS) and the central nervous system (CNS), including midbrain dopaminergic neurons,[7,8] locus coeruleus noradrenergic neurons,[9] spinal motoneurons,[10,11] and distinct subpopulations of peripheral sensory, sympathetic, and parasympathetic neurons.[12,13] These findings have generated immense interest in the possible therapeutic applications of GDNF in neurodegenerative conditions such as Parkinson's disease and amyotrophic lateral sclerosis.

Analysis of GDNF-deficient mice has demonstrated a critical role for GDNF in development of the enteric nervous system and in kidney organogenesis.[14–16] Interestingly, there were no severe deficits in dopaminergic neurons or motoneurons in these animals, suggesting a level of redundancy and the possibility that other factors are also important in regulating the development of these neuronal populations.

NTN was the second member of this family of neurotrophic factors to be identified and was isolated from Chinese hamster ovary cells, based on its ability to promote the survival of sympathetic neurons.[17] NTN is 40% identical to GDNF. Although the full range of its trophic effects is not yet known, it promotes the survival of sympathetic, nodose, and dorsal root ganglia neurons in vitro. A third member, PSP, has recently been identified using degenerate polymerase chain reaction (PCR).[18] PSP is 40% identical to GDNF and NTN. This factor promotes survival of midbrain dopaminergic neurons and motoneurons in vitro and in vivo following experimental lesions. However, PSP does not support the survival of either sympathetic neurons or dorsal root ganglia (DRG) cells.

4.3   RECEPTORS FOR THE GDNF FAMILY

Members of the GDNF family signal via a receptor complex. This consists of RET, a tyrosine kinase receptor, which acts as a signal-transducing domain and a member of the GFRα family of GPI-linked receptors (GFRα1 to 4), which act as ligand-binding domains.[12,19–30] Either GFRα1 or GFRα2 in conjunction with RET can mediate GDNF or NTN signaling, although GDNF is thought to bind preferentially to GFRα1 and NTN to GFRα2. The fact that there is significant crosstalk between GDNF/NTN and their respective GFRα receptors was recently demonstrated by findings from GFRα1-deficient mice. Results from GDNF-, RET-, and GFRα1-deficient mice indicate that these are all essential for the development of the kidney and enteric nervous system.[14–16,31–33] However, although RET and GDNF are required for the development of a number of peripheral ganglia (cervical and nodose), these are virtually unaffected in GFRα1-deficient mice, suggesting that GDNF must be acting via another receptor component (GFRα2) in supporting these populations. The receptor components by which PSP acts are as yet unknown. Fibroblasts transfected with RET in combination with GFRα1 or GFRα2 did not respond to PSP,[18] suggesting that this factor uses either different or additional receptor

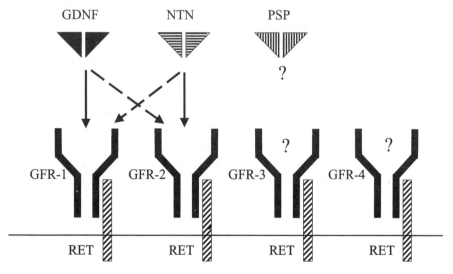

Figure 4.1   Schematic illustration of the interaction of the GDNF family with their receptors. Members of the GDNF family signal via a receptor complex. This consists of RET, a tyrosine kinase receptor, which acts as a signal-transducing domain and a member of the GFRα family of GPI-linked receptors (GFRα1 to 4) which act as ligand-binding domains. GDNF is thought to bind preferentially to GFRα1 and NTN to GFRα2 although there is some crosstalk in this interaction. The receptor for PSP is unknown and the ligand-binding specificities of GFRα3 and 4 are also unknown.

components. The endogenous ligands acting at GFRα3 and GFRα4 are also as yet unknown. A schematic illustration of the interaction of members of the GDNF family with their receptors is shown in Figure 4.1.

4.4   TROPHIC FACTOR DEPENDENCE OF SENSORY NEURONS DURING DEVELOPMENT

Sensory neurons can be broadly divided into a number of anatomical and functional subgroups. There is marked specificity in terms of the trophic dependence of these subgroups of sensory neurons: NT3 acts as a target-derived factor for large-diameter afferents, mostly sensitive mechanoreceptors.[34–36] The role of BDNF in the development of peripheral sensory neurons is less clear. It may be a target-derived survival factor for some placode-derived primary sensory neurons, such as those of the nodose ganglia. For spinally projecting sensory neurons, however, it may fulfil an autocrine or paracrine role.[37,38] NGF is critical in the development of small-diameter DRG cells, which possess unmyelinated axons, terminate in the superficial laminae of the spinal cord, and respond principally to nociceptive stimuli.[39–41] During development it appears that all small-diameter neurons express trkA and are dependent for survival on NGF.[42] However, during the postnatal period, about one-half of the nociceptors (those that are marked by their ability to bind the lectin isolectin-B4 (IB4) down-regulate trkA expression[43,44] so that in the adult they do not express detectable levels of the low-affinity neurotrophin receptor p75 nor any known trk receptor. The reasons for this down regulation are at present unclear, although modulating NGF levels in the periphery apparently has no impact on this change.[44] There is therefore the possibility that during this period these neurons lose their NGF dependence and become dependent on another trophic factor.

In the mouse, between E10 and E12, GDNF mRNA is expressed at high levels in restricted regions of the proximal limb buds where axons converge and enter the limb. Between E14 and E16 GDNF is expressed in nonneuronal cells along peripheral nerves, in the dermis, and in some muscles.[45] This pattern of expression is consistent with GDNF acting as a trophic factor for sensory neurons during axon outgrowth and the period of naturally occurring cell death. GDNF can support the survival of a population of embryonic sensory neurons in vitro, and interestingly, the size of this population increases as development proceeds.[13,46] A physiological role for GDNF during sensory neuron development is supported by the fact that at P0 there is already a significant (20%) loss of DRG cells in GDNF-deficient mice.[14] GDNF can also prevent cell death in sensory neurons in vivo following neonatal axotomy.[47]

RET, the signal-transducing domain of the GDNF receptor, is expressed by DRG cells early in development (E11.5 in the mouse[48]). RET is initially expressed in large-diameter DRG cells, which innervate hair follicles and terminate in deep laminae of the spinal cord. As development proceeds (and through the postnatal period) the small-diameter DRG cells, which are marked by their ability to bind IB4, begin to express RET, during the exact period when the same cells are losing their NGF sensitivity by down-regulating trkA expression.[43,44] With emerging RET expression these neurons become sensitive to GDNF, and at this time GDNF promotes the survival of IB4-binding neurons in vitro.[48] The postnatal period therefore represents a period when IB4-binding DRG cells switch from NGF to GDNF dependence. A significant proportion of large-diameter DRG cells express RET and therefore would be expected to be GDNF sensitive. The developmental role of GDNF on these neurons is as yet unknown.

NTN is expressed in a number of peripheral tissues and can support a population of embryonic sensory neurons in vitro.[17] However, whether this represents a specific population (e.g., IB4 binding) of DRG cells is unknown. An NTN knockout would provide more information on the developmental role of this protein. Unlike GDNF and NTN, PSP does not have survival-promoting effects on embryonic sensory neurons in vitro. It is also expressed at extremely low levels in the periphery and is inefficiently spliced.[18] In summary, there is growing evidence that GDNF and NTN do play a role in sensory neuron development, but a detailed analysis of knockout animals will be required for a full description of their actions.

4.5 ACTIONS OF GDNF IN THE ADULT

4.5.1 Expression of GDNF Family Receptor Components

GDNF family receptor components (RET and GFRα1, 2, and 3) continue to be expressed in subsets of adult primary sensory neurons in the adult. As described above, expression of these proteins rises in DRG neurons in the postnatal period, and by the age of 2 weeks, the adult pattern is, in essence, established. That is, RET is expressed by about 60% of neurons (Fig. 4.2), and GFRα1, 2, and 3 are found in about 40, 30, and 40% of neurons, respectively.[49,50] RET and GFRα1 are expressed in subpopulations of both small- and large-diameter DRG cells; however, GFRα2 and 3 are expressed almost exclusively by small-diameter DRG cells.

The cells of the adult DRG can be broadly subdivided into three minimally overlapping subgroups based on their histochemical and functional properties (Fig. 4.3). First, about one-third of neurons, the classically defined "large

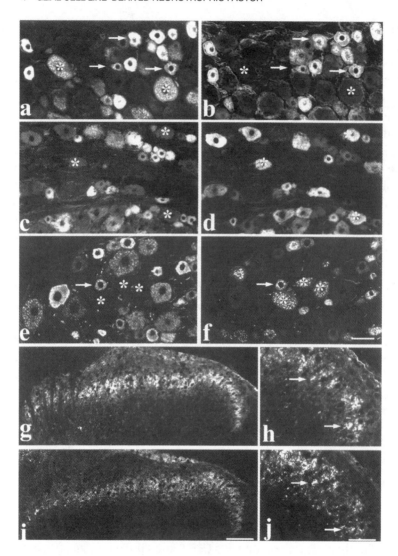

Figure 4.2   Colocalization of RET immunoreactivity with neurochemical markers in DRG cells and spinal cord. (a–f) Dual labeling showing RET immunofluorescence (a, c, e) combined with IB4 labeling (b), trkA immunofluorescence (d), and CGRP immunofluorescence (f) in DRG cells. Arrows indicate extensive colocalization of RET and IB4 in small-diameter cells (a, b). Note that all IB4 cells show RET immunoreactivity. However, several RET-positive cells do not bind IB4 (asterisks). RET labeling is not evident in many trkA cells (c, d). Asterisks denote trkA cells that are not colabeled for RET. Similarly, few CGRP expressing DRG cells are RET immunoreactive (e, f); asterisks indicate cells that do not express RET but are labeled for CGRP. The arrow indicates a cell, which is dual labeled. (g–j) Low (g, i) and high (h, j) magnification micrographs showing RET immunofluorescence (g, h) and IB4 (i, j) double labeling in the dorsal horn of the spinal cord. Labeling is most intense in inner lamina II. Arrows in (h) and (j) indicate individual double-labeled axons. Scale bars: 50 μm (a–f), 100 μm (g, i), and 30 μm (h, j). (See Ref. 50.)

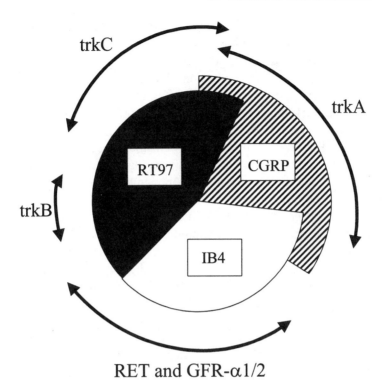

Figure 4.3   Pie chart summarizing the expression of neurotrophin and GDNF receptor components in spinal sensory neurons. The figure shows three principal subgroups of primary afferents. The first is the population of classically defined large light neurons, known to possess predominantly myelinated axons. These cells can be marked by their immunoreactivity for neurofilaments using antibodies such as N52. The other cells form the classically defined small dark population, known to possess predominantly unmyelinated axons. About one-half of the C fibers express the neuropeptide CGRP, and the other half express the enzyme TMP and bind the lectin IB4. The former group of C fibers have NGF receptors, while the latter have GDNF receptor components.

light" population, are rich in neurofilament and can be identified immunocytochemically with neurofilament antibodies such as RT97 and N52. These cells have myelinated axons (A fibers) and are known to be mostly sensitive mechanoreceptors. The remaining two-thirds of DRG neurons are the classically defined "small dark" neurons, known mostly to possess unmyelinated axons (C fibers). In most species, including rat, mouse, monkey, and humans, more than 90% of these cells are nociceptive in nature. These small cells can be subdivided into two groups of approximately equal size. One subgroup is marked by the expression of calcitonin gene–related peptide (CGRP). These cells express both p75 and trkA, receptors for NGF. The remaining small cells have a distinct chemical phenotype. They are nonpeptidergic, bind the lectin

IB4, and express the enzyme activities fluoride-resistant acid phosphatase (FRAP) and thiamine monophosphatase (TMP). These cells have recently been found to selectively express the purinoreceptor P2X$_3$.[51,52]

Strikingly, a high level of expression of all three GDNF receptor components is found in nonpeptidergic IB4-binding DRG cells (Figs. 4.2 and 4.3). Thus virtually all IB4-binding cells express RET mRNA and protein. The majority of these cells (79%) also express the ligand-binding domains for GDNF: GFRα1 or GFRα2. In some IB4 cells these receptor components are expressed independently, but a significant population coexpress GFRα1 and GFRα2. In contrast, GDNF receptor components are found in only a few of the CGRP/trkA expressing small DRG cells. The IB4-binding DRG neurons do not in general express NGF or, indeed, any neurotrophin receptors.[53] Hence there appears to be a clear dichotomy in C-fiber properties: In the adult animal, about one-half of these cells express receptor components for NGF, and the other half, components for GDNF. A subgroup of the large neurofilament-rich DRG neurons express RET and GFRα1 and hence are likely to be GDNF sensitive. The expression of GFRα3 has not yet been related to these different histochemical subtypes of sensory neurons (although it is expressed principally in small-diameter DRG cells).

As described previously with receptors for other trophic factors, there appears to be a high degree of plasticity in GDNF receptor expression following nerve injury. Interestingly, different receptor components are differentially regulated[49] (Fig. 4.4). Two weeks following axotomy there is an increase in the proportion of DRG cells that express RET and GFRα1 (to 75% and 70% of DRG cells, respectively), so that virtually all large-diameter DRG cells express these receptor components. There remains, however, a population of small-diameter DRG cells (probably those that express trkA) which do not express these receptor components. The expression of GFRα3 also increases following axotomy (from 40% to 66% of DRG cells), and this increase occurs principally within small-diameter DRG cells. Ligand signaling via GFRα3 may therefore be expected to have interesting properties in that it may be neuroprotective for a large population of small-diameter DRG cells following nerve injury. Conversely, GFRα2, which is also selectively expressed within small-diameter DRG cells, is down-regulated following axotomy (from 30% to 12% of DRG cells). Treatment with exogenous GDNF can reverse many of these changes in receptor component expression following axotomy.

In summary, GDNF receptor components are expressed in a population of both small- and large-diameter DRG cells. Within small-diameter DRG cells, they are expressed by a population of neurons which are nonpeptidergic, IB4 binding, and do not express trk receptors and hence are unresponsive to the neurotrophins. Plasticity in GDNF family receptor component expression fol-

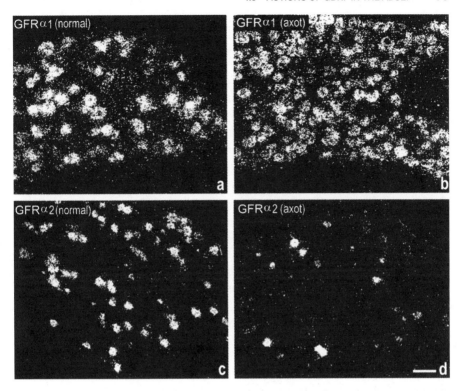

Figure 4.4   Dark field photomicrographs of sections of L4/5 DRG in normal animals (a, c) and following axotomy (b, d) after hybridization with probes for GFRα1 (a, b) and GFRα2 (c, d). Note that following axotomy there is a large increase in the proportion of DRG cells that express GFRα1 and a reduction in the proportion that express GFRα2. Scale bar: 100 μm.

lowing nerve injury implies that the sensitivity of sensory neurons to different members of the GDNF/NTN/PSP family will change (i.e., there will be increased sensitivity to GDNF and reduced sensitivity to NTN).

4.5.2   Biological Effects of GDNF on Sensory Neurons

The distribution of trophic factor receptors, described above, suggests that C fibers in the adult are likely to be sensitive to either NGF or GDNF. There is now a large body of evidence showing that the peptidergic small cells (expressing trkA) are indeed strongly affected by the availability of NGF. Exogenous NGF has a range of actions on nociceptive systems (as reviewed in Ref. 2): It produces pain and hyperalgesia when given to humans and rats. It can sensitize and activate C fibers. Following retrograde transport to the cell bodies of trkA expressing C fibers, it increases the expression of CGRP, substance P, and, perhaps more surprisingly, BDNF, in these neurons.[54,55]

Perhaps as a consequence of these altered levels, exogenous NGF can also facilitate spinal transmissions of C-fiber activity.[56] NGF can also reverse some of the effects of axotomy in trkA-expressing neurons, such as the down-regulation of substance P and CGRP.[2] Conversely, reducing endogenous NGF levels produces complementary changes in nociceptive systems: It leads to behavioral hypoalgesia and electrophysiologically, to reduced sensitivity of some C fibers to noxious heat and the algogen bradykinin.[2,57] It also produces modest decreases in peptide expression in appropriate C fibers. An important question, therefore, is whether GDNF exerts a similar range of effects on the IB4-binding population of C fibers.

4.5.3   Neuroprotective Effects of GDNF on DRG Cells

In vitro, GDNF has been demonstrated to support the survival of IB4-binding DRG cells during the neonatal period and can promote neurite outgrowth from these neurons in the adult.[48,58] To investigate the trophic actions of GDNF in vivo, we have used sciatic axotomy as a standard model of nerve injury. Following such injury, a series of reactive changes are seen in the peripherally damaged neurons both in cell bodies in the fourth and fifth lumbar dorsal root ganglia (DRG) and in the central terminals of these afferents in the dorsal horn of the spinal cord. These changes include the down-regulation of markers in both populations of small sensory neurons. Within the peptidergic population of small-diameter afferents there is reduced expression of CGRP, and within the nonpeptidergic population there is reduced binding of IB4 and reduced activity of the enzyme TMP. We therefore set out to ask if appropriate trophic factor support could reverse these axotomy effects.[50] We delivered NGF, GDNF, or vehicle intrathecally (at a dose of 1.2 or 12 µg/day) via miniosmotic pumps continuously for 14 days, starting the treatment concomitantly with a unilateral sciatic nerve section. At the end of the 14 days of treatment we assessed histochemically the expression of these markers in DRG cells. NGF completely prevented the down-regulation of CGRP within sensory neurons following nerve injury but had no significant effect on IB4 or TMP numbers (Fig. 4.5). Strikingly, a complementary pattern of effect was seen with GDNF. TMP activity was restored to normal levels, and about an 80% rescue was seen in IB4 binding (Fig. 4.5). CGRP levels were unaffected by this treatment. The "rescue" effects of NGF and GDNF occurred in a dose-dependent fashion. It has recently been demonstrated that the purinoreceptor $P2X_3$ is selectively expressed within the IB4-binding population of small-diameter afferents. The expression of this receptor is also reduced following nerve injury, and again this change can be prevented by treatment with GDNF.[52]

Another effect of peripheral axotomy, seen apparently in all classes of peripheral neuron, is a slowing of axonal conduction velocity. This effect is

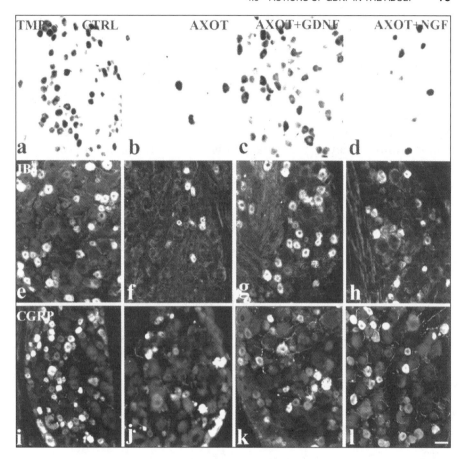

Figure 4.5   Histochemistry for TMP (a–d), IB4 labeling (e–h), and CGRP immunofluorescence (i–l) in dorsal root ganglia of control animals (a, e, i), animals with unilateral sciatic nerve section (b, f, j), animals with unilateral sciatic nerve section combined with intrathecal GDNF treatment (12 μg/day; c, g, k), and animals with unilateral sciatic nerve section combined with intrathecal NGF treatment (12 μg/day; d, h, l). Sciatic nerve section causes a loss of TMP (b) and IB4 (f) labeling, which is prevented by GDNF treatment (c, g) but not by NGF (d, h). In contrast, the loss of CGRP staining caused by sciatic nerve section (j) is prevented by NGF (l) but not by GDNF (k). Scale bar: 50 μm.

probably secondary to a decrease in axonal caliber, itself arising because of a decrease in the expression of structural proteins such as neurofilament. This rather nonspecific effect is a useful outcome measure because it occurs ubiquitously with injury—the specificity of putative neuroprotective effects can be seen against a background of widespread change. We have recently used this measure to assess GDNF and NGF actions.[50] We measured the distribution of C-fiber conduction velocity in normal animals by recording from fine filaments of the L5 dorsal root and electrically stimulating the peripheral tibial nerve with supramaximal shocks. In most strands of dorsal root, one or more C-fiber potentials (i.e., those conducting at less than 2 m/s) are elicited. We accumulated a representative sample of these fibers in each animal and then constructed a cumulative sum plot, as shown in Figure 4.6. Here, the median conduction velocity is indicated by reading across from the 50% value on the ordinate. For normal animals it was about 0.85 m/s. In similar experiments undertaken on animals 2 weeks after peripheral axotomy of the tibial nerve, the entire distribution of conduction velocities is shifted significantly to the left (Fig. 4.6), with about a 25% drop in median velocity. As shown in Figure 4.6, either NGF or GDNF delivered in-

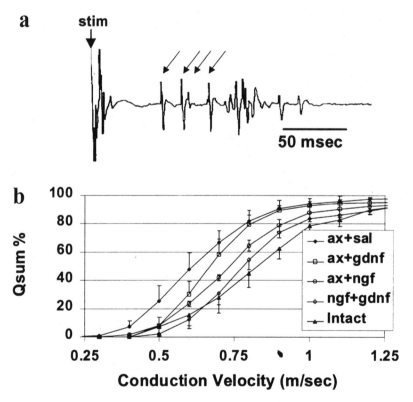

Figure 4.6   The conduction velocity (CV) of C fibers projecting through the tibial nerve was measured by stimulation of that nerve electrically and recording and averaging activity in fine strands of the L5 dorsal root. (a) Representative recording from an animal in which the tibial nerve had been cut and tied 2 weeks previously and continuously treated with intrathecal GDNF and NGF (each at 12 μg/day). Arrows show examples of individual C-fiber potentials occurring in response to the stimulation. (b) Cumulative sum plots showing the average CV distributions constructed from groups of animals receiving different treatment. Error bars show SEM. Note that axotomy results in a significant slowing of C fibers (seen as a leftward shift in the Qsum plots) and NGF and GDNF both partially prevent this slowing. (See Ref. 50.)

trathecally as before at 12 μg/day for 2 weeks partially (and significantly) reversed the expected drop in conduction velocity. Again this is consistent with the notion that each factor affects only a subgroup of primary sensory C fibers. In further support of this notion, animals treated with a mixture of GDNF and NGF (at the same dose) showed a further rescue of conduction velocity, and in this case the distribution is not significantly different from that seen in normal animals.

4.5.4 Neuroprotective Actions of GDNF Within the Dorsal Horn

A very similar rescue of primary afferent phenotype was apparent at the level of central terminals within the dorsal horn. In normal animals TMP is seen as a thin band of staining in lamina IIinner (IIi). After axotomy (as expected from the changes in DRG somata, described above), the area of central terminals occupied by sciatic afferents (the medial three-fourths of the dorsal horn at this spinal level) is almost completely devoid of TMP activity (Fig. 4.7). Treatment of animals with GDNF following axonomy resulted in TMP levels that were apparently normal. In contrast, NGF was much less effective at restoring TMP levels, although partial effects were seen. Similarly, GDNF but not NGF could prevent the reduction in IB4 binding within the dorsal horn. CGRP levels were rescued, as expected, by NGF but not by GDNF. The known overlap between the different markers[53] probably accounts for the limited nonselective effects seen, but the clear conclusion is that NGF and GDNF have distinct and complementary neuroprotective actions on the two classes of nociceptive afferent neurons.

A final effect of axotomy we discuss here relates to anatomical reorganization of afferent terminals within the dorsal horn. An injury response that may be related to the emergence of neuropathic pain is the sprouting of the central terminals of large myelinated fibers. These afferents, known to be almost exclusively a population of tactile mechanoreceptors, normally terminate most profusely in the deep dorsal horn laminae. Importantly, bulk transport methods and intraaxonal filing of single fibers reveals that they rarely form synaptic boutons in lamina II. A few days after peripheral axotomy, however, these afferent fibers sprout centrally and begin to form inputs in lamina II.[59,60] This change may allow inputs from innocuous mechanoreceptors to gain access to nociceptive spinal systems and may contribute to the phenomenon of touch-evoked pain that occurs in neuropathic states. There is reason to believe that this anatomical remodeling is secondary to atrophic changes in central C-fiber terminals. Part of this evidence is that capsaicin can induce this central change; this change can apparently occur in the absence of damage to A fibers.[61] Moreover, the central terminations of sciatic C fibers are rostrocaudally and mediolaterally more restricted than those of A

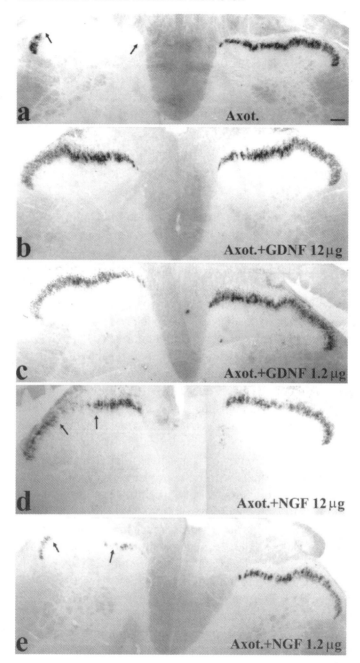

Figure 4.7   Histochemistry for TMP at the level of L4 in the dorsal horn of an animal with unilateral (left side) sciatic nerve section (top), and animals with unilateral sciatic nerve section combined with continuous intrathecal GDNF or NGF treatment (1.2 or 12 μg/day). Sciatic nerve section causes a loss of TMP in the sciatic termination territory within lamina IIi, which is prevented by GDNF treatment. Scale bar: 100 μm. (See Ref. 50.)

fibers, and the sprouting that occurs following peripheral axotomy is restricted to the area where damaged C fibers are present.[60]

We have reported that NGF but not BDNF or NT3 can prevent the injury-induced sprouting of A fibers.[62] Recently, we have asked whether GDNF also has this capacity. We delivered GDNF intrathecally as above, at a dose of 12 μg/day, to animals with sciatic axotomy. We labeled the central terminals of A fibers using the anterograde transport of the B-subunit of cholera toxin. The sprouting that was apparent in control animals (axotomy alone) was completely blocked by GDNF. These results further suggest that sprouting occurs as a secondary consequence of damage to C fibers. One suggestion has been that damaged C fibers release some positive factor that induces A-fiber sprouting. However, if this is the case, our findings suggest that subthreshold amounts would have to derive from both the NGF- and GDNF-sensitive subgroups. An alternative interpretation might be that A fibers sprout as a result of competition for synaptic space between damaged A and C fibers and that either group of C fibers is sufficient to provide a barrier to sprouting if they are maintained by an appropriate trophic factor. In any case, the fact that GDNF is sufficient to prevent dorsal horn remodeling after axonal injury supports the case for its therapeutic use in the treatment of some forms of peripheral neuropathy.

4.6 FUNCTIONAL ROLE OF GDNF

As described above, GDNF has a powerful neuroprotective action on sensory neurons. GDNF can prevent a number of changes in IB4-binding DRG cells and the A-fiber sprouting that occurs following axotomy. Such changes may have a role in the evolution of neuropathic pain, so GDNF administration may be useful in treatment of this condition. This is a possibility we will investigate in the future. It would, of course, be interesting to investigate the neuroprotective actions of other members of the GDNF family, such as NTN, but this has not yet been possible, due to the insoluble nature of this protein.

As described above, NGF has important sensitizing actions on nociceptive afferents, and increased NGF levels are important in the generation of inflammatory pain. An intriguing possibility is that GDNF may have similar actions on the IB4-binding population of nociceptive afferents. We have found that unlike NGF, the acute peripheral administration of GDNF has no effect on sensory thresholds (unpublished observations). So although GDNF can exert important trophic effects on the IB4-binding population of sensory neurons (e.g., following nerve injury), it does not appear to have acute sensitizing actions on these neurons. It may, however, have a more tonic neuromodulatory role on these neurons. It has recently been shown that in vitro

GDNF can increase both the thermal sensitivity and the TTX-resistant sodium current in IBR-binding DRG cells.[63] It will be interesting to know whether GDNF has similar actions in vivo and also to determine whether GDNF can regulate the chemical sensitivity of IB4-binding DRG cells (in terms of their ATP sensitivity, for instance). One important question that is as yet unanswered is: What is the role of endogenous GDNF? To study this, some kind of pharmacological antagonism is required, which is as yet unavailable.

4.7   CONCLUSIONS

In this chapter we have reviewed some new data relating to the effects of trophic factors on adult nociceptive neurons. We show in figure 4.8 that spinal C fibers can be subdivided into two distinct groups, one sensitive to NGF and the other to GDNF (Fig. 4.8). The properties of these two groups differ markedly in other ways: The former group selectively express the neuropep-

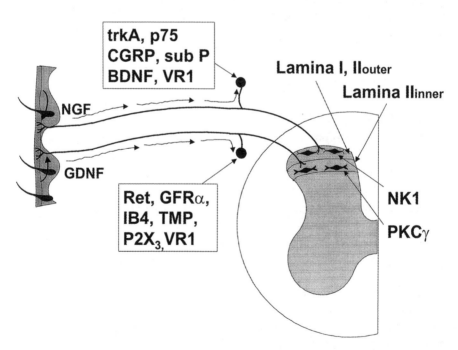

Figure 4.8   Two distinct subgroups of cutaneous C fibers can be recognized, one sensitive to NGF and the other to GDNF. These two groups differ in many ways, including the expression of neuromodulators and receptors and in their anatomical terminations in the dorsal horn. It is not yet clear if these two groups have distinct physiological responsiveness or if they might have different functional roles in chronic pain states. (See Ref. 64.)

tides CGRP and substance P and project to lamina I and IIouter (IIo) of the dorsal horn. The second group does not express these sensory neuropeptides, but is marked histochemically by expression of the enzyme TMP and their ability to bind the lectin IB4. These cells also selectively express the purinoreceptor $P2X_3$ and, distinctly, terminate in lamina IIi of the dorsal horn. Both of these groups express the recently cloned capsaicin receptor VR1,[65] although there may be a higher level of expression in the peptidergic NGF-sensitive group.[66] What is less clear is whether these two groups have distinct functions. There are several reasons for believing that most neurons in both groups are nociceptors. First, more than 90% of C fibers in rat, mouse, monkey, and humans are nociceptive. Second, both populations are sensitive to the algesic agent capsaicin (even in the adult animal). Third, noxious stimuli can induce release of CGRP and substance P from the former group and ATP analogs, likely to act on the latter group can produce pain when injected into humans and nocifensive responses when injected into animals. It is an intriguing possibility that NGF- and GDNF-sensitive nociceptors differ in the types of stimuli they respond to and may play different roles in chronic pain states.

REFERENCES

1. Lindsay, R. M. (1996). Role of neurotrophins and trk receptors in the development and maintenance of sensory neurons: an overview [review]. Philos. Trans. R. Soc. Lond. B Biol. Sci. 351:364–373.

2. McMahon, S. B., and Bennett, D. L. H. (1995). Growth factors and pain. In: Pharmacology and clinical pharmacology of pain, ed. Dickenson, A., and Besson, J. M., Springer-Verlag, New York.

3. McMahon, S. B., Bennett, D. L. H., Priestley, J. V., and Shelton, D. L. (1995). The biological effects of endogenous NGF in adult sensory neurons revealed by a trkA-IgG fusion molecule. Nature Med. 1(8):774–780.

4. Woolf, C. J., Safieh-Garabedian, B., Ma, Q. P., Crilly, P., and Winter, J. (1994). Nerve growth factor contributes to the generation of inflammatory sensory hypersensitivity. Neuroscience 62:327–331.

5. McMahon, S. B., and Priestley, J. V. (1995). Peripheral neuropathies and neurotrophic factors: animal models and clinical perspectives [review; 77 refs.]. Curr. Opin. Neurobiol. 5:616–624.

6. Lin, L. F., Doherty, D. H., Lile, J. D., Bektesh, S., and Collins, F. (1993). GDNF: a glial cell line–derived neurotrophic factor for midbrain dopaminergic neurons [see comments]. Science 260:1130–1132.

7. Beck, K. D., Valverde, J., Alexi, T., Poulsen, K., Moffat, B., Vandlen, R. A., Rosenthal, A., and Hefti, F. (1995). Mesencephalic dopaminergic neurons protected by GDNF from axotomy-induced degeneration in the adult brain [see comments]. Nature 373:339–341.

8. Tomac, A., Lindqvist, E., Lin, L. F., Ogren, S. O., Young, d., Hoffer, B. J., and Olson, L. (1995). Protection and repair of the nigrostriatal dopaminergic system by GDNF in vivo [see comments]. Nature 373:335–339.

9. Arenas, E., Trupp, M., Akerud, P., and Ibanez, C. F. (1995). GDNF prevents degeneration and promotes the phenotype of brain noradrenergic neurons in vivo. Neuron 15:1465–1473.

10. Henderson, C. E., Phillips, H. S., Pollock, R. A., Davies, A. M., Lemeulle, C., Armanini, M., Simmons, L., Moffet, B., Vandlen, R. A., Simpson, L. C., et al. (1994). GDNF: a potent survival factor for motoneurons present in peripheral nerve and muscle [see comments]. Science 266:1062–1064. Published erratum appears in Science Feb. 10, 1995; 267(5199):777.

11. Yan, Q., Matheson, C., and Lopez, O. T. (1995). In vivo neurotrophic effects of GDNF on neonatal and adult facial motor neurons [see comments]. Nature 373:341–344.

12. Buj-Bello, A., Adu, J., Piñón, L. G., Horton, A., Thompson, J., Rosenthal, A., Chinchetru, M., Buchman, V. L., and Davies, A. M. (1997). Neurturin responsiveness requires a GPI-linked receptor and the Ret receptor tyrosine kinase. Nature 387:721–724.

13. Trupp, M., Ryden, M., Jornvall, H., Funakoshi, H., Timmusk, T., Arenas, E., and Ibanez, C. F. (1995). Peripheral expression and biological activities of GDNF, a new neurotrophic factor for avian and mammalian peripheral neurons. J. Cell Biol. 130:137–148.

14. Moore, M. W., Klein, R. D., Fariñas, I., Sauer, H., Armanini, M., Phillips, H., Reichardt, L. F., Ryan, A. M., Carver-Moore, K., and Rosenthal, A. (1996). Renal and neuronal abnormalities in mice lacking GDNF. Nature 382:76–79.

15. Pichel, J. G., Shen, L., Sheng, H. Z., Granholm, A. C., Drago, J., Grinberg, A., Lee, E. J., Huang, S. P., Saarma, M., Hoffer, B. J., Sariola, H., and Westphal, H. (1996). Defects in enteric innervation and kidney development in mice lacking GDNF. Nature 382:73–76.

16. Sanchez, M. P., Silos-Santiago, I., Frisen, J., He, B., Lira, S. A., and Barbacid, M. (1996). Renal agenesis and the absence of enteric neurons in mice lacking GDNF. Nature 382:70–73.

17. Kotzbauer, P. T., Lampe, P. A., Heuckeroth, R. O., Golden, J. P., Creedon, D. J., Johnson, E. M. J., and Milbrandt, J. (1996). Neurturin, a relative of glial-cell-line–derived neurotrophic factor. Nature 384:467–470.

18. Milbrandt, J., de Sauvage, F. J., Fahrner, T. J., Baloh, R. H., Leitner, M. L., Tansey, M. G., Lampe, P. A., Heuckeroth, R. O., Kotzbauer, P. T., Simburger, K. S., Golden, J. P., Davies, J. A., Vejsada, R., Kato, A. C., Hynes, M., Sherman, D., Nishimura, M., Wang, L. C., Vandlen, R. Moffat, B., Klein, R. D., Poulsen, K., Gray C., Garces, A., and Johnson, E. M. J. (1998). Persephin, a novel neurotrophic factor related to GDNF and neurturin. Neuron 20:245–253.

19. Jing, S., Wen, D., Yu, Y., Holst, P. L., Luo, Y., Fang, M., Tamir, R., Antonio, L., Hu, Z., Cupples R., Louis, J. C., Hu, S., Altrock, B. W., and Fox, G. M. (1996).

GDNF-induced activation of the ret protein tyrosine kinase is mediated by GDNFR-α, a novel receptor for GDNF. Cell 85:1113–1124.

20. Jing, S., Yu, Y., Fang, M., Hu, Z., Holst, P. L., Boone, T., Delaney, J., Schultz, H., Zhou, R., and Fox, G. M. (1997). GFRα-2 and GFRα-3 are two new receptors for ligands of the GDNF family. J. Biol. Chem. 272:33111–33117.

21. Creedon, D. J., Tansey, M. G., Baloh, R. H., Osborne, P. A., Lampe, P. A., Fahrner, T. J., Heuckeroth, R. O., Milbrandt, J., and Johnson, E. M., (1997). Neurturin shares receptors and signal transduction pathways with glial cell line–derived neurotrophic factor in sympathetic neurons. Proc. Natl. Acad. Sci. USA 94:7018–7023.

22. Baloh, R. H., Tansey, M. G., Golden, J. P., Creedon, D. J., Heuckeroth, R. O., Keck, C. L., Zimonjic, D. B., Popescu, N. C., Johnson, E. M. J., and Milbrandt, J. (1997). TrnR2, a novel receptor that mediates neurturin and GDNF signaling through Ret. Neuron 18:793–802.

23. Klein, R. D., Sherman, D., Ho, W. H., Stone, D., Bennett, G. L., Moffat, B., Vandlen, R., Simmons, L., Gu, Q., Hongo, J. A., Devaux, B., Poulsen, K., Armanini, M., Nozaki, C., Asai, N., Goddard, A., Phillips, H., Henderson, C. E., Takahashi, M., and Rosenthal, A. (1997). A GPI-linked protein that interacts with Ret to form a candidate neurturin receptor. Nature 387:717–721. Published erratum appears in Nature Mar. 12, 1998; 392(6672):210.

24. Sanicola, M., Hession, C., Worley, D., Carmillo, P., Ehrenfels, C., Walus, L., Robinson, S., Jaworski, G., Wei, H., Tizard, R., Whitty, A., Pepinsky, R. B., and Cate, R. L. (1997). Glial cell line–derived neurotrophic factor–dependent RET activation can be mediated by two different cell-surface accessory proteins. Proc. Natl. Acad. Sci. USA 94:6238–6243.

25. Naveilhan, P., Baudet, C., Mikaels, A., Shen, L., Westphal, H., and Ernfors, P. (1998). Expression and regulation of GFRα3, a glial cell line–derived neurotrophic factor family receptor. Proc. Natl. Acad. Sci. USA 95:1295–1300.

26. Worby, C. A., Vega, Q. C., Chao, H. H., Seasholtz, A. F., Thompson, R. C., and Dixon, J. E. (1998). Identification and characterization of GFRα-3, a novel coreceptor belonging to the glial cell line–derived neurotrophic receptor family. J. Biol. Chem. 273:3502–3508.

27. Baloh, R. H., Gorodinsky, A., Golden, J. P., Tansey, M. G., Keck, C. L., Popescu, N. C., Johnson, E. M. J., and Milbrandt, J. (1998). GFRα3 is an orphan member of the GDNF/neurturin/persephin receptor family. Proc. Natl. Acad. Sci. USA 95:5801–5806.

28. Thompson, J., Doxakis, E., Piñón, L. G., Strachan, P., Buj-Bello, A., Wyatt, S., Buchman, V. L., and Davies, A. M. (1998). GFRα-4, a new GDNF family receptor. Mol. Cell. Neurosci. 11:117–126.

29. Treanor, J. J., Goodman, L., de Sauvage, F., Stone, D. M., Poulsen, K. T., Beck, C. D., Gray, C., Armanini, M. P., Pollock, R. A., Hefti, F., Phillips, H. S., Goddard, A., Moore, M. W., Buj-Bello, A., Davies, A. M., Asai, N., Takahashi, M., Vandlen, R., Henderson, C. E., and Rosenthal, A. (1996). Characterization of a multicomponent receptor for GDNF [see comments]. Nature 382:80–83.

30. Durbec, P., Marcos-Gutierrez, C. V., Kilkenny, C., Grigoriou, M., Wartiowaara, K., Suvanto, P., Smith, D., Ponder, B., Costantini, F., Saarma, M., et al. (1996). GDNF signaling through the Ret receptor tyrosine kinase [see comments]. Nature 381:789–793.

31. Schuchardt, A., D'Agati, V., Larsson-Blomberg, L., Costantini, F., and Pachnis, V. (1994). Defects in the kidney and enteric nervous system of mice lacking the tyrosine kinase receptor Ret [see comments]. Nature 367:380–383.

32. Cacalano, G., Farinas, I., Wang, L. C., Hagler, K., Forgie, A., Moore, M., Armanini, M., Phillips, H., Ryan, A. M., Reichardt, L. F., Hynes, M., Davies, A. M., and Rosenthal, A. (1998). GFRα1 is an essential receptor component for GDNF in the developing nervous system and kidney. Neuron 21:53–62.

33. Enomoto, H., Araki, T., Jackman, A., Heuckeroth, R. O., Snider, W. D., Johnson, E. M. J., and Milbrandt, J. (1998). GFRα1–deficient mice have deficits in the enteric nervous system and kidneys. Neuron 21:317–324.

34. Ernfors, P., Lee, K. F., Kucera, J., and Jaenisch, R. (1994). Lack of neurotrophin-3 leads to deficiencies in the peripheral nervous system and loss of limb proprioceptive afferents. Cell 77:503–512.

35. Farinas, I., Jones, K. R., Backus, C., Wang, X. Y., and Reichardt, L. F. (1994). Severe sensory and sympathetic deficits in mice lacking neurotrophin-3. Nature 369:658–661.

36. Airaksinen, M. S., Koltzenburg, M., Lewin, G. R., Masu, Y., Helbig, C., Wolf, E., Brem, G., Toyka, K. V., Thoenen, H., and Meyer, M. (1996). Specific sub-types of cutaneous mechanoreceptors require neurotrophin-3 following target innervation. Neuron 16:287–295.

37. Schecterson, L. C., and Bothwell, M. (1992). Novel roles for neurotrophins are suggested by BDNF and NT-3 mRNA expression in developing neurons. Neuron 9:449–463.

38. Acheson, A., Conover, J. C., Fandl, J. P., DeChiara, T. M., Russell, M., Thadani, A., Squinto, S. P., Yancopoulos, G. D., and Lindsay, R. M. (1995). A BDNF autocrine loop in adult sensory neurons prevents cell death [see comments]. Nature 374:450–453.

39. Carroll, S. L., Silos-Santiago, I., Frese, S. E., Ruit, K. G., Milbrandt, J., and Snider, W. D. (1992). Dorsal root ganglia neurons expressing trk are selectively sensitive to NGF deprivation in utero. Neuron 9:779–788.

40. Ruit, K. G., Elliott, J. L., Osborne, P. A., Yan, Q., and Snider, W. D. (1992). Selective dependence of mammalian dorsal root ganglion neurons on nerve growth factor during embryonic development. Neuron 8:573–587.

41. Crowley, C., Spencer, S. D., Nishimura, M. C., Chen, K. S., Pitts-Meek, S., Armanini, M. P., Ling, L. H., McMahon, S. B., Shelton, D. L., Levinson, A. D., et al. (1994). Mice lacking nerve growth factor display perinatal loss of sensory and sympathetic neurons yet develop basal forebrain cholinergic neurons. Cell 76:1001–1011.

42. Silos-Santiago, I., Molliver, D. C., Ozaki, S., Smeyne, R. J., Fagan, A. M., Barbacid, M., and Snider, W. D. (1995). Non-TrkA–expressing small DRG neurons are lost in TrkA deficient mice. J. Neurosci. 15:5929–5942.

43. Bennett, D. L. H., Averill, S., Clary, D. O., Priestley, J. V., and McMahon, S. B. (1996). Postnatal changes in the expression of the trkA high affinity NGF receptor in primary sensory neurons. Eur. J. Neurosci. 8:2204–2208.

44. Molliver, D. C., and Snider, W. D. (1997). Nerve growth factor receptor TrkA is down-regulated during postnatal development by a subset of dorsal root ganglion neurons. J. Comp. Neurol. 381:428–438.

45. Wright, D. E., and Snider, W. D. (1996). Focal expression of glial cell line–derived neurotrophic factor in developing mouse limb bud. Cell Tissue Res. 286:209–217.

46. Buj-Bello, A., Buchman, V. L., Horton, A., Rosenthal, A., and Davies, A. M. (1995). GDNF is an age-specific survival factor for sensory and autonomic neurons. Neuron 15:821–828.

47. Matheson, C. R., Carnahan, J., Urich, J. L., Bocangel, D., Zhang, T. J., and Yan, Q. (1997). Glial cell line–derived neurotrophic factor (GDNF) is a neurotrophic factor for sensory neurons: comparison with the effects of the neurotrophins. J. Neurobiol. 32:22–32.

48. Molliver, D. C., Wright, D. E., Leitner, M. L., Parsadanian, A. S., Doster, K., Wen, D., Yan, Q., and Snider, W. D. (1997). IB4-binding DRG neurons switch from NGF to GDNF dependence in early postnatal life. Neuron 19:849–861.

49. Bennett, D. L. H., Boucher, T., Armanini, M. P., Phillips, H. S., McMahon, S. B., and Shelton, D. L. (1998). RET, GFRα-1, 2 and 3 expression within sensory neurons innervating different targets and the response to nerve injury. Soc. Neurosci. Abst. 24:1545.

50. Bennett, D. L. H., Michael, G. J., Ramachandran, N., Munson, J. B., Averill, S., Yan, Q., McMahon, S. B., and Priestley, J. V. (1998). A distinct subgroup of small DRG cells express GDNF receptor components and GDNF is protective for these neurons after nerve injury. J. Neurosci. 18:3059–3072.

51. Vulchanova, L., Riedl, M. S., Shuster, S. J., Stone, L. S., Hargreaves, K. M., Buell, G., Surprenant, A., North, R. A., and Elde, R. (1998). $P2X_3$ is expressed by DRG neurons that terminate in inner lamina II. Eur. J. Neurosci. 10:3470–3478.

52. Bradbury, E. J., Burnstock, G., and McMahon, S. B. (1998). The expression of $P2X_3$ purinoceptors in sensory neurons: effects of axotomy and glial-derived neurotrophic factor. Mol. Cell. Neurosci. 12:256–268.

53. Averill, S., McMahon, S. B., Clary, D. O., Reichardt, L. F., and Priestley, J. V. (1995). Immunocytochemical localization of trkA receptors in chemically identified subgroups of adult rat sensory neurons. Eur. J. Neurosci. 7:1484–1494.

54. Apfel, S. C., Wright, D. E., Wiiderman, A. M., Dormia, C., Snider, W. D., and Kessler, J. A. (1996). Nerve growth factor regulates the expression of brain

derived neurotrophic factor mRNA in the peripheral nervous system. Mol. Cell. Neurosci. 7:134–142.

55. Michael, G. J., Averill, S., Nitkunan, A., Rattray, M., Bennett, D. L., Yan, Q., and Priestly, J. V. (1997). Nerve growth factor treatment increases brain-derived neurotrophic factor selectively in Trk-A-expressing dorsal root ganglia cells and in their central terminations within the spinal cord. J. Neurosci. 17:8476–8490.

56. Thompson, S. W., Dray, A., McCarson, K. E., Krause, J. E., and Urban, L. (1995). Nerve growth factor induces mechanical allodynia associated with novel A fibre-evoked spinal reflex activity and enhanced neurokinin-1 receptor activation in the rat. Pain 62:219–231.

57. Bennett, D. L. H., Koltzenburg, M., Priestley, J. V., Shelton, D. L., and McMahon, S. B. (1998). Endogenous nerve growth factor regulates the sensitivity of nociceptors in the adult rat. Eur. J. Neurosci. 10:1282–1291.

58. Leclere, P., Ekstrom, P., Edstrom, A., Priestley, J., Averill, S., and Tonge, D. A. (1998). Effects of glial cell line–derived neurotrophic factor on axonal growth and apoptosis in adult mammalian sensory neurons in vitro. Neuroscience 82:545–558.

59. Woolf, C. J., Shortland, P., and Coggeshall, R. E. (1992). Peripheral nerve injury triggers central sprouting of myelinated afferents. Nature 355:75–78.

60. Woolf, C. J., Shortland, P., Reynolds, M., Ridings, J., Doubell, T, and Coggeshall, R. E. (1995). Reorganization of central terminals of myelinated primary afferents in the rat dorsal horn following peripheral axotomy. J. Comp. Neurol. 360:121–134.

61. Mannion, R. J., Doubell, T. P., Coggeshall, R. E., and Woolf, C. J. (1996). Collateral sprouting of uninjured primary afferent A-fibers into the superficial dorsal horn of the adult rat spinal cord after topical capsaicin treatment to the sciatic nerve. J. Neurosci. 16:5189–5195.

62. Bennett, D. L. H., French, J., Priestley, J. V. P., and McMahon, S. B. (1996). NGF but not NT-3 or BDNF prevents the A fiber sprouting into lamina II of the spinal cord that occurs following axotomy. Mol. Cell. Neurosci. 8(4):211–220.

63. Stucky, C. L., and Lewin, G. R. (1998). Nerve growth factor (NGF) increases the heat current in isolectin-B4 (IB4)–negative sensory neurons. Soc. Neurosci. Abst. 24:1043.

64. Snider, W. D., and McMahon, S. B. (1998). Tackling pain at the source: new ideas about nociceptors [review; 15 refs.]. Neuron 20:629–632.

65. Tominaga, M., Caterina, M. J., Malmberg, M. B., Rosen, T. A., Gilbert, H., Skinner, K., Raumann, B. E., Basbaum, A. I., and Julius, D. (1998). The cloned capsaicin receptor integrates multiple pain-producing stimuli. Neuron 21:531–543.

66. Michael, G. J., and Priestley, J. V. (1998). Expression of mRNA for vanilloir receptor (VR1) in sensory ganglia and its downregulation following axotomy. Soc. Neurosci. Abst. 24:1842.

CHAPTER 5

Molecular Approaches to the Study of Pain

RICHARD J. MANNION, MICHAEL COSTIGAN, AND CLIFFORD J. WOOLF

Massachusetts General Hospital and Harvard Medical School
Boston, Massachusetts

5.1 INTRODUCTION

Clinical pain can be produced by two processes. The first is an activation of nociceptors by persistent intense peripheral stimuli. Although this has been the mechanism assumed to be the primary or exclusive cause of pain by most clinicians, it represents only a fraction of clinical pain, particularly that produced at the onset of tissue-damaging stimuli. Most of the pain and sensitivity characteristic of clinical pain is in fact a manifestation of the modifiability of the nervous system. Alterations in the performance of the somatosensory system as a consequence of functional, chemical, and structural changes in primary sensory and dorsal horn neurons following activity, inflammation, or nerve damage are now well recognized as being the key factor in the generation of pain.[1–5] The challenge now is to identify these changes and investigate their initiation and maintenance. Molecular biological techniques can be used to address three aspects of pain generation. Genes that are uniquely expressed in nociceptor neurons and which contribute to their specialized function can be identified; these so far include receptors[6,7] and ion channels[8,9] (see Chapter 9). The signal molecules that act on sensory neurons to induce changes in their function or phenotype can be identified; these include growth factors,[10,11] cytokines,[12,13] and neurokines.[14] Finally, the actual changes in the phenotype of the neurons in clinical pain states can be determined and their contribution to the pathophysiology of pain elucidated.[15,16]

Molecular Basis of Pain Induction, Edited by John N. Wood
ISBN 0-471-34607-1   Copyright © 2000 by Wiley-Liss, Inc. All rights reserved.

A study of the molecular components of the generation of pain offers the prospect of increased understanding of how the pain is produced. In addition, diagnostic markers specific for particular processes may be discovered (e.g., for nerve damage), enabling therapy to be targeted specifically to the underlying mechanism. Finally, this approach is very likely to lead to the discovery of new targets for drug development. The aim of this chapter is to highlight techniques that can be used to analyze changes in the expression of known genes as well as approaches that can be used to discover novel genes, particularly within primary sensory neurons. There is no "pain" gene, but it is obvious that molecular biological techniques offer the possibility of enormous progress in advancing our understanding of how pain is produced with the realistic prospect of improved management of this condition.

5.2   INVESTIGATING CANDIDATE MOLECULES IN PAIN MODELS

Inflammatory and neuropathic pain both involve alterations in the local chemical environment of primary sensory neurons which trigger signaling pathways within the neurons, many of which result in a change in the rate of transcription of key molecules with subsequent up- or down-regulation of their expression. A key challenge is to define the changes that occur in known candidate genes as well as to identify and investigate unknown genes whose regulation may contribute to the pathophysiological processes underlying the pain. Such alterations can be investigated by looking at changes in the levels of mRNA, which reflect altered rates of gene transcription or posttranscriptional changes in the stability or editing of the mRNA transcript. An alternative strategy is to look at all the proteins expressed by a particular tissue, which is now possible with very small samples using mass spectroscopy. Posttranslational modifications to proteins are also key points of modulation, and acylation, glycosylation, and phosphorylation are all capable of dramatically altering protein function in the absence of any change in gene transcription. In this chapter, however, we only discuss strategies designed to investigate alterations in, or the presence of, particular species of mRNA.

5.2.1   Northern Blots

The expression of mRNAs encoding specific molecules can be monitored using a number of techniques. In the most commonly used method, Northern blotting, total RNA is prepared from tissue, electrophoresed on an agarose gel, transferred to a nitrocellulose membrane, and probed with a labeled nucleotide sequence complementary to that of the molecule under investigation. It allows both the estimation of mRNA transcript size and relative quantification of the amounts of a specific mRNA in different tissue samples on the same blot. A limitation of this technique is that relatively large amounts of total RNA are required (10 to 15 µg total RNA). Different types of nucleic acid probes can be used to identify the species of mRNA under investigation—cDNA probes, RNA probes (riboprobes) and oligonucleotide probes—each type with its own merits and drawbacks. cDNA and riboprobes have high specific activity because they are longer in length than oligoprobes; riboprobes produce the most stable hybrids (RNA–RNA) and thus the stringency of the hybridization conditions can be increased, improving specificity. A feature of cDNA probes, because of their double-stranded nature, is reannealing within the hybridization buffer, which decreases the amount of probe available for the mRNA. To improve the sensitivity of oligoprobes, a complex mixture of oligonucleotides targeted against different regions of the same mRNA can be used.

A fundamental concern in Northern blotting is to ensure equal loading of total RNA within each lane on the gel. Using spectophotometry, approximately equal amounts of total RNA can be calculated before loading, and this can be roughly quantified by observing the ethidium bromide staining intensity of ribosomal RNA following electrophoresis. The best control for loading is to probe the blot twice, once with the probe for the molecule of interest, then second, using a probe for an mRNA that is not regulated by the treatment under investigation. Any Northern blot that has not been equalized in this way cannot be interpreted with confidence. Commonly used "control" probes are cyclophilin, glyceraldehyde-3-phosphate dehydrogenase (GAPDH), and actin, although these are not appropriate for all experiments. Actin, for example, is up-regulated along with other cytoskeletal molecules in primary sensory neurons after peripheral nerve injury as part of the regenerative response.[17] An example of a Northern blot is shown in Figure 5.1. Transcripts representing as little as 0.001% of the total mRNA pool can readily be analyzed by Northern blotting[18]; for analysis of very rare transcripts, Northern blots using poly-A RNA can be prepared. Most eukaryotic mRNAs possess a poly-A tail, allowing messenger RNA to be isolated from total RNA using oligo-dT column chromatography or oligo-dT beads. Messenger RNA represents approximately 1% of total cellular RNA[19] and 1 to 2 µg of poly-A RNA is typically loaded on a Northern blot as opposed to 10 to 15 µg total RNA, increasing the amount of mRNA present about tenfold.

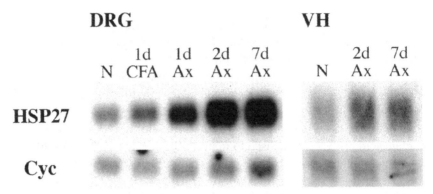

Figure 5.1   Northern blot for HSP-27 mRNA in the rat DRG after sciatic nerve section, show-ing an ninefold up-regulation by 2 and 7 days after nerve injury (DRG 2d, 7d Ax), without an equivalent change at 1 or 7 days after inflammation of the hindpaw (1d CFA and results not shown). A more slight up-regulation was seen in the ventral segment of the spinal cord at 2 and 7 days (VH 2d, 7d Ax) due to an up-regulation of HSP27 within the motor neuron cell bodies (results not shown). The same blot has been probed with cyclophilin (whose levels are known not to change in the DRG after sciatic axotomy) to normalize the blot for RNA loading differ-ences between lanes. N = levels of HSP27 mRNA in naive unoperated animal. (Modified from Ref. 57.)

5.2.2   In Situ Hybridization

Although Northern blots are commonly employed to study changes in the lev-els of particular mRNAs, they offer no information on the cellular localiza-tion of the mRNA, which in a heterogeneous population of cells, such as a dorsal root ganglion (DRG) may be neurons, Schwann cells, or fibroblasts. In situ hybridization (ISH) allows localization and comparative quantitation of mRNA transcripts at a cellular level. A labeled probe complementary to the molecule of interest is generated (the same issues apply in terms of choice of probe as in Northern blotting), then hybridized with the cellular mRNA tran-script in sections of tissue. Although radioactive ISH is more sensitive, non-isotopic protocols are now widely used. These protocols, predominantly using the plant steroid digoxygenin (dig) to label nucleotide probes followed by im-munohistochemical detection of dig, are quicker, cheaper, and more discrete than isotopic ISH (Fig. 5.2).

5.2.3   RNase Protection Assays

One disadvantage of both Northern blots and ISH is that of sensitivity. It is likely that particular molecules involved in nociception within DRG neu-rons, the peripheral nerve, the dorsal horn, or the skin may have a very low copy number of mRNA. RNase protection can be used to determine transcript levels where amounts of total cellular RNA are limiting and a high degree of sensitivity is required. Total RNA is prepared from the tissue of interest and hybridized with a radiolabeled riboprobe; then all remaining single-stranded RNA is digested with RNase. Only double-stranded RNA is protected from the RNase; these products can then be run out on a sequencing gel and quantified with autoradiography. This protocol requires up to 10 µg of total RNA per sample and is at least tenfold more sensitive than standard Northern blots.[18] As only short sequences need be used as probes, this method also allows expression analysis of specific splice forms of the same gene within the same tissue. One point to note for RNase protection is that the probe must be exactly complementary to the sequence under investigation, otherwise it will be degraded during the highly sensitive RNase step. Therefore, probes generated by polymerase chain reaction (PCR) using standard Taq polymerase may not be suitable for this method unless fully sequenced.

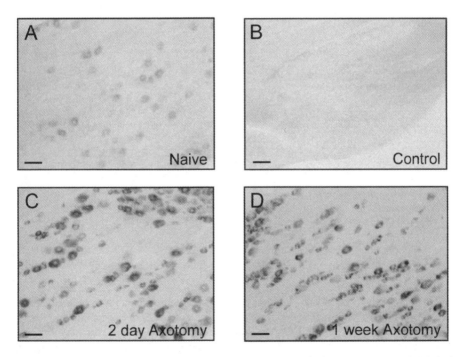

Figure 5.2 In situ hybridization for HSP27 mRNA in the rat DRG using a nonisotopic labeled riboprobe protocol in naive animals (A), then 2 days and 1 week after sciatic nerve section (C, D). Sense strand controls show no staining (B). In the naive animals, low-level HSP27 mRNA is present in medium-sized to large cells (A) 2 days and 1 week postaxotomy; however, marked up-regulation of HSP27 is evident in the medium-sized and large neurons as well as the de novo high-level expression in small cells (C, D). Scale bars: 100 µm. (Modified from Ref. 57.)

5.2.4 Reverse Transcription Polymerase Chain Reaction

When looking at changes in the levels of very low abundance mRNA, reverse transcriptase polymerase chain reaction (RT-PCR) is the method of choice. Several protocols are available for quantifying mRNA levels by RT-PCR: Comparative PCR allows semiquantitative determination of mRNA levels reasonably simply and easily[20] (Fig. 5.3). Messenger RNA is prepared from total RNA and reverse transcribed using oligo-d(T) or random hexamer primers to form first-strand cDNA. Specific forward and reverse primers designed both against the molecule of interest (the target) and a normalization template (the control) are used to PCR-amplify the first-

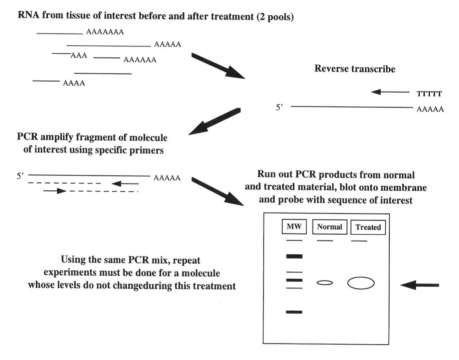

Figure 5.3 Schematic diagram highlighting the basic methodology for comparative PCR. RNA is taken from the tissue under investigation (e.g., the DRG in naive animals and after hindpaw inflammation). Both RNA populations are reverse transcribed with random hexamers or oligo-d(T) primers. Specific primers targeted against the molecule under investigation are then used on both populations of cDNA to PCR amplify a fragment of that molecule. The same number of cycles are used for each cDNA population. The PCR reactions are then electrophoresed on an agarose gel and DNA is stained with ethidium bromide. As an additional control, the DNA can be blotted onto nitrocellulose membrane and probed with the sequence under investigation to ensure that the correct sequence has been PCR amplified (see Fig. 5.4).

N   24h i 24h c 72h i 72h c 1wk i 1wk c 2wk i 2wk c

Substance P

Cyclophilin

Figure 5.4   Southern blot showing comparative PCR for substance P expression in the DRG after injection of complete Freund's adjuvant into the hindpaw of the rat. The PCR products were electrophoresed and blotted onto nitrocellulose membrane before being probed for substance P and exposed to autoradiographic film. Primers for cyclophilin were also used to control for differences in amounts of cDNA in the PCR reaction. Substance P is up-regulated in the ipsilateral (i) DRG but not the contralateral DRG.

strand cDNA samples. By controlling the number of PCR cycles so that the kinetics of amplification remain within the exponential phase, linear amplification can be achieved and the relative levels of a particular mRNA species can be compared between the multiple samples. One key control is to use a common PCR master mix to amplify both the target and the control species. This mixture should contain all the PCR reagents necessary for amplification (except the primers for either target or control sequence). Target and control amplifications should be performed at the same time on the same PCR amplification block, so that all amplification conditions are controlled for. Figure 5.4 shows an example of comparative PCR with appropriate controls.

A far more accurate but more labor-intensive technique is internal control quantitative PCR,[21,22] allowing absolute numbers of mRNA transcripts in a sample to be determined. In this protocol, a competitor cDNA is produced that is identical in sequence to the target mRNA, except that it possesses a small deletion in the amplified portion of the molecule. Synthetic RNA (sRNA) is produced from the competitor cDNA and is mixed in known quantities with a standard amount of total RNA. Because the competitor sRNA is reverse transcribed with the target RNA, differences in the efficiency of reverse transcription between different reactions are controlled for. During the PCR reaction that follows, the target and competitor cDNA contain the same primer binding sites as well as a homologous sequence, and consequently, each sequence competes for the available reagents (primers and nucleotides) with equal efficiency. Variations in the amplification efficiency of the target and control are therefore avoided. Target and competitor PCR products are separated by gel electrophoresis, and absolute levels of the target mRNA within the total RNA sample are obtained by comparing the ratio of target and competitor PCR products[23] (Fig. 5.5).

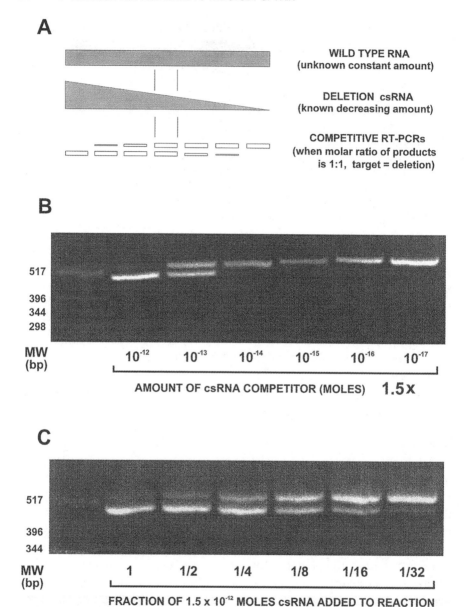

Figure 5.5   Competitive RT-PCR quantification of rat $\alpha 1$ type IV collagen transcript levels. (A) Schematic diagram of a competitive RT-PCR reaction scheme. A constant amount of wild-type RNA is mixed with a series of decreasing amounts of synthetic deletion competitor RNA (scRNA) in separate tubes. Competitive RT-PCR reactions are then performed and the PCR products resolved by gel electrophoresis. When the molar ratio of target and deletion amplification products are equal, the initial concentration of target and deletion transcripts are equal. (B) A ten-fold serial dilution of Rα1DEL csRNA (1.5×10^{-12} to 1.5×10^{-17} mol) was competed against a constant amount of a rat total kidney RNA sample (1 μg). (C) A twofold serial dilution of

5.3   SEARCHING FOR NEW DIFFERENTIALLY REGULATED GENES

Choosing candidate molecules such as the neuropeptides substance P or calcitonin gene–related peptide, receptors such as the μ opiate receptor or γ-aminobutyric acid (GABA) receptors, sodium ion channels or growth-associated genes, and monitoring their expression in different models of clinical pain has dramatically furthered our understanding of how primary sensory neurons adapt to injury or inflammation. However, it is likely that many molecules whose expression is regulated in neuropathic and inflammatory models are either not yet known or have not yet been studied in these cells. Advances in molecular technology have led to the development of a number of techniques that can be used to isolate and clone these molecules. Essentially, these techniques can be split into two categories: non-library-based or open systems, and library-based or closed systems, where differentially regulated genes are cloned from cDNA and more recently, oligonucleotide libraries. Whichever methods are used to obtain the clones, verification of their differential regulation by a method independent of the original screening protocol is essential (such as with Northern blotting or in situ hybridization), as all of these techniques tend to identify some false positives.

5.4   LIBRARY-BASED TECHNIQUES

The conventional method used to isolate genes differentially expressed in different or in the same tissue after different treatments is the differential screening of a cDNA library. A library, preferably generated from the tissue of interest, is plated out and duplicate filter lifts are taken and hybridized with two cDNA probes.[19] Each probe is a radiolabeled reverse transcription product generated from poly-A or total RNA taken from normal and treated tissue, and therefore each probe represents a complex mixture of cDNAs complementary to all the transcripts present within that RNA type. The source of RNA used to produce each probe is dependent on the experiment being performed, but may represent two differing cell types[24] or a control and experimental state of the same tissue or cell line.[25,26] Differentially expressed clones are identified as plaques that display altered levels of hybridization between

---

Rα1DEL csRNA was competed against 1 μg of rat total kidney RNA. This experiment was designed in order that the csRNA concentrations bracketed the estimation of deletion/target equivalence made by the tenfold dilution shown in (B). The initial csRNA concentration was 1.5×10^{-12} mol and was reduced in six twofold steps to span a 32-fold range in deletion concentration.

the two cDNA probes. They are picked from the plates, the cDNAs are isolated, and their differential expression is subsequently confirmed.

One disadvantage of conventional differential screening is that relatively large amounts of poly-A or total RNA are needed to produce the cDNA probes (1 to 5 µg of poly-A RNA for some paradigms) and in many models, generating these quantities of RNA is not feasible. mPCR is a method that attempts to overcome this problem.[27] Rather than using a complex cDNA probe generated from reverse transcribing RNA to screen a library, mPCR generates a complex probe by PCR-amplifying mRNA-derived double-stranded cDNA, thus producing a PCR product representative of the original mRNA population[27] (Fig. 5.6). PCR amplification allows large amounts of mPCR product to be produced from small quantities of RNA (100 ng total RNA), which are then radiolabeled and used as probes for cDNA library differential screening.[27] One advantage of closed screening techniques is that both up- and down-regulated cDNAs can be targeted in the same screen. The drawback of differential library-based screening is that of limited sensitivity, resulting in the identification of predominantly abundant clones with large changes in expression. Also, if a clone is not present in the library used, then whatever the extent of its expression change, it cannot be isolated using these techniques—hence the term *closed system.*

An adaptation of conventional differential cDNA library screening is to enrich your library with up- or down-regulated clones by making a subtracted cDNA library before carrying out the screening process.[24,28] A well-constructed subtracted library will contain a greater proportion of regulated clones, increasing the likelihood of a successful differential screen[29,30] (see Section 5.5.2 for details on cDNA subtraction).

If genes are required that code for molecules performing a particular function (e.g., a previously characterized ion channel or a new neurite inhibitory molecule), functional screening of expression libraries can be useful. A cDNA library is made in an expression vector and pools of the library, normally around 10,000 to 20,000 clones per pool, are systematically transfected into a cell line. Clones are expressed by the transfected cells, which can then be screened for a particular function. The vector can be isolated and the clone identified from those cells that display the ability to perform the function associated with the coveted gene. An expression cloning strategy was recently used with great success to clone the capsaicin receptor, vanilloid receptor-1 (VR1).[7] Based on the fact that capsaicin causes a large influx of calcium into cells that express its receptor, a DRG cDNA library was expressed in HEK293 cells which were subsequently screened for calcium influx after capsaicin treatment using the fluorescent calcium–sensitive dye Fura-2. Positive cells were taken and rescreened before the vector was isolated and its 3-kilobase insert identified as VR1.

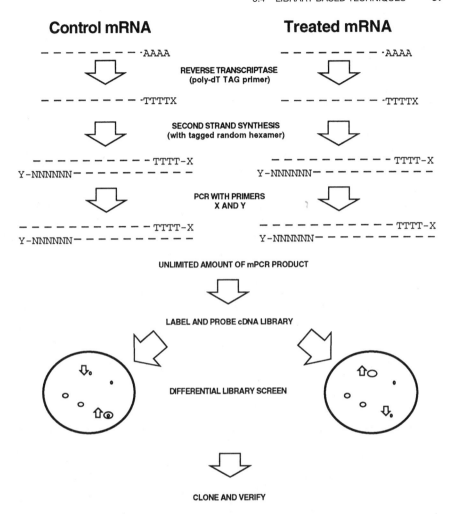

Figure 5.6   Schematic diagram highlighting the basic methodology for mPCR. Total cellular RNA is taken from the tissue under investigation. Both RNA populations are reverse transcribed with tagged oligo-d(T) primers. Second-strand cDNA synthesis is performed with a tagged random hexamer primer. Unlimited amounts of mPCR products, representing complex mixtures of the original cDNAs present in each sample, can be amplified by PCR with primers complementary to the two incorporated tags. These mPCR products are then labeled and used to screen a cDNA differentially using standard protocols.

Many pharmaceutical and biotechnology companies are currently using large-scale differential screening and library sequencing strategies to uncover genes that are regulated in different disease states with the aim of identifying novel targets for diagnostics and treatment. One approach adopted by the company Affymetrix is to screen oligonucleotide libraries differentially.

High-density arrays of oligonucleotides are generated on silica micro chips.[31] The sequence of each oligonucleotide is specific to an individual gene, and multiple oligonucleotides are produced for each gene. In the first protocol described,[31] total RNA was reverse transcribed in the presence of fluorescently labeled nucleotides to produce a complex labeled cDNA probe. The probe was then hybridized with the oligonucleotide microarrays, the silica chips were washed at high stringency and automatically scanned by confocal laser, and signals were quantified. This novel method has a number of potential advantages: the most important being that there is no initial cloning step as there is in making a cDNA library—only the gene sequence is required—and as a number of total genome sequencing projects near completion, in theory at least, the expression levels of every gene within a particular organism may be assayed by this method. Other advantages include the investigation of gene families, splice variants, and polymorphic allele analysis of genetic traits.

A number of biotechnology companies are involved in enormous cDNA library sequencing projects. This type of project produces millions of sequences known as expressed sequence tags (ESTs). ESTs are generally short sequences that represent parts of novel sequences within a library. Through the sequencing of two or more cDNA libraries, it is possible to subtract the two libraries electronically to find sequences specific to a particular tissue/treatment (e.g., PC12 cells before and after nerve growth factor treatment).[32] Briefly, thousands of randomly selected clones from a cDNA library are partially sequenced from the 3' and 5' ends using a high-throughput sequencer to produce a collection of ESTs which are then compared with ESTs from another library using sophisticated bioinformatic software packages. Differentially regulated genes can be identified by comparing the number of times a particular gene sequence appears in one library relative to the other, and the differential regulation of these sequences can then be confirmed by Northern blots.

The serial analysis of gene expression (SAGE) technique[33,34] is a method that uses similar electronic subtraction technology. Libraries are created containing concatenated 9 to 11 base-pair (bp) sequence tags isolated from the 3' end of each gene in a population of reverse-transcribed cDNA. To assemble sequence tag concatemers, total RNA is reverse transcribed with a biotinylated oligo-dT primer. Second-strand cDNA is synthesized and each preparation is cut with a frequent-cutting (4-bp recognition sequence) restriction endonuclease. The 3' fragment of each gene is then isolated using streptavadin beads that bind to biotin. This preparation is then split into two fractions and separate linkers are ligated on to each cDNA sample via the frequent-cutter restriction site. Each linker contains a distinct PCR primer site and a common type IIS restriction site (type IIS restriction enzymes cleave

DNA at a defined position up to 20 bp away from their restriction site). Digestion with this enzyme releases the linker sequence and a short piece of the cDNA; it is this sequence that makes up the SAGE tag. The two pools of SAGE tags with differing linkers are then ligated to one and other. PCR with primers targeted against sequences in either linker then ensures representative amplification of all the SAGE tags.[33] Once amplified, the SAGE tags are digested with the frequent-cutting enzyme used originally to remove the linkers (PCR primer sites). The tags are then ligated to one another to produce concatemers of 50 or more SAGE sequences, and each concatemer is then cloned and sequenced. Theoretically, nine base pairs is enough to distinguish between every cDNA in the gene pool, offering an unparalleled ability to perform high-throughput screening of short ESTs, because each concatenated clone represents at least 50 different genes as opposed to just the one in standard EST analysis.[34] Using this technology, hundreds of thousands of individual sequences can be analyzed rapidly, representing many thousand genes. This technique has been used very successfully to isolate 14 genes from over 7000 transcripts analyzed that are up-regulated in a colorectal carcinoma cell line in response to p53-induced apoptosis.[35]

5.5   NON-LIBRARY-BASED TECHNIQUES

5.5.1   Differential Display and Related Techniques

The open approaches are a more diverse group of techniques, the main advantage being that any source of RNA, either tissue or a cell line, can be studied without being restricted by the identity of clones in a particular library. Differential display is a PCR-based transcriptional assay devised by Liang and Pardee.[36–39] Messenger RNA is purified from total RNA and reverse-transcribed with poly-d(T) primers anchored at their 3′ end. First-strand cDNA is then amplified with PCR using arbitrary 5′ primers and anchored 3′ oligo-d(T) primers with radiolabeled nucleotides (^{35}S and more recently, ^{33}P) at low annealing temperatures. PCR products, which are a mixture of sequences of different lengths, are run out on a 6% polyacrylamide denaturing gel and visualized by autoradiography. Using RNA from two (or more) different sources to generate PCR products, for example, rat lumbar DRG neurons before and after treatment with NGF,[40] the two ladders of different lengths of DNA can be compared. Most of the bands should be common to both display ladders, representing mRNA sequences present in both cell populations. Any differences are potentially genes whose expression is regulated by the treatment of interest. This technique, therefore, relies critically on reproducibility of ladders for the same pools of cDNA. The band of interest is eluted from the dried polyacrylamide and PCR-amplified with the original primers before being subcloned, sequenced, and its differential expression validated.

An adaptation of differential display is RNA fingerprinting.[41-44] Here, messenger RNA is purified from total RNA, reverse-transcribed, and PCR-amplified using arbitrary primers alone instead of the oligo-d(T) and arbitrary primer used by Liang and Pardee in the original protocol. In the Liang and Pardee procedure the length of products is limited to about 500 base pairs of their 3' end because the PCR products are electrophoresed on a sequencing gel, which may not be of sufficient length to reach coding region (mRNAs have on average 500 bases of 3' untranslated region between coding region and their polyadenylated tail). With RNA fingerprinting, the limit on product size is still 500 base pairs, but because reverse transcription is achieved with arbitrary primers, they can bind anywhere along the mRNA transcript, greatly increasing the chance of amplifying sequence corresponding to coding region and therefore increasing the likelihood of being able to identify the product from a database. Much effort has been put into working out the number of primer combinations, and therefore PCR reactions necessary to sample greater than 95% of the mRNA population under study (over 300 PCR reactions for each set of RNA from some calculations).[45] However, these calculations are purely theoretical and can only be applied to techniques that use oligo-d(T) primers to reverse transcribe. It is likely that they both overestimate the number of different primer combinations required to sample abundant mRNAs and underestimate the number required for rare mRNAs.[42]

Many adaptations of the original differential display and RNA fingerprinting protocols have since been published, aimed predominantly at reducing the number of false positives that have plagued this technique. Sokolov and Prockop[46] published an alternative technique where polyA mRNA is prepared from total RNA and reverse-transcribed with fully degenerate random hexamers. PCR amplification of resultant first-strand cDNA is achieved using arbitrary 10 to 28mers, and no radioactive label is used. Rather, the PCR products are electrophoresed on a 2% low-melting-point agarose gel and stained with ethidium bromide (Fig. 5.7). Bands representing candidate "differentially expressed molecules" are then excised from the gel and subcloned directly into a TA cloning vector. Further PCR amplification of individual bands using the original primers is not necessary (a step required in traditional differential display and RNA fingerprinting, where some workers have reported up to 70% failure of bands to reamplify). This technique is therefore much less laborious, using far fewer combinations of primers, and avoids the use of radioactivity during PCR. However, it produces only 15 to 30 bands per lane on the agarose gel, compared to the 50 to 100 on sequencing gel, mean-

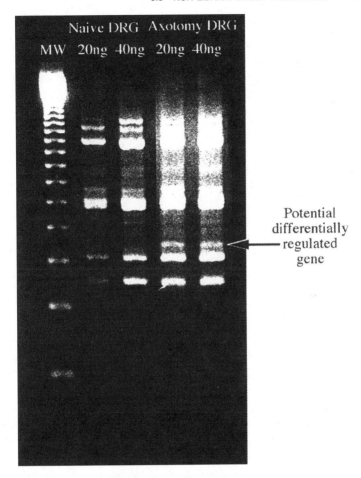

Figure 5.7 Example of a typical differential display gel using the protocol taken from Sokolov and Prockop.[46] The arrow is pointing at a band that is present after axotomy but not in normal DRGs. A step taken to reduce the chance of false positives is to perform the PCR amplification with two different concentrations of cDNA for each condition, and only bands present in both lanes are picked as potentially regulated sequences.

ing that a much lower number of potentially regulated genes are observed. Another limitation of this protocol stems from the fact that fewer PCR amplification primer combinations are used; this results in reduced sampling of the mRNA population and therefore less likelihood of finding differentially expressed genes, particularly those with a low copy number per cell.[46] In practice, however, studies that have employed this technique have identified a number of differentially regulated genes that they have been unable to detect using Northern blots, an indicator of relative abundance, and have subsequently had to use semiquantitative PCR to validate differential expression.[47]

Despite criticisms about the potential effectiveness of differential display and RNA fingerprinting to identify any differentially regulated genes other than those of high abundance,[48] a number of studies have revealed differentially expressed mRNAs expressed at low levels (e.g., Ref. 47) and molecules expressed only in a subpopulation of the cells under investigation.[49] A major advantage of this approach is that many different RNA types can be analyzed simultaneously.

5.5.2   Subtractive Hybridization

Subtractive hybridization (SH) is an alternative technique employed to reveal regulated mRNAs. SH was developed in the 1980s to produce subtracted cDNA libraries but was inapplicable as a tool in studying many biological events because of the vast amount of polyA mRNA required (around 5 to 10 μg). Taking advantage of PCR as a tool for amplification has meant that SH can now be applied to biological events where mRNA is a limited resource. A PCR-based SH protocol developed from the original Brady protocol[50] has been used in our laboratory to identify genes differentially regulated in neuropathic and inflammatory models of pain. This method (outlined in Fig. 5.8) is powerful, capable of dissecting out molecular differences in gene expression between single cells.[28,50] Others have used SH protocols to identify genes specific to DRG neurons[29] and within the proximal nerve stump following axotomy.[51,52]

Briefly, SH aims to isolate sequences present in an experimental (tracer) mRNA sample but not in the control (driver) mRNA sample. Two pools of mRNA corresponding to the tracer and driver are extracted from, for example, rat dorsal root ganglia before and after peripheral nerve injury, and reverse-transcribed with poly-d(T) primers to produce short lengths of first-strand cDNA, largely representative of the 3′ untranslated region of the mRNA transcript. A polyA tail is added to the 3′ end of the single-stranded cDNA using terminal transferase and dATP, and each tailed cDNA population is then amplified by PCR using a single tagged primer to generate pools of double-stranded DNA.[53] The driver pool is photobiotinylated and hybridized with the tracer pool in the ratio 20:1. Under these conditions tracer sequences common to the driver pool will hybridize with the excess biotinylated driver cDNA. The biotinylated DNA hybrids are removed by adding streptavidin followed by extraction with phenol. Up-regulated genes whose sequences are present in the tracer but poorly represented in the driver will not be extracted and can be recovered by PCR. This pool of cDNAs (H1), the product of the first subtraction, is now reused as tracer and rehybridized with a 20-fold excess of the driver pool to obtain the H2 pool, which is subtracted once more to obtain the H3 pool (Fig. 5.8).

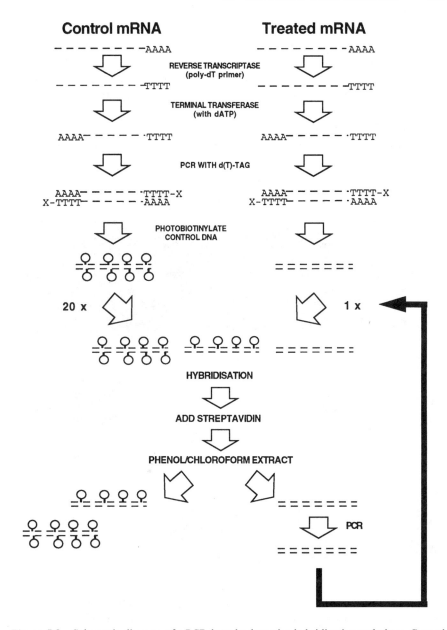

Figure 5.8   Schematic diagram of a PCR-based subtractive hybridization technique. Control and treated mRNA are reverse transcribed from total RNA using a poly-dT primer. A poly-A tail is then added to the 3′ end of the single-stranded cDNA using terminal transferase. Universal amplification of all the cDNA in each population (control and treated) is performed with a poly-dT tag primer. An excess of control PCR product DNA is then photobiotinylated and is hybridized with unlabeled treated DNA at a ratio of 20:1. All common hybrids are removed by streptavidin addition and phenol chloroform extraction. The subtracted DNA population is then resubtracted with another 20-fold excess of biotinylated control cDNA.

The effectiveness of this approach is illustrated in Figure 5.9. We have used this technique to look for genes up-regulated after peripheral axotomy, and intraplantar complete Freund's adjuvant.[55,56] We have cloned multiple genes regulated in the DRG by peripheral axotomy and inflammation, ranging from 2- to 10-fold up- or down-regulated (confirmed by Northern blotting) and we are currently analyzing these clones further. One gene regulated in the DRG after axotomy that we have discovered in this way is the heat shock protein HSP27, which may have a role in preventing programmed cell

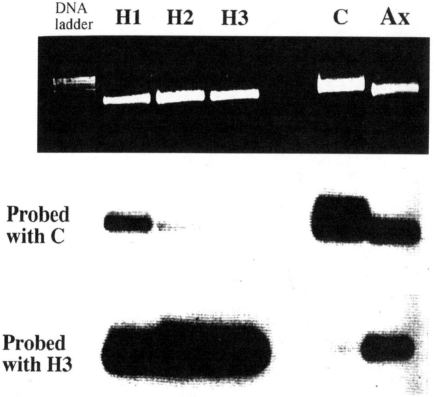

Figure 5.9   Southern blot analysis of PCR products produced by subtractive hybridization. PCR products were run 2 cm into an 1% agarose gel and blotted onto nitrocellulose membrane. Untreated control (C) and 48-h postsciatic nerve axotomy (Ax) DRG total RNA were used to produce PCR products (see the text for details). H1 is the amplification product of the first subtraction of "axotomy minus control" DNA. H2 is the product of the second subtraction of H1 minus control, and H3 is the product of H2 minus control. The blot was probed with the original control DNA. The control probe does not hybridize with H2 or H3 products, showing that these DNA products contain very few sequences common to the control population. The blot was stripped and reprobed with the product of the third subtraction (H3). The H3 product hybridizes with the axotomy DNA product but not the control DNA, confirming that H3 has been enriched for axotomy-induced sequences.

death of sensory and motor neurons after peripheral nerve injury[57] (Figs. 5.1 and 5.2).

One of the major disadvantages of SH of cDNA is that the subtraction product often contains a proportion of clones that are not regulated but remain in the pool. This is thought to be due to some unhybridized single-stranded tracer cDNAs remaining in the reaction and escaping subtraction. Modifying the hybridization conditions, such as the length of time or temperature, can help to reduce highly abundant sequences from the subtracted pool.[54]

5.5.3 Degenerate PCR

The use of degenerate primers and low-stringency homology screening using PCR to clone novel members of particular families of molecules such as ion channels are now standard molecular procedures. We have applied degenerate primer screening to a DRG cDNA library with the aim of cloning novel sodium channels. Primers were designed to conserved sequences within the 3′ coding region of the brain II, heart, skeletal muscle, and glial voltage-gated sodium channels. These primers were used to PCR a sodium channel pan-specific probe from rat genomic DNA. A rat DRG cDNA library was then used to assemble a novel full-length clone, which when expressed in HEK293T cells, encoded a functional channel tetrodotoxin-resistant (TTXr) voltage-gated sodium channel. Due to the fact that this clone shared 63% amino acid sequence homology to the only other cloned sensory-neuron-specific TTXr sodium channel (SNS)[8] and that its expression pattern was sensory neuron specific, too, we have named this sodium channel SNS2.[58]

We have also applied degenerate PCR screening to DRG cDNA with the goal of cloning novel zinc finger proteins regulated in inflammatory and neuropathic models. Zinc finger proteins are molecules that contain one or more zinc finger DNA binding domains, occurring in repeated tandem arrays. The proteins that contain these arrays can act as transcription factors or RNA binding proteins. Degenerate primers were designed against highly conserved regions of the zinc finger domain, and PCR was performed on cDNA prepared from DRG at low annealing temperatures to produce a ladder of DNA sequences, representing multiple zinc finger domains (Fig. 5.10). We have then used mPCR screening strategies to identify quickly whether any of these molecules are regulated by inflammation in the hindpaw or sciatic nerve injury.

Recently, the use of degenerate PCR primers against families of transcription factors has been used in a modified differential display protocol. Rather than using arbitrary primers for PCR amplification from first-strand cDNA, degenerate primers designed against specific families (e.g., helix-loop-helix proteins have been used in an attempt to clone members of that family whose

DNA   PCR
ladder products

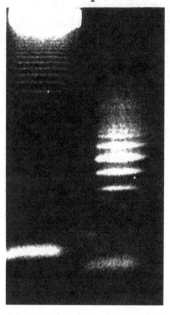

Figure 5.10 Example of PCR products generated from using degenerate primers designed against conserved sequences either side of zinc finger domains, using cDNA generated from DRG mRNA. The smallest band represents one zinc finger domain, the next band two, then three, and so on. PCR products were cloned, sequenced, and mPCR screened to recognize whether any were regulated in the DRG after particular treatments.

expression is regulated by the treatment of interest.[47] Transcription factors are of interest in the etiology of chronic pain, as they act as the molecular switches within the cell, changing a cell's phenotype from that which is seen under normal conditions to that seen in a given pathology (i.e., inflammatory pain).[59]

5.6   CONCLUSIONS

Molecular biological techniques offer a powerful approach for dissecting out the mechanisms that operate to produce pain. Its full potential can, however, be realized only if combined with nonmolecular techniques where the function of identified genes can be studied. The capacity to transfect cells with a gene or with antisense to the gene integrates cell biology with molecular biology while transgenic mutations provide the means to combine systems neurobiology with molecular biology. Measuring changes in the level of a particular species of mRNA in sensory neurons or, indeed, cloning a novel gene expressed in these cells is just the beginning. The formidable task ahead is to devise a strategy for identifying the functional or pathophysiological role of these genes. Once this is in place we will be truly well on the way to understanding the molecular basis of pain.

REFERENCES

1. Woolf, C. J. (1995). Somatic pain: pathogenesis and prevention. Br. J. Anaesth. 75:169–176.
2. Woolf, C. J. (1996). Phenotypic modification of primary sensory neurones: the role of nerve growth factor in the production of persistent pain. Philos. Trans. R. Soc. Lond. B 351:441–448.
3. Woolf, C. J., and Doubell, T. P. (1994). The pathophysiology of chronic pain: increased sensitivity to low threshold Aβ-fibre inputs. Curr. Opin. Neurobiol. 4:525–534.
4. McMahon, S. B., Lewin, G. R., and Wall, P. D. (1993). Central hyperexcitability triggered by noxious inputs. Curr. Opin. Neurobiol. 3:602–610.
5. Dubner, R., and Ruda, M. A. (1992). Activity-dependent neuronal plasticity following tissue injury and inflammation. TINS 15(3):96–103.
6. Chen, C. C., Akopian, A. N., Sivilotti, L., Colquhoun, D., Burnstock, G., and Wood, J. N. (1995). A P2X purinoceptor expressed by a subset of sensory neurons. Nature 377:428–431.
7. Caterina, M. J., Schumacher, M. A., Tominaga, M., Rosen, T. A., Levine, J. D., and Julius, D. (1997). The capsaicin receptor: a heat-activated ion channel in the pain pathway. Nature 389:816–824.
8. Akopian, A. N., Sivilotti, L., and Wood, J. N. (1996). A tetrodotoxin-resistant voltage-gated sodium channel expressed by sensory neurons. Nature 379:257–262.
9. Sangameswaran, L., Delgado, S. G., Fish, L. M., Koch, B. D., Jakeman, L. B., Stewart, G. R., Sze, P., Hunter, J. C., Eglen, R. M., and Herman, R. C. (1996). Structure and function of a novel voltage-gated, tetrodotoxin-resistant sodium channel specific to sensory neurons. J. Biol. Chem. 271:5953–5956.
10. Woolf, C. J., Safieh-Garabedian, B., Ma, Q.-P., Crilly, P., and Winter, J. (1994). Nerve growth factor contributes to the generation of inflammatory sensory hypersensitivity. Neuroscience 62:327–331.
11. McMahon, S. B., Bennett, D. L. H., Priestley, J. V., and Shelton, D. L. (1995). The biological effects of endogenous NGF in adult sensory neurones revealed by a trkA IgG fusion molecule. Nature Med. 1:774–780.
12. Safieh-Garabedian, B., Poole, S., Allchorne, A., Winter, J., and Woolf, C. J. (1995). Contribution of interleukin-1β to the inflammation-induced increase in nerve growth factor levels and inflammatory hyperalgesia. Br. J. Pharmacol. 115:1265–1275.

13. Woolf, C. J., Allchorne, A., Safieh-Garabedian, B., and Poole, S. (1997). Cytokines, nerve growth factor and inflammatory hyperalgesia: the contribution of tumour necrosis factor α. Br. J. Pharmacol. 121:417–424.

14. Patterson, P. H. (1994). Leukemia inhibitory factor, a cytokine at the interface between neurobiology and immunology. Proc. Natl. Acad. Sci. USA 91:7833–7835.

15. Leslie, T. A., Emson, P. C., Dowd, P. M., and Woolf, C. J. (1995). Nerve growth factor contributes to the upregulation of GAP-43 and preprotachykinin A mRNA in primary sensory neurons following peripheral inflammation. Neuroscience 67:753–761.

16. Neumann, S., Doubell, T. P., Leslie, T. A., and Woolf, C. J. (1996). Inflammatory pain hypersensitivity mediated by phenotypic switch in myelinated primary sensory neurones. Nature 384:360–364.

17. Fawcett, J. W., and Keynes, R. J. (1990). Peripheral nerve regeneration. Annu. Rev. Neurosci. 13:43–60.

18. Sambrook, J., Fritsch, E. F., and Maniatis, T. (1989). Molecular cloning: a laboratory manual, Cold Spring Harbor Laboratory Press, Cold Spring Harbor, N.Y.

19. Ausubel, F. M., Brent, R., Kingston, R. E., Moore, D. D., Seidman, J. G., Smith, J. A., and Struhl, K. (1991). Current protocols in molecular biology, Vol. 1(1), Greene Publishing Associates and Wiley-Interscience, New York.

20. Kendall, G., and Latchman, D. S. (1996). Polymerase chain reaction for RNA analysis. A companion to Methods Enzymol. 10:279–282.

21. Wang, A. M., Doyle, M. V., and Mark, D. F. (1989). Quantitation of mRNA by the polymerase chain reaction. Proc. Natl. Acad. Sci. USA 86:9717–9721.

22. Gilliland, G., Perrin, S., Blanchard, K., and Bunn, H. F. (1990). Analysis of cytokine mRNA and DNA: detection and quantitation by competitive polymerase chain reaction. Proc. Natl. Acad. Sci. USA 87:2725–2729.

23. Souze, F., Ntodou-Thome, A., Tran, C. Y., Rostene, W., and Forgez, P. (1996). Quantitative RT-PCR: limits and accuracy. Biotechniques 21:280–285.

24. Tedder, T. F., Streuli, M., Schlossman, S. F., and Saito, H. (1988). Isolation and structure of a cDNA encoding the B1 (CD20) cell-surface antigen of human B lymphocytes. Proc. Natl. Acad. Sci. USA 85:208–212.

25. May, P. C., Lampert-Etchells, M., Johnson, S. A., Poirier, J., Masters, J. N., and Finch, C. E. (1990). Dynamics of gene expression for a hippocampal glycoprotein elevated in Alzheimer's disease and in response to experimental lesions in rat. Neuron 5:831–839.

26. Leonard, D. G., Ziff, E. B., and Greene, L. A. (1987). Identification and characterization of mRNAs regulated by nerve growth factor in PC12 cells. Mol. Cell. Biol. 7:3156–3167.

27. Kendal, G., Ensor, E., Crankson, H. D., and Latchman, D. S. (1996). Nerve growth factor treatment of sensory neuron primary cultures causes elevated levels of the mRNA encoding the ATP synthase β-unit as detected by a novel PCR-based differential cloning method. Eur. J. Biochem. 236:360–364.

28. Dulac, C., and Axel, R. (1995). A novel family of genes encoding putative pheromone receptors in mammals. Cell 83:195–206.

29. Akopian, A. N., and Wood, J. N. (1995). Peripheral nervous system–specific genes identified by subtractive cDNA cloning. J. Biol. Chem. 270:21264–21270.

30. Klar, A., Baldassare, M., and Jessell, T. M. (1992). F-spondin: a gene expressed at high levels in the floor plate encodes a secreted protein that promotes neural cell adhesion and neurite extension. Cell 69:95–110.

31. Schena, M. (1996). Genome analysis with gene expression microarrays. Bioessays 18:427–431.

32. Lee, N. H., Weinstock, K. G., Kirkness, E. F., Earle-Hughes, J. A., Fuldner, R. A., Marmaros, S., Glodek, A., Gocayne, J. D., Adams, M. D., Kerlavage, A. R., Fraser, C. M., and Venter, J. C. (1995). Comparative expressed-sequencing analysis of differential gene expression profiles in PC-12 cells before and after nerve growth factor treatment. Proc. Natl. Acad. Sci. USA 92:8303–8307.

33. Velculescu, V. E., Zhang, L., Vogelstein, B., and Kinzler, K. W. (1995). Serial analysis of gene expression. Science 270:484–487.

34. Adams, M. D. (1996). Serial analysis of gene expression: ESTs get smaller. Bioessays 18:261–262.

35. Polyak, K., Xia, Y., Zwieler, J. L., Kinzler, K. W., and Vogelstein, B. (1997). A model for p53-induced apoptosis. Nature 389:300–305.

36. Liang, P., and Pardee, A. B. (1997). Differential display: a general protocol. Methods Mol. Biol. 85:3–11.

37. Liang, P., and Pardee, A. B. (1995). Recent advances in differential display. Curr. Opin. Immunol. 7:274–280.

38. Liang, P., Bauer, D., Averboukh, L., Warthoe, P., Rohrwild, M., Muller, H., Strauss, M., and Pardee, A. B. (1995). Analysis of altered gene expression by differential display. Methods Enzymol. 254:304–321.

39. Liang, P., Zhu, W., Zhang, X., Guo, Z., O'Connell, R. P., Averboukh, L., Wang, F., and Pardee, A. B. (1994). Differential display using one-base anchored oligo-dT primers. Nucleic Acids Res. 22:5763–5764.

40. Kendall, G., Crankson, H., Ensor, E., Lublin, D. M., and Latchman, D. S. (1996). Activation of the gene encoding decay accelerating factor following nerve growth factor treatment of sensory neurons is mediated by promoter sequences within 206 bases of the transcriptional start site. J. Neurosci. Res. 45:96–103.

41. McClelland, M., Chada, K., Welsh, J., and Ralph, D. (1993). Arbitrary primed PCR fingerprinting of RNA applied to mapping differentially expressed genes. EXS 67:103–115.

42. McClelland, M., Matheiu-Daude, F., and Welsh, J. (1995). RNA fingerprinting and differential display using arbitrarily primed PCR. Trends Genet. 11:242–246.

43. Welsh, J., Chada, K., Dalal, S. S., Cheng, R., Ralph, D., and McClelland, M. (1992). Arbitraily primed PCR fingerprinting of RNA. Nucleic Acids Res. 20:4965–4970.

44. McClelland, M., and Welsh, J. (1994). RNA fingerprinting by arbitrarily primed PCR. PCR Methods Appl. 4:S66–S81.

45. Bauer, D., Muller, H., Reich, J., Riedel, H., Ahrenkiel, V., Warthoe, P., and Strauss, M. (1993). Identification of differentially expessed mRNA species by an improved display technique (DDRT-PCR). Nucleic Acids Res. 21:4272–4280.

46. Sokolov, B. P., and Prockop, D. J. (1994). A rapid and simple PCR-based method for isolation of cDNAs from differentially expressed genes. Nucleic Acids Res. 22:4009–4015.

47. Zoidl, G., Blanchard, A. D., Zoidl, C., Dong, Z., Brennan, A., Parmantier, E., Mirsky, R., and Jessen, K. R. (1997). Identification of transciptionally regulated mRNAs from mouse Schwann cell precursors using modified RNA fingerprinting methods. J. Neurosci. Res. 49:32–42.

48. Bertioli, D. J., Schlichter, U. H., Adams, M. J., Burrows, P. R., Steinbiss, H. H., and Antoniw, J. F. (1991). An analysis if differential display shows a strong bias towards high copy number mRNAs. J. Gen. Virol. 72:1801–1809.

49. Livesey, F., O'Brien, J., Li, M., Smith, A., Murphy, L., and Hunt, S. (1997). A Schwann cell mitogen accompanying regeneration of motor neurons. Nature 390:614–618.

50. Brady, G., Bilia, F., Knox, J., Hoang, T., Kirsch, I. R., Voura, E. B., Miyamoto, N., Boehmelt, G., and Iscove, N. N. (1995). Analysis of gene expression in a complex differentiation hierarchy by global amplification of cDNA from single cells. Curr. Biol. 5:909–922.

51. De Leon, M., Welcher, A. A., Suter, U., and Shooter, E. M. (1991). Identification of transcriptionally regulated genes after sciatic nerve injury. J. Neurosci. Res. 29:437–448.

52. Gillen, C., Gleichmann, M., Spreyer, P., and Muller, H. W. (1995). Differently expressed genes after peripheral nerve injury. J. Neurosci. Res. 42:159–171.

53. Brady, G., Barbara, M., and Iscove, N. N. (1990). Representative in vitro cDNA amplification from individual hemopoietic cells and colonies. Methods Mol. Cell Biol. 2:17–25.

54. Wang, Z., and Brown, D. D. (1991). A gene expression screen. Proc. Natl. Acad. Sci. USA 88:11505–11509.

55. Chong, M.-S., Reynolds, M. L., Irwin, N., Coggeshall, R. E., Emson, P. C., Benowitz, L. I., and Woolf, C. J. (1994). GAP-43 expression in primary sensory neurons following central axotomy. J. Neurosci. 14(7):4375–4384.

56. Chong, M.-S., Fitzgerald, M., Winter, J., Hu-Tsai, M., Emson, P. C., Weise, U., and Woolf, C. J. (1992). GAP-43 mRNA in rat spinal cord and dorsal root ganglia neurons: developmental changes and re-expression following peripheral nerve injury. Eur. J. Neurosci. 4:883–895.

57. Costigan, M., Mannion, R. J., Kendall, G., Lewis, S. E., Campagna, J. A., Coggeshall, R. E., Meridith-Middleton, J., Tate, S., and Woolf, C. J. (1998). Heat shock protein 27: developmental regulation and expression after peripheral nerve injury. J. Neurosci. 18:5891–900.

58. Tate, S., Benn, S., Hick, C., Trezise, D., John, V., Mannion, R. J., Costigan, M., Plumpton, C., Grose, D., Gladwell, Z., Kendall, G., Dale, K., Bountra, C., and Woolf, C. J. (1998). Two sodium channels contribute to the TTX-R sodium current in primary sensory neurons. Nature Neurosci. 1:653–655.

59. Woolf, C. J., and Costigan, M. (1999). Translational and post-translational plasticity and the generation of inflammatory pain. Proc. Natl. Acad. Sci. USA 96:7723–7730.

CHAPTER 6

Sensory Neuron–Specific Ion Channels and Receptors

ARMEN N. AKOPIAN, CHIH-CHENG CHEN, VERONIKA SOUSLOVA,
KENJI OKUSE, AND JOHN N. WOOD

University College
London

6.1   INTRODUCTION

Drugs with analgesic effects act on broadly expressed receptors [e.g., opioid receptors, neuronal nicotinic receptors, 5HT3 (5-hydroxytryptamine receptors) or enzymes (e.g., cyclooxygenases). As these drug targets are involved in a variety of physiological functions quite apart from pain transmission or modulation, it has proved difficult to develop compounds that retain analgesic activity without some undesirable side effects on other physiological systems. Two approaches have been used to try to overcome this problem. A direct approach developed by Tamas Bartfai and his collaborators involves the synthesis of heteromeric bivalent drugs that bind to two distinct receptor populations that are exposed on the tissue of interest: in this case, nociceptors or neurons involved in pain pathways. As high-affinity binding depends on the co-expression of different receptor subtypes on the tissue of interest [e.g., neurokinin-1 (NK1) and N-methyl D-aspartate (NMDA) receptors on second-order sensory neurons], a measure of specificity can be developed. Thus far, no clinically useful entities have been described using this approach, despite its theoretical attractions for analgesic drug development as well as other indications.

A second approach described here is to define genes that are only expressed in neurons involved in pain pathways. The logic of this approach is that genes expressed specifically by particular cell types are likely to play a specialized functional role. Below we describe the exploitation of molecular genetics to identify potential novel analgesic drug targets expressed in nociceptive sensory neurons.

6.2   Difference Cloning

The hunt for sensory neuron–specific genes has involved a variety of difference and homology cloning methods followed by in situ and Northern blot analysis of distribution patterns, as well as expression cloning exercises that have led to the identification of dorsal root ganglia (DRG)-specific receptors such as the capsaicin receptor VR1 (vanilloid receptor-1) (Chapter 9). In this chapter we describe the use of difference and homology cloning methods to identify sensory neuron–specific channels and receptors that may play important roles in nociception.

The construction of a representative cDNA library from relatively small amounts of tissue is a prerequisite for difference cloning and requires sensitive screening protocols to isolate interesting clones. Development of the photobiotin/streptavidin subtractive hybridization technique[1] has led to the identification of transcripts specifically expressed even in very small numbers of cells.[2,3] The basis of this technique is to complex cDNA from the tissue of interest with RNA from a variety of other tissues that has been coupled to biotin. The common transcripts present in all tissues can be solvent extracted after addition of streptavidin, and a tiny amount of cDNA encoding transcripts present only in the tissue of interest are left to be amplified and cloned. More recently, differential screening of single-cell libraries has become a feasible and productive technique and has led to the identification of a new class of putative pheromone receptors.[4] The major problem with the use of the polymerase chain reaction (PCR) to generate libraries is the overrepresentation of small transcripts, because of their more efficient amplification. One approach to overcoming this difficulty is to amplify larger transcripts in pools of cDNA for more PCR cycles. Another important factor in the production of a representative library is the choice of the "driver" RNA that is used to remove irrelevant transcripts. Both the spectrum of transcripts as well as their abundance in the subtracted library are influenced by the driver RNA, because the relative proportion of various DRG-specific genes may be altered by different levels of subtraction. Commonly expressed motifs [e.g., nucleotide binding sites, src-homology domains (SH_2) or PSD-95/discs-large/ZO-I (PDZ) domains] are also likely to lead to the depletion of tissue-specific transcripts that contain such sequences no matter what tissue is used to "subtract" irrelevant transcripts. Using such a technique described in detail elsewhere,[5] a substantial number of DRG-specific clones were identified using differential screening. We review here the properties of some clones encoding ion channels that may be significant in nociception.

6.3 SENSORY NEURON SODIUM CHANNELS

Two clones encoding a voltage-gated (SNS) and an atypical voltage-gated sodium channel α subunit (NaG or SCL-11) have been cloned from a DRG difference library.[6,7] The functional voltage-gated sodium channels (VGSCs) present in both the peripheral and central nervous system comprise a large membrane-spanning α-subunit of 260 kD which comprises four repeated domains of six transmembrane segments (Fig. 6.1). In addition, there are associated regulatory subunits: a β1 subunit of 36 kD and a covalently associated β2 subunit of 33 kD.[8–12] There is indirect evidence that a number of different β2 subunits exist.[11] The α-subunit mRNAs can direct the translation of functional channels.[8] However, the accessory β1 and β2 subunits enhance functional channel expression in *Xenopus* oocytes and regulate the kinetic properties of expressed channels. In addition, the β2 subunit may play a role in anchoring the protein at particular locations within the cell.[10]

The functional voltage-gated sodium channel α-subunit SNS (also homology cloned and named PN3 by Sangemeswaran et al.[13]) is particularly interesting, as it corresponds to an unusual type of sodium channel present in small-diameter sensory neurons that is resistant to the puffer fish poison tetrodotoxin (TTX). Evidence for functional heterogeneity of sodium channels in sensory neurons has relied on kinetic analysis and the use of TTX to define channels in terms of resistance to block. At least three kinetically and pharmacologically distinct VGSCs have been described in DRG sensory neurons in this way.[14–16] One of these channels is insensitive to micromolar

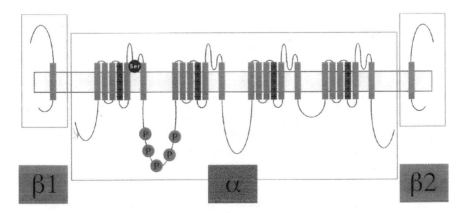

Figure 6.1 Sodium channel structure.

concentrations of TTX and exhibits a low single-channel conductance, slow activation and inactivation kinetics, and a more depolarized threshold of activation than other VGSCs.[17,18] Ogata and Tatebayashi[19] analyzed the pattern of expression of sodium channels in adult rat DRG cultures. Large-diameter neurons (mean 46 ± 1.4 μm) expressed TTX-sensitive sodium currents, whereas small-diameter neurons (mean diameter 25.9 ± 1.3 μm) expressed exclusively TTX-insensitive (TTXi) sodium currents under the recording conditions used. A third of the neurons tested, with a mean diameter intermediate between the large and small populations, expressed both types of current. There are obvious anomalies between such recordings from the somata of sensory neurons in vitro and recordings from sensory neuron fibers in vivo, which appear to be TTX sensitive. These observations may be reconciled by the axotomized nature of sensory neurons in culture and the differential distribution of expression of sodium channel subtypes in vivo.

Mounting evidence suggests that the TTXr sodium channel plays a unique role in the transmission of nociceptive information to the spinal cord. Thus bradykinin-dependent release of calcitonin gene–related peptide (CGRP), as well as the depolarization of dorsal horn cells elicited through C-fiber activation, was apparently insensitive to peripherally applied TTX.[20] However, a more prevalent view is that in most nerves, essentially all electrically evoked depolarisations leading to both A- and C-fiber-mediated action potential propagation are TTX sensitive, and the role of SNS may be to regulate the threshold of activation of small-diameter sensory neurons.

The sodium channel transcripts present in dorsal root ganglia have been explored by Northern blots and PCR (Table 6.1). The neuronal forms type I and II are present, while the embryonic type III reappears after axotomy. Both SNS and the TTXs channel PN1 are present at high levels in peripheral neurons. PN1, type I, NaCh6, and type II TTXs-sensitive transcripts occur in descending order of abundance. The atypical (see below) sodium channel NaG is expressed predominantly by Schwann cells but is also found in sensory neurons. Only the small-diameter sensory neuron–specific SNS subunit is present exclusively in small-diameter sensory neurons, however. This pattern of distribution has been demonstrated by in situ hybridization and RT-PCR examination of a range of tissues. In addition, the destruction of small-diameter sensory neurons by capsaicin, which acts predominantly on nociceptors, leads to loss of the SNS transcript.[6] These observations, combined with the resistance to TTX block (IC_{50} 60 mM), support the view that SNS underlies the TTXi currents observed in C fibers and small-diameter neurons. The molecular basis for the TTX insensitivity exhibited by SNS has recently been addressed by site-directed mutagenesis experiments. A critical residue in the pore of the channel of TTX-sensitive VGSCs that is normally hydrophobic is transformed to a serine in SNS. When this single amino acid position is altered to

Poppies in October

Even the sun-clouds this morning cannot manage such skirts.
Nor the woman in the ambulance
Whose red heart blooms through her coat so astoundingly —

A gift, a love gift
Utterly unasked for
By a sky

Palely and flamily
Igniting its carbon monoxides, by eyes
Dulled to a halt under bowlers.

O my God, what am I
That these late mouths should cry open
In a forest of frost, in a dawn of cornflowers.

Sylvia Plath

TABLE 6.1   Sodium Channels of DRG

Name	Gene	Chromosome		Functional
Type I	SCN1a	2	X03638	Yes
Type II	SCN2a	2	X03639	Yes
Type IIa		2		Yes
Type III	SCN3a	2	Y00766	Yes
SM1	SCN4a	11	JN0007	Absent
SM2	SCN5a	9	A33996	Absent
NaCh6	SCN8a	15	U59966	Yes
PN1, HneNa	SCN9a	2	X82835	Yes
SNS	SCN10a	9	X92184	Yes
NaG/SCL11	SCN7a		Y09164	?
NaN	SCN11a?	9	AF059030	Yes

phenylalanine, sensitivity to TTX is increased dramatically (IC_{50} 2 nM).[21] These studies confirm earlier ideas about the TTX-binding site in sodium channel atria based on mutagenesis studies of the cardiac sodium channel.

Gold et al.[22] and England et al.[23] have demonstrated the functional modulation of TTXi VGSC activity in sensory neurons by inflammatory mediators that are known to lower pain thresholds. Prostaglandin E_2, adenosine, and serotonin all increased the magnitude of INa, shifted its conductance–voltage relation in a hyperpolarizing direction, and increased the rates of activation and inactivation of sodium channels in small-diameter sensory neurons in culture. Such data suggest that TTXi sodium currents play an important role in regulating pain thresholds. This topic is covered in detail in Chapter 12.

As well as the inflammatory mediators investigated in these studies, there is now good evidence that NGF is a key regulator of nociceptive thresholds[24]; its application has been shown to cause dramatic decreases in thermal thresholds of pain perception in animal models and NGF levels rise in damaged tissue (Chapter 3). NGF is known to act through the high-affinity receptor trkA to increase the TTXi sodium flux in PC12 cells in culture,[25] and Omri and Meiri[26] have also demonstrated the induction of Na currents by NGF in DRG neurons in serum-free medium. More recently, very good evidence that NGF up-regulates the expression of the SNS transcript in vivo has been obtained using minipumps to deliver NGF to axotomized neurons in rat.[27] In these experiments, the increase in mRNA levels was correlated with increased TTXi current densities in acutely dissociated DRG neurons from the same animals. The same group has shown that injection of carageenan, which causes the release of inflammatory mediators, including NGF, also increases the expression of SNS mRNA, again supporting a role for TTXr in nociception.[28] In vitro studies of embryonic rat DRG cultures have shown that other sodium channel α- and β1-subunit expression is up-regulated by NGF using a semi-quantitative in situ hybridization method [29] After 4 days in vitro in the absence of NGF, sodium channel α-subunit II mRNA was expressed at moderate levels in E16 rat DRG neurons, and the transcripts for sodium channel α-subunits I and III, NaG, and β1 subunit were undetectable. With the addition of NGF, DRG neurons expressed moderate levels of sodium channel αI and αIII subunits and high levels of αII transcript. Sodium channel β1 mRNA was also up-regulated by NGF to a high level of expression.

Although SNS does not appear to be completely dependent on NGF for expression, there is an up-regulation of both the transcript and the protein, together with the appearance of an unusual, and apparently nonfunctional, splice variant on addition of NGF to sensory neurons in culture.[30] In addition, a soluble factor released by Schwann cells that may well be NGF seems to be involved in the up-regulation of SNS expression.[31] Given the restricted expression of trkA on the neuronal subpopulation that is principally concerned with nociception, NGF regulation of sodium channels, particularly SNS, may play a role in regulating inflammatory pain thresholds. Interestingly, IB4-positive GDNF-sensitive small-diameter sensory neurons also express SNS, raising the possibility that other factors, such as GDNF, may regulate SNS expression in this class of nociceptor. In support of this view, GDNF has been found to up-regulate TTXr current in small-diameter sensory neurons and rescue the expression of SNS and NaN (see below) in axotomized sensory neurons. NGF, in contrast, up-regulates SNS but not NaN (34). In contrast to the up-regulation of TTXr currents and SNS transcripts with inflammatory mediators, a variety of manipulations that lead to neuropathic pain (ligature-induced and diabetic neuropathies) lead to a down-regulation of SNS expression. This suggests that SNS may play a more significant role in inflammatory rather than neuropathic pain states.

The recently described antihyperalgesic agent BW2040W92[32] appears to be a use-dependent blocker of TTXr activity in sensory neurons, and some of its antihyperalgesic actions may be ascribed to SNS block, although the compound also acts on TTXs channels. These observations provide further indirect support for a role for SNS in setting pain thresholds. As the unique low-affinity TTX binding site in the SNS channel atrium has been partially defined, substituted guanidines specifically directed against SNS could provide an additional approach to selective channel block.[21] A direct approach to determining the functional significance of SNS is to ablate the expression of the channel in a null mutant mouse and measure the behavioral and electrophysiological consequences. Studies of such mice demonstrate that all TTXr activity found in sensory neurons in culture is encoded by SNS.[33] The behavioral correlates of a loss of SNS expression are of major interest in terms of nociceptive processing. Behavioral analysis depends on careful manipulation of genetic backgrounds by repeated back-crosses to produce congenic strains, as well as the assessment of any compensatory developmental changes that may occur in *sns* null mutants to obtain meaningful data. Analysis of SNS null mutants back-crossed onto a C57B16 background supports a role for SNS in pain pathways. Null mutants show deficits in thermoreception and the development of inflammatory pain. Strikingly, behavioral responses to noxious mechanical stimulation were completely abolished.[33]

A new sodium channel transcript named NaN has been identified in small-diameter sensory neurons.[34] The channel contains the appropriate sodium selectivity filters and voltage sensor motifs, although it has three less positively charged residues than SNS has in its S4 domains. Very interestingly, the channel expresses a serine residue at the same position of the TTX binding site as SNS, suggesting that the channel is likely to be TTX resistant. There is evidence that the transcript encodes a functional channel, but analysis of SNS null mutants (which have no slow sensory neuron TTXr currents) argues against a major role for NaN as a TTXi sodium channel in nociception.[33,66]

An additional full-length sodium channel transcript related to the glial sodium channel NaG, named SCL11,[7] was also isolated from the subtracted rat DRG library described above. The full-length clone has less than 50% identity to functional VGSC α subunits and does not appear to form a functional channel, consistent with the work by Tamkun and colleagues,[35] who were also unable to express functional sodium channels with the structurally related $hNa_v2.1$ and $mNa_v2.3$ proteins. There are grounds to believe that SCL11, as well as $hNa_v2.1$ and $mNa_v2.3$, may be neither voltage-gated nor sodium channels, because sodium selectivity filters and voltage sensors are all absent in these proteins. In addition, the regions implicated in fast inactivation are also lost. SCL11 mRNA shows an unusual pattern of expression, being found not only in neurons and Schwann cells in DRG, but also in lung, sciatic nerve, pituitary, bladder and vas deferens, spleen, and liver, as in cortex, cerebellum, and hippocampus. The significance of the atypical, apparently nonfunctional sodium channels is uncertain. As no functional activities are known for these channels, it is not possible to explore their physiological role with antagonists. The production and analysis of a null mutant is thus an attractive approach to defining the role of both SCL11 and other members of this putative cation channel family.

6.4 SENSORY NEURON ATP-GATED ION CHANNELS

An additional DRG-specific ion channel was identified in the same subtracted library and encoded an adenosine 5′-triphosphate (ATP)-gated cation channel named P2X3.[36] Burnstock[37] first proposed a role for ATP as a neurotransmitter, and in 1977 it was found that injection of ATP in human blister bases can evoke pain,[38] consistent with a direct action of ATP on nociceptive sensory neurons. This explanation for the pain-inducing actions of ATP is supported by electrophysiological studies that have shown that many DRG sensory neurons respond to ATP with elevated intracellular free calcium concentrations or depolarizing responses.[39–42] These effects are probably mediated by the P2X class of ATP-gated ion channels that have all been shown to be expressed by DRG neurons (Table 6.2). Such receptors comprise a family of glycosylated proteins of apparent molecular weight about 60 kD that have intracellular N- and C-terminal domains; two membrane-spanning hydrophobic domains, the second of which lines the channel pore; and a large extracellular domain. The subunits are encoded by different genes, although alternatively spliced transcripts of particular subtypes also occur. The channels are 35 to 50% identical at the amino acid level and are permeant to both monovalent and divalent cations. These channels show some similarities with amiloride-sensitive sodium channel subunits and *Caenorhabditis elegans* degenerins but have a distinct pattern of expression of conserved cysteine residues in the predicted extracellular domain of the proteins.[44] Seven different P2X receptors have been cloned and expressed in *Xenopus* oocytes and their distribution analyzed by in situ hybridization. Six known P2X-subtype mRNA transcripts have been found to be expressed in sensory neurons of the dorsal root, nodose, and trigeminal ganglia (reviewed in Ref. 45). However, only one subtype, P2X3, is expressed selectively in small-diameter sensory neurons that generally subserve a nociceptive function. An electrophysiological analysis of the properties of the expressed P2X3 channel showed many similarities with rat sensory neurons in culture. Thus the channel rapidly desensitized and was activated by ATP congeners with the same rank order of potency as that described for sensory neurons in culture [at low concentrations, 2-methyl-thio-ATP >> ATP > α,β-methylene-ATP > γ-thio-ATP > 2'-deoxy-ATP > cytidine triphosphate (CTP) > adenosine diphosphate (ADP) >> uridine 5'-triphosphate (UTP) β,γ-methylene-ATP > guanosine triphosphate (GTP)]. Indirect evidence for heteromultimeric channels in sensory neurons has been provided by coexpression studies of distinct P2X subunits in *Xenopus* oocytes. Some nodose ganglion cells desensitize slowly in response to α,β-methylene-ATP.[42] However, the oocyte-expressed P2X3 receptor desensitizes rapidly. If P2X2 (first identified in PC12 cells) is coexpressed with P2X3 in oocytes, a slowly desensitizing form of the receptor is formed.[46] This evidence is consistent with, but does not prove, that heteromultimeric receptors exist in sensory neurons. Structural studies using cross-linking reagents suggest that monomeric receptors exist as trimers, unlike any other known class of ion channels.[47] Recent evidence suggests that P2X3 is expressed exclusively by c-ret-positive GDNF-sensitive sensory neurons which comprise a subset of the nociceptor population.[48] Developmental analysis showed that P2X$_3$ transcripts

TABLE 6.2 Tissue Distribution of Rat P2X Receptors[a]

	$P2X_1$	$P2X_2$	$P2X_3$	$P2X_4$	$P2X_5$	$P2X_6$	$P2X_7$
Brain	+[b]	+	−	+	+	+	+
Spinal cord	+	+	−	+	+	+	+
Sensory ganglia	+	+	+	+	+	+	na
Superior cervical ganglia	+	+	−	+	−	+	na
Smooth muscle	+	+	−	+	−	−	na
Skeletal muscle	−(h)	−	−	+(h)	na	na	na
Heart	−(h)	−	−	+	+	+	na
Thymus	+	na	na	+	−	−	−
Spleen	+	−	−	+	−	−	+
Salivary gland	−	−	−	+	−	−	na
Bronchial epithelium	−	−	−	+	−	+	na
Lung	+	−	−	+	−	+	+
Kidney	+(h)	−	−	+	−	−	na
Liver	+(fh)	−	−	+(h)	−	+	na
Adrenal medulla	−	+	−	+	−	+	na
Pituitary	na	+	−	+	−	+	na
Testis	+	+	na	+	−	+	na

[a] na, Not available; h, data from human being; fh, data from fetal human.
[b] Neonatal rat brain only, not in the adult.[43]

are expressed as early as the period of sensory neurogenesis (E11.5 in the rat). In E12.5 rat, $P2X_3$ transcripts are found in somatovisceral primary sensory neurons, including neurons of trigeminal, facial, petrosal, nodose, and dorsal root ganglia, but not in other kinds of primary sensory neurons, such as olfactory epithelia, retina, and trigeminal mesencephalic nuclei.

Evidence of a role for P2X3 in nociception comes from physiological studies of conscious rats following subplantar injection of ATP and the ultrapotent congener α,β-methylene-ATP, which shows some selectivity for P2X3. Hindpaw lifting and licking occurred in animals injected subplantar with α,β-methylene-ATP. Nociceptive behaviors were dose-related; desensitization with a subplantar injection of capsaicin abolished all pain-related behavior in animals subsequently injected with α,β-methylene-ATP.[49]

A specific role of P2X3 is nociception is thus an interesting possibility given its selective expression pattern on nociceptive neurons. Nondesensitising P2X receptors seem to be present on dorsal horn neurons and probably correspond to P2X2, P2X4, and P2X6 receptor subtypes.[50] Recent studies on spinal cord splices confirm that ATP applied to DRG neuron spinal cord cocultures stimulates glutamate release.[51] Interestingly, an expression-cloned mechanoreceptor that corresponds to a P2Y1 receptor has been reported. The same authors found that tissue distortion caused by mechanical stimulation could also activate P2X3 through the release of ATP from distended cells, suggesting a possible role for P2X3 in mechanical as well as chemotransduction.[52]

The hypothesis that P2X3 receptors have a specialized role in nociception has been further embellished by a group who showed that $P2X_3$-immunostaining and ATP-induced inward current indeed appear in fluorescence-traced nociceptors of rat tooth pulp.[53] However, the fact that P2X3 is present in motor neurons of mice (but not rats) suggests that specific P2X3 antagonists may have effects other than acting as analgesics. The rapid hydrolysis of ATP to adenosine is a complication in interpreting the role of ATP in pain production, because adenosine also has a role in pain modulation in rodents and humans and null mutant mice for the adenosine receptor A_{2a} have recently been shown to have increased nociceptive thresholds.[53]

6.5   SENSORY NEURON PROTON-GATED CHANNELS

Proton-gated channels associated with sensory neurons are of particular interest because low pH is an important component in the induction of inflammatory pain.[54] The potentiation of action of a number of inflammatory mediators by protons has been demonstrated by the Reeh laboratory and is discussed in more detail in Chapter 9. An unusual nondesensitizing proton-gated calcium current has been described in sensory neurons in culture, and it has been suggested that a related channel could be the capsaicin receptor. There is increasing support for this view, as the cloned capsaicin receptor VR1 is activated at low pH (Chapter 9). Recently, a new set of cation (predominatly sodium)-selective ion channels gated by protons has been described in sensory neurons, which may contribute to such currents.[56] A proton-gated cation channel named ASIC (acid-sensing ion channel) expressed throughout the nervous system was the first channel to be identified.[57] The ASIC channels also comprise a two-transmembrane subunit with some topological similarities to the P2X receptors but with distinct primary sequences that place them in the familiy of amiloride-sensitive ENAc channels. The family has expanded to include the MDEG channels, renamed ASIC2a and 2b, and a related clone expressed in DRG sensory neurons named DRASIC or ASIC3[57–61] (and see below). Interestingly, all the ASIC clones have highly conserved extracellular cysteine residues, suggesting that as with the P2X class of receptors, the overall topology of the extracellular domain is similar within this particular class of receptor. Recent studies have provided compelling evidence that the members of the ENac family are tetramers, when heterologously expressed, in contrast to the trimeric P2X receptors.[62]

Using homology cloning techniques, the ASIC homolog (DRASIC) was found to be present in sensory neurons.[58] The orginal claim was that DRASIC is expressed exclusively in sensory neurons, but there is now some evidence that it is expressed in spinal cord and other central nervous system (CNS) locations at lower levels.[61] In addition, two splice variants of an additional channel named MDEG (mammalian degenerin homolog-1) have been identified. MDEG1 is a functional proton-gated ion channel, but MDEG2 is a splice variant that does not function except as a heteromultimer with ASIC or DRASIC. Interestingly, the properties of DRASIC/MDEG2 heteromultimers are distinct from DRASIC, with altered kinetics and ionic permeabilities, providing strong evidence that members of the ENaC family may form heteromultimers of, presumably, four subunits in total.[60] MDEG1 and 2 are also known as ASIC2a and ASIC2b. Only Asic2b is found in sensory neurons.[56]

An ASIC-related clone with distinct 5′ and 3′ UTRs named ASICα and a splice variant with a unique 5′ region and the same C terminal and 3′ UTR as ASICα named ASICβ have also been identified by homology cloning. ASICβ has a unique 172-amino acid N-terminal region with a putative first transmembrane domain that is homologous to DRASIC channel sequence.[61] A single ASICα 3.2-kb transcript is expressed in sensory neurons and other tissues. A similar-sized transcript is expressed by ASICβ in DRG alone and is present only in a subset of small-diameter sensory neurons. The functional properties of ASICβ are subtly different to those of other members of this family (Table 6.1). Unlike ASICα, both DRASIC and ASICβ show fast and slow components of proton-evoked channel opening. However, the slow response of ASICβ is less marked than with DRASIC and is unaffected by the application of amiloride, which blocks the fast component in both channels but potentiates the slow component in DRASIC. Like ASICα, ASICβ discriminates poorly between cations, since the reversal potential for the pH-gated current in ASICβ expressing COS cells was some 50 mV more negative than would be expected for a "pure" sodium conductance (+22 mV versus a calculated ENa of +73 mV). ASICβ shows some calcium permeability, since increasing extracellular calcium enhances the size of currents, while ASICα is markedly inhibited even with physiological levels of extracellular calcium. Interestingly, in sensory neurons in culture, proton-evoked ion fluxes are calcium permeant,[63] which implies that either the capsaicin-gated cation channel or a novel combination of ASIC subunits mediate proton-evoked fluxes. Identification of sensory neuron-specific channels that alone or in combination account for a long-lasting component of proton-evoked cation flux provides another potential new route to the development of anti-inflammatory analgesic drugs. The possibility that some of the proton-gated channels may participate in mechanosensitive ion channel complexes should also be considered (see Chapter 7).

6.6 FUTURE DIRECTIONS

Difference, expression, and homology cloning have led to the identification of a number of selectively expressed ion channels and receptors that may prove to be useful analgesic drug targets. A better understanding of the regulatory sequences that specify sensory neuron–specific gene expression may also be useful in designing screens for modulators that alter channel expression rather than function. Tissue–specific gene ablation using the cre-lox system will also allow us to examine the contribution of broadly expressed genes to nociceptive pathways.[64] Taking these various approaches together, it is clear that the application of molecular genetics to the study of sensory neurobiology has been valuable and informative, and should lead to useful treatments for pain disorders in the immediate future.

REFERENCES

1. Sive, H. L., and St. John, T. (1988). A simple subtractive hybridisation technique employing photoactivatable biotin and phenol extraction. Nucleic Acids Res. 16:10937.

2. Klar, A., Baldassare, M., and Jessell, T. M. (1992). F-spondin: a gene expressed at high levels in the floor plate encodes a secreted protein that promotes neural cell adhesion and neurite extension. Cell 69(1):95–110.

3. Wang, X., Barone, F. C., White, R. F., and Feuerstein, G. Z. (1998). Subtractive cloning identifies tissue inhibitor of matrix metalloproteinase-1 (TIMP-1) increased gene expression following focal stroke. Stroke 29(2):516–520.

4. Dulac, C., and Axel, R. (1995). A novel family of genes encoding putative pheromone receptors in mammals. Cell 83(2):195–206.

5. Akopian, A. N., and Wood, J. N. (1995). Peripheral nervous system–specific genes identified by subtractive cDNA cloning. J. Biol. Chem. 270:21264–21270.

6. Akopian, A. N., Sivilotti, L., and Wood J. N. (1996). A tetrodotoxin-resistant sodium channel expressed by C-fibre associated sensory neurons. Nature 379, 257–262.

7. Akopian, A. N., Souslova, V., Sivilotti, L., and Wood, J. N. (1997). Structure and distribution of a broadly-expressed atypical sodium channel. FEBS Lett. 400:183–187.

8. Kallen, R. G., Cohen, S. A., and Barchi, R. L. (1993). Structure, function and expression of voltage-dependent sodium channels. Mol. Neurobiol. 7:383–428.

9. Yang, N., George, A. L., and Horn, R. (1996). Molecular basis of charge movement in voltage-gated sodium channels. Neuron 16:113–122.

10. Isom, L. L., Ragsdale, D. S., De Jongh, K. S., Westenbroek, R. E., Reber, B. F., Scheuer, T., and Catterall, W. A. (1995). Structure and function of the β_2 subunit

of brain sodium channels, a transmembrane glycoprotein with a CAM motif. Cell 83:433–442.

11. Isom, L. L., and Catterall, W. A. (1996). Na⁺ channel subunits and Ig domains. Nature 383:307–308.

12. Goldstein, S. A. N. (1996). A structural vignette common to voltage sensors and conduction pores; canaliculi. Neuron 16:717–722.

13. Sangameswaran, L., Delgado, S. G., Fish, L. M., Koch, B. D., Jakeman, L. B., Stewart, G. R., Sze, P., Hunter, J. C., Eglen, R. M., and Herman, R. C. (1996). Structure and function of a novel voltage-gated TTX-resistant sodium channel specific to sensory neurons. J. Biol. Chem. 271:5953–5956.

14. Caffrey, J. M., Eng, D. L., Black, J. A., Waxman, S. G., and Kocsis, J. D. (1992). Three types of sodium channels in adult rat dorsal root ganglion neurons. Brain Res. 592:283–297.

15. Nowycky, M. N. (1992). Voltage-gated ion channels in DRG neurons. In Sensory neurons, ed. Stone, S. Academic Press, London.

16. Rizzo, M. A., Kocsis, J. D., and Waxman, S. G. (1994). Slow sodium conductances of dorsal root ganglion neurons: intraneuronal homogeneity and interneuronal heterogeneity. J. Neurophysiol. 72:2796–2815.

17. Roy, M. L., and Narahashi, T. (1992). Differential properties of TTX-sensitive and TTX-resistant sodium currents in rat dorsal root ganglion neurons J. Neurosci. 12:2104–2111.

18. Elliott, A. A., and Elliott, J. R. (1993). Characterization of TTX-sensitive and TTX-resistant sodium currents in small cells from adult rat dorsal root ganglia. J. Physiol. (Lond.) 463:39–56.

19. Ogata, N., and Tatebayashi, H. (1992). Ontogenic development of the TTX-sensitive and TTX-insensitive Na channels in neurons of the rat dorsal root ganglia. Dev. Brain Res. 65:93–100.

20. Jeftinija, S. (1994). Bradykinin excites tetrodotoxin-resistant primary afferent fibres. Brain Res. 665:69–76.

21. Sivilotti, L., Okuse, K., Akopian, A. N., Moss, S., and Wood, J. N. (1997). A single serine residue confers tetrodotoxin insensitivity on the rat sensory-neuron–specific sodium channel SNS. FEBS Lett 409(1):49–52.

22. Gold, M. S., Reichling, D. B., Shuster, M. J., and Levine, J. D. (1996). Hyperalgesic agents increase a tetrodotoxin-resistant Na current in nociceptors. Proc. Natl. Acad. Sci. USA 93:1108–1112.

23. England, S., Bevan, S., and Docherty, R. J. (1996). PGE2 modulates the tetrodotoxin-resistant sodium current in neonatal rat DRG neurones via the cAMP-protein kinase A cascade. J. Physiol. 495(2):429–440.

24. Wood, J. N., and Perl, E. R. (1999). Pain. Curr. Opin. Genet. Dev. 9:328–332.

25. Rudy, B., Kirschenbaum, B., Rukenstein, A., and Greene, L. A. (1987). NGF increases the number of functional Na channels and induces TTX-resistant Na channels in PC12 cells. J. Neurosci. 7:1613–1625.

26. Omri, G., and Meiri, H. (1990). Characterisation of sodium currents in sensory neurons cultured in serum-free defined medium with and without NGF. J. Membr. Biol. 115:13–29.

27. Dib-Hajj, S. D., Black, J. A., Cummins, T. R., Kenney, A. M, Kocsis, J. D, and Waxman S. G. (1998). Rescue of α-SNS sodium channel expression in small dorsal root ganglion neurons after axotomy by nerve growth factor in vivo. J. Neurophysiol. 79(5):2668–2676.

28. Tanaka, M., Cummins, T. R., Ishikawa, K., Dib-Hajj, S. D., Black, J. A., and Waxman S. G. (1998). SNS Na$^+$ channel expression increases in dorsal root ganglion neurons in the carrageenan inflammatory pain model. Neuroreport 9(6):967–972.

29. Zur, K. B., Oh, Y., Waxman, S. G., and Black, J. A. (1995). Differential up-regulation of sodium channel α- and β1–subunit mRNAs in cultured embryonic DRG neurons following exposure to NGF. Brain Res. Mol. Brain Res. May; 30(1): 97–105.

30. Okuse, K., Akopian, A. N., Souslova, V., McMahon, S., and Wood, J. N. (1997). NGF induces trans-splicing of the SNS sodium channel. Soc. Neurosci. Abst. 363(8).

31. Hinson, A. W., Gu, X. Q., Dib-Hajj, S., Black, J. A., and Waxman, S. G. (1997). Schwann cells modulate sodium channel expression in spinal sensory neurons in vitro. Glia 21(4):339–349.

32. Trezise, D. J., John, V. H., and Xie, X. M. (1998). Voltage- and use-dependent inhibition of Na$^+$ channels in rat sensory neurones by 4030W92, a new antihyperalgesic agent. Br. J. Pharmacol. July; 124(5):953–963.

33. Akopian, A. N., Souslova, V., England, S., Okuse, K., Ogata, N., Ure, A., Smith, J., Kerr, B. J., McMahon, S., Boyce, S., Hill, R., Stanfa, L., Dickenson, A., and Wood, J. N. (1999). The tetrodotoxin-resistant sodium channel SNS plays a specialised role in pain pathways. Nature Neurosci. 2:541–548.

34. Dib-Hajj, S. D., Tyrrell, L., Black, J. A., and Waxman, S. G. (1998). NaN, a novel voltage-gated Na channel, is expressed preferentially in peripheral sensory neurons and down-regulated after axotomy. Proc. Natl. Acad. Sci. USA 95(15): 8963–8968.

35. George, A. L. Jr., Knittle, T. J., and Tamkun, M. M. (1992). Molecular cloning of an atypical voltage-gated sodium channel expressed in human heart and uterus: evidence for a distinct gene family. Proc. Natl. Acad. Sci. USA 89(11): 4893–4897.

36. Chen, C.-C., Akopian, A. N., Sivilotti, L., Colquhoun, D., Burnstock, G., and Wood, J. N. (1995). A P2X purinoceptor expressed by a subset of sensory neurons. Nature 377:428–431.

37. Burnstock, G., Campbell, G., Satchell, D., and Smythe, A. (1970). Evidence that adenosine triphosphate or a related nucleotide is the transmitter substance released by non-adrenergic inhibitory nerves in the gut. Br. J. Pharmacol. 40:668–688.

38. Bleehen, T., and Keele, C. A. (1977). Observations on the algogenic actions of adenosine compounds on the human blister base preparation. Pain 4:367–377.

39. Jahr, C. E., and Jessell, T. M. (1983). ATP excites a subpopulation of rat dorsal horn neurons. Nature 304:730–733.

40. Bean, B. P. (1992). Pharmacology and electrophysiology of ATP-ativated ion channels. Trends Pharmacol. Sci. 13:87–90.

41. Bouvier, M. M., Evans, M. L., and Benham, C. D. (1991). Calcium influx induced by stimulation of ATP receptors on neurones cultured from dorsal root ganglia. Eur. J. Neurosci. 3:285–291.

42. Khakh, B. S., Humphrey, P. P., and Surprenant, A. (1995). Electrophysiological properties of P2X-purinoceptors in rat superior cervical, nodose and guinea-pig coeliac neurones. J. Physiol. 484:385–395.

43. Kidd, E. J., Grahames, C. B. A., Simon, J., Michel, A. D., Barnard, E. A., and Humphrey, P. P. A. (1995). Localization of P2X purinoceptor transcripts in the rat nervous system. Mol. Pharmacol. 48:569–573.

44. Chalfie, M., Driscoll, M., and Huang, M. (1993). Degenerin similarities. Nature 361(6412):504.

45. Buell, G., Collo, G., and Rassendren, F. (1996). P2X receptors: an emerging channel family. Eur. J. Neurosci. 8:2221–2228.

46. Lewis, C., Neidhart, S., Holy, C., North, R. A., Buell, G., and Surprenant, A. (1995). Heteropolymerization of P2X receptor subunits can account for ATP-induced current in sensory neurons. Nature 377:432–435.

47. Nicke, A., Bäumert, H. G., Rettinger, J., Eichele, A., Lambrecht, G., Mutschler, E., and Schmalzing, G. (1998). P2X1 and P2X3 receptors form stable trimers: a novel structural motif of ligand-gated ion channels. EMBO J. 17:3016–3028.

48. Bennett, D. L., Michael, G. J., Ramachandran, N., Munson, J. B., Averill, S., Yan, Q., McMahon, S. B., and Priestley, J. V. (1998). A distinct subgroup of small DRG cells express GDNF receptor components and GDNF is protective for these neurons after nerve injury. J Neurosci. 18(8):3059–3072.

49. Bland-Ward, P. A., and Humphrey, P. (1997). Acute nociception mediated by hindpaw P2X receptor activation in the rat. Br. J. Pharmacol. Sept.; 122(2): 365–371.

50. Bardoni, R., Goldstein, P. A., Lee, C. J., Gu, J. G., and MacDermott, A. B. (1997). ATP P2X receptors mediate fast synaptic transmission in the dorsal horn of the rat spinal cord. J. Neurosci. 15; 17(14):5297–5303.

51. Gu, J. G., and MacDermott, A. B. (1997). Activation of ATP P2X receptors elicits glutamate release from sensory neuron synapses. Nature 389(6652):749–753.

52. Nakamura, F., and Strittmatter, S. M. (1996). P2Y1 purinergic receptors in sensory neurons: contribution to touch-induced impulse generation. Proc. Natl. Acad. Sci. USA 93:10465–10470.

53. Cook, S. P., Vulchanova, L., Hargreaves, K. M., Elde, R., and McCleskey, E. W. (1997). Distinct ATP receptors on pain-sensing and stretch-sensing neurons. Nature 387:505–508.

54. Ledent, C., Vaugeois, J. M., Schiffmann, S. N., Pedrazzini, T., El Yacoubi, M., Vanderhaeghen, J. J., Costentin, J., Heath, J. K., Vassart, G., and Parmentier, M. (1998). Aggressiveness, hypoalgesia and high blood pressure in mice lacking the adenosine A2a receptor. Nature 388(6643):674–678.

55. Steen, K. H., Steen, A. E., and Reeh, P. W. (1995). A dominant role of acid pH in inflammatory excitation and sensitisation of nociceptors in rat skin, in vitro. J. Neurosci. 15:3982–3989.

56. Waldmann, R., and Lazdunski, M. (1998). $H^{(+)}$-gated cation channels: neuronal acid sensors in the NaC/DEG family of ion channels. Curr. Opin. Neurobiol. 8(3):418–424.

57. Waldmann, R., Champigny, G., Bassilana, F., Heurteaux, C., and Lazdunski, M. (1997). A proton-gated cation channel involved in acid-sensing. Nature 386:173–177.

58. Waldmann, R., Basilana, F., de Weille, J., Champigny, G., Heurteaux, C., and Lazdunski, M. (1997). Molecular cloning of a non-inactivating proton-gated Na^+ channel specific for sensory neurons. J. Biol. Chem. 272:20975–20978.

59. Garcia-Anoveros, J., Derfler, B., Neville-Golden, J., Hyman, B. T., and Corey, D. P. (1997). BNaC1 and BNaC2 constitute a new family of human neuronal sodium channels related to degenerins and epithelial sodium channels. Proc. Natl. Acad. Sci. USA 94:1459–1464.

60. Lingueglia, E., de Weille, J. R., Bassilana, F., Heurteaux, C., Sakai, H., Waldmann, R., and Lazdunski, M. (1997). A modulatory subunit of acid sensing ion channels in brain and dorsal root ganglion cells. J. Biol. Chem. 272:29778–29783.

61. Chen, C.-C., England, S., Akopian, A. N., and Wood, J. N. (in press). A sensory neuron specific proton-gated cation channel. Proc. Natl. Acad. Sci. USA 95:10240–10245.

62. Coscoy, S., Lingueglia, E., Lazdunski, M., and Barbry, P. (1998). The Phe–Met–Arg–Phe–amide—activated sodium channel is a tetramer. J. Biol. Chem. 273(14):8317–8322.

63. Wood, J. N., and Docherty, R. (1997). Chemical activators of sensory neurons. Annu. Rev. Physiol. 59:457–482.

64. Kuhn, R.., Schwenk, F., Aguet, M., and Rajewsky, K. (1995). Inducible gene targeting in mice. Science 269(5229):1427–1429.

65. Fjell, J., Cummins, T. R., Dib-Hajj, S. D., Fried, K., Black, J. A., and Waxman, S. G. (1999). Differential role of GDNF and NGF in the maintenance of two TTX-resistant sodium channels in adult DRG neurons. Brain Res. Mol. Brain Res. 67(2):267–282.

66. Tate, S., Benn, S., Hick, C., Trezise, D., John, V., Mannion, R. J., Costigan, M., Plumpton, C., Grose, D., Gladwell, Z., Kendall, G., Dale, K., Bountra, C., and Woolf, C. J. (1998). Two sodium channels contribute to the TTX-R sodium current in primary sensory neurons. Nat. Neurosci. 1(8):653–655.

CHAPTER 7

Sensory Neuron Mechanotransduction: Regulation and Underlying Molecular Mechanisms

GARY R. LEWIN AND CHERYL L. STUCKY

Max-Delbrück-Center for Molecular Medicine
Berlin

7.1   INTRODUCTION

Sensory neurons in the dorsal root ganglia are specialized to detect various forms of mechanical, chemical, and thermal stimuli that affect peripheral tissues such as skin and muscle. Many years of work using electrophysiological techniques to measure the stimulus-response properties of sensory neurons have shown that almost all somatic sensory neurons respond to mechanical stimuli and, in addition, some respond to other modalities, such as heat and algogenic chemicals.[1] Although a considerable amount is known about the mechanical response properties of different classes of mammalian sensory neurons, such as their mechanical threshold for a response, their optimal type of stimulus, and their frequency and pattern of firing, surprisingly little is known about factors that regulate these properties and, more basically, how a mechanical stimulus is actually transduced into a receptor potential in the nerve membrane.[2]

Recent work indicates that the specification of cutaneous sensory neurons to detect and transmit different types of mechanical stimuli, such as vibration, indentation of the skin, movement of hair follicles, and noxious mechanical stimuli is controlled by the availability of neurotrophic factors during development.[3,4] These soluble factors include nerve growth factor (NGF), brain-derived neurotrophic factor (BDNF), neurotrophin-3 (NT3),

Molecular Basis of Pain Induction, Edited by John N. Wood
ISBN 0-471-34607-1   Copyright © 2000 by Wiley-Liss, Inc. All rights reserved.

Low-threshold Mechanoreceptors

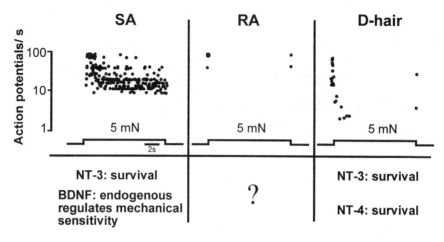

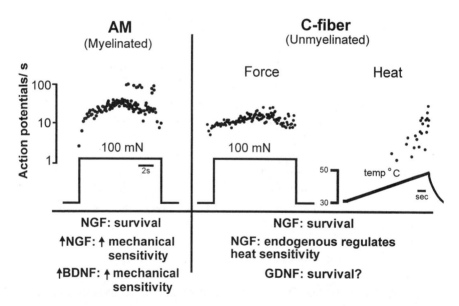

Figure 7.1 Specific neurotrophins regulate specific classes of sensory neurons. All types of functionally defined cutaneous sensory neurons are shown together with the neurotrophins that are known to influence them. For each type of neuron, a typical response to a mechanical or thermal stimulus is shown, and each dot represents one action potential. Slowly adapting (SA) fibers respond throughout a sustained force, whereas rapidly adapting (RA) fibers respond only at the onset or offset of the stimulus. D-hair receptors respond to very low intensity stimuli (<1 mN) and fire with high frequency at the onset and offset of the stimulus. A mechano-nociceptors (AM) and C-fiber nociceptors respond throughout a high-intensity force, and some

and neurotrophin-4 (NT4), and each supports the survival of a functionally distinct subtype of sensory neuron during development (Fig. 7.1). Thus nociceptors, particularly those responding to heat, require NGF during development for survival,[5,6] but other low-threshold mechanoreceptors, for example, slowly adapting mechanoreceptors, require NT3 for survival.[7] In some cases, the deletion of two different neurotrophic factors can lead to the loss of the same type of afferent neuron. For example, recent studies with knockout mice have shown that fibers that innervate vellus hair follicles (D-hair receptors) require both NT3 and NT4 for survival.[7,8] More specifically, our studies now suggest that during the early postnatal period, D-hair receptors require NT3 for survival, and after 3 weeks of age, they switch their dependence over to NT4 (C.L. Stucky and G.R. Lewin, unpublished observations). On another level, the availability of some neurotrophins controls the expression of specific physiological attributes of sensory neurons such as mechanical and heat sensitivity.[6,9–12]

To learn more about how a mechanical stimulus applied to peripheral tissue is actually transduced into a receptor potential in the nerve membrane, we have begun to identify target genes that may code for putative constituents of the mechanotransduction apparatus in mammals. One approach we have taken is to use the recent body of evidence on the mechanotransduction molecules of the nematode worm *Caenorhabditis elegans*. *C. elegans* possesses only six touch receptive neurons, and many induced gene mutations in these touch neurons lead to mechanical insensitivity. In the past several years, these mutations in *C. elegans* have been mapped to novel genes (mec genes), and several have close structural homologs in vertebrates.[13,14] We have asked whether the vertebrate homologs are selectively expressed in mechanosensitive sensory neurons in the mouse. In the future, genetic approaches in mice, such as the overexpression or deletion of specific genes, combined with electrophysiological techniques that allow one to record from and characterize functionally distinct mechanoreceptors,[7,15] should reveal whether these mammalian homologs of *C. elegans* mec genes play a physiological role in vertebrate mechanotransduction. Once the proteins responsible for mechano-electrical transduction are identified in vertebrates, the detailed biophysical and molecular mechanisms through which we experience tactile and nociceptive stimuli can be addressed.

C fibers also respond to noxious heat. During development, each type of neuron depends on specific neurotrophins for survival and function.[3] For example, nociceptors depend primarily on NGF for both survival and function; SA fibers simultaneously require two different neurotropins for survival and mechanical sensitivity, and D hairs require both NT3 and NT4 for survival but require NT3 during the early postnatal period and NT4 later.

7.2   SITES OF SENSORY MECHANOTRANSDUCTION

Early physiological studies of mechanoreception in vertebrates carried out in the 1960s and 1970s established some basic principles of how mechanical stimuli are transformed into a train of action potentials.[16] These studies showed that after a mechanical stimulus is applied to peripheral tissue, a generator or receptor potential is set up in the sensory neuron that subsequently leads to the initiation of action potentials. This receptor potential, which is thought to be due to a depolarizing, nonspecific cation conductance,[2] has been measured in a variety of types of mechanoreceptors, including sensory axons that innervate Pacinian corpuscles and muscle spindles.[17,18]

An important point to establish is whether or not all aspects of mechanotransduction are intrinsic properties of the sensory neuron. One issue is whether or not the specialized endings of mechanoreceptors possess all or part of the transducer complex that converts mechanical force into receptor potentials. One specialized cutaneous end organ that has been studied extensively is the Merkel cell, which is innervated by slowly adapting type I (SAI) mechanoreceptors.[19] The roles that Merkel cells and SAI receptors play in mechanotransduction have been studied for many years, yet they continue to be a source of controversy. Several groups have used chemical and/or phototoxic methods to selectively eradicate Merkel cells before testing SAI fibers for mechanical function,[20–22] but the outcome of these experiments has differed between laboratories. Some investigators have concluded that the mechanosensory function of SAI fibers is severely impaired after destruction of the Merkel cells[20,21] whereas others find that SAI fibers are normal in mechanosensitivity.[23] Two problems with these studies are that it is difficult with many morphological techniques to prove that Merkel cells are completely gone and that chemical and phototoxic methods can directly damage the nerve terminals. Therefore, Mills and Diamond[24] conducted a detailed study in which they eradicated Merkel cells and then carefully mapped the receptive fields of individual SAI fibers that were normal in responsiveness and found that not a single Merkel cell was present in the receptive fields of normal SAI fibers. This evidence strongly indicates that the Merkel cell cannot possess the mechanotransducer. Furthermore, a recent study has been performed with a knockout mouse in which Merkel cells are lost postnatally without the use of invasive techniques that could damage nerve terminals. Since Merkel cells express the low-affinity neurotrophin receptor p75,[25] one possibility is that the p75 receptor is important for the development and survival of Merkel cells. Therefore, the development of Merkel cells was analyzed in mice lacking p75. Merkel cells in the hairy skin of these mice developed normally and were present in normal numbers until 2 weeks of age. However, by 2 months, Merkel cells were virtually gone, yet the SAI fibers survived and had completely normal mechanical sensitivity.[26] Together, these studies provide strong evidence that mechanotransduction in SAI fibers is intrinsic to sensory neurons.

A second piece of evidence which indicates that mechanotransduction is intrinsic to sensory neurons is that unmyelinated and myelinated nociceptors, of which nearly all respond to high-intensity mechanical stimuli, do not have specialized end organs but instead, terminate as free endings in peripheral tissues. Thus, nociceptive mechanical stimuli are presumably transduced in the nerve terminal.

Third, sensory neurons that are dissociated from their normal target tissues are still capable of responding to mechanical stimuli. Following axotomy, the cut ends of large myelinated sensory axons within the neuroma retain some mechanical sensitivity.[27] The fact that the sensitivity of neurons within the neuroma is less than that of neurons in their native environment may be due either to a lower density of mechanosensory sites on the axon compared to the native nerve terminal or to the down-regulation of mechanotransduction proteins, since it is known that after axotomy, the expression of many proteins are up- or down-regulated. Furthermore, Korschorke and colleagues[27] showed that mechanical sensitivity in the neuroma is dependent on anterograde axonal transport, a finding which suggests that proteins intrinsic to the nerve are transported from the soma to maintain a functional mechanosensor in the terminal.

Another model in which sensory neurons are separated from their peripheral targets is cultured or dissociated sensory neurons. Indeed, somatic and visceral sensory neurons isolated in culture appear to show physiological responses to mechanical stimuli.[28,29] These responses however, are probably far from being a true reflection of the physiological receptor potential seen in situ because such responses in cultured cells may merely reflect mechanical damage induced by culture conditions, dissociation procedures, or mechanical stimulus applied directly to the neuronal membrane. An additional concern is that most of these in vitro studies have used calcium imaging techniques to measure neuronal responses because intracellular and patch clamp recordings are difficult to maintain during a mechanical stimulus applied to the cell soma (but see Cunningham et al.[30]). Although calcium may be one cation that contributes to the endogenous receptor potential, the major ion is probably sodium.[2]

7.3 MECHANICAL SENSITIVITY OF SENSORY NEURONS MODULATED BY EXTRINSIC FACTORS

Although the evidence reviewed above suggests that sensory mechanotransduction is an intrinsic property of the neuron, it is still possible that the sensitivity of the process is modulated by factors outside the sensory terminal or membrane. Two types of extrinsic factors might be envisaged. The first is that of soluble factors such as neurochemicals, neurohormones, or neurotrophins, which might modulate the mechanosensory complex either by local receptor-mediated mechanisms at the terminal membrane or through uptake, transport, and gene transcription. As we shall see below, evidence exists for such modulatory events. The second type of extrinsic factor might be extracellular matrix molecules, which may bind directly to the mechanosensory complex in the nerve membrane, anchoring it to the local environment. This idea is strongly supported by genetic evidence from the nematode worm *C. elegans,* where such molecules have been shown to play a crucial role in mechanotransduction.[31–33]

A large body of evidence indicates that soluble factors such as inflammatory chemicals can modulate the response properties of sensory neurons to natural stimuli such as heat and chemicals, and thereby contribute to the sensory phenomenon of hyperalgesia, which accompanies peripheral injury and inflammation.[34] In terms of mechanical hyperalgesia, many studies have investigated whether the sensitization of peripheral neurons, central neurons, or both plays a major role. The general consensus today is that mechanical hyperalgesia is due predominantly to the sensitization of spinal neurons to the constant barrage of input from sensory neurons,[35] and the effects of inflammatory chemicals on the mechanical threshold of nociceptive neurons are relatively small.[36] What is more dramatic is that some visceral and somatic unmyelinated afferents are almost completely insensitive to mechanical stimuli under normal circumstances but gain mechanical sensitivity rapidly following exposure to an inflammatory stimulus.[34] For example, some unmyelinated somatic neurons that are mechanically insensitive exhibit novel responses to mechanical stimuli shortly after exposure to itch-inducing chemicals, suggesting that this class of neurons underly itch sensation.[37] Many visceral sensory neurons innervating tissue such as the bladder are normally quite insensitive to mechanical stimuli, but shortly after exposure to an inflammatory stimulus, the majority become mechanically sensitive.[38,39] Interestingly, one of the mediators that appears to be involved in this process is nerve growth factor (NGF). NGF is increased during inflammation[5] and has been shown to mimic some of the acute increases in mechanical sensitivity that occur during inflammation of the bladder.[40] NGF appears to exert its effects on the mechanosensitivity of visceral afferent fibers without initiating novel or increased gene transcription because the effects occur within minutes.[40] NGF is not the only example of acute effects of neurotrophins since other members of the neurotrophin family have also been shown to induce fast local changes in neurons, although the signaling mechanisms underlying these effects are still unclear.[41] In both somatic and visceral fibers, the time course of the appearance of mechanosensitivity suggests that a latent mechanotransducer at the terminals of these fibers is tonically suppressed under normal conditions and is activated after exposure to soluble factors. Furthermore, this short time course of action implies that complex local regulatory mechanisms exist that control whether or not such afferent fibers are capable of responding to peripheral stimuli.

Apart from the acute influences of soluble mediators on sensory afferent fibers, it has become clear in recent years that the mechanosensitivity of some receptors may be regulated chronically by the presence of neurotrophic factors that activate the trk family of tyrosine kinase receptors. In the first studies of this kind, it was found that treatment of rats with NGF during the first 2 weeks of life led to an extremely long-lasting sensitization of myelinated mechanociceptors.[9] The effects of NGF were specific for these nociceptors, presumably because the high-affinity receptor for NGF, trkA, is expressed by nociceptive neurons in the postnatal period and beyond.[42] The sensitization of these neurons to mechanical stimuli outlasted the NGF treatment by at least 4 weeks. Since NGF is known to induce axon sprouting in some systems,[43] the mechanical sensitization may have been due to an increase in the density of terminals that express mechanotransduction sites. Alternatively, NGF may have up-regulated the production of certain proteins required for mechanotransduction such that more mechanosensitive sites were expressed on existing terminals or that the existing mechanosensitive sites were more sensitive. It is not clear, however, whether the presence of more transduction sites would necessarily lower the mechanical threshold for a given neuron. It has long been assumed that action potentials need to be initiated at only one site in the peripheral terminal of a sensory afferent fiber. It thus follows that the mechanical threshold for a particular neuron may depend on the average threshold at each mechanotransduction site within a given neuron.

A second, more direct example of a neurotrophin-regulating mechanical threshold is that of the role of brain-derived neurotrophic factor (BDNF) during the postnatal period. Mice homozygous for the deletion of the BDNF gene display a small loss in dorsal root ganglion neurons; however, it is still unclear which neurons die in these animals.[44,45] Our investigations have shown that many neurons expressing full-length trk B transcripts are still present in the BDNF knockout mice (P. Carroll and G.R. Lewin, unpublished observations). Furthermore, an extensive electrophysiological and anatomical analysis of cutaneous sensory neurons revealed that none of the neurons with myelinated axons require BDNF for survival. In fact, this analysis revealed that one subtype of mechanoreceptor, the slowly adapting type I fiber (SAI) that innervates Merkel cells in the touch dome, was severely impaired in its mechanical sensitivity. SAI fibers normally have very low thresholds for activation, but in BDNF-deficient animals, SAI fibers are extremely insensitive to mechanical stimuli. The deficit in mechanosensitivity was equally severe

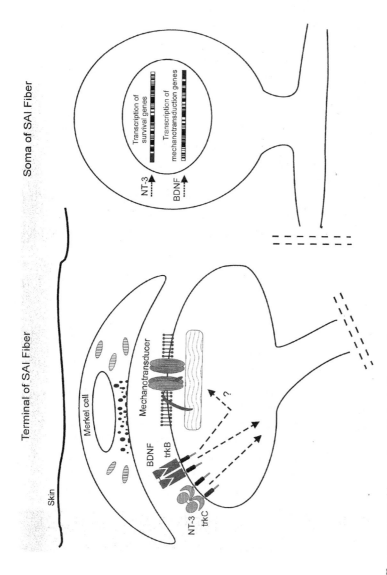

Figure 7.2 Different neurotrophins can have distinct effects on the same sensory neuron. During development, SA fibers require NT3 for survival and at the same time, require BDNF for mechanical sensitivity. Both of these neurotrophin effects are most likely mediated by uptake, transport, and modulation of gene transcription. It is also feasible that the tyrosine kinase receptors may directly modulate the mechanotransducer complex at the terminal, although there is no direct evidence for this. It is interesting to note that although both NT3 and BDNF bind to tyrosine kinase receptors that activate very similar intracellular signaling systems, these two neurotrophins elicit very different biological effects in the same neuron at the same time.

in mice hetero- and homozygous for the mutation, indicating that only small reductions in the level of BDNF produce the phenotype. Thus the concentration of BDNF appears to be limiting under normal conditions. This effect was specific in that no other attributes of the neurons were affected, including conduction velocity, maximum firing frequency, or the morphology of the Merkel cell–neurite complex. Furthermore, we showed that exogenous BDNF given to BDNF-deficient mice from birth to 2 weeks of age could completely rescue the mechanical insensitivity of SAI fibers.[12] These data strongly indicate that BDNF normally functions to regulate the sensitivity of SA fibers to mechanical stimuli because increasing or decreasing the availability of BDNF respectively increases or decreases the mechanical sensitivity of SA fibers. We postulated that BDNF exerts these effects through activation of the trkB receptor, which then regulates the expression of downstream genes that are required for normal mechanotransduction. Indeed, recent experiments have shown that fully functional trkB receptors are required to maintain SA receptor mechanosensitivity.[46] It is of particular interest that trkB receptors are required for the mechanical sensitivity of SAI fibers because these same fibers require another neurotrophin, neurotrophin-3 (NT3), for survival at the same time.[7] These data then suggest that two tyrosine kinase receptors, trkB and trkC, mediate completely separate functions simultaneously in the same cell (Fig. 7.2) (see also Ref. 47).

7.4   MUTAGENESIS EXPERIMENTS IN *C. ELEGANS*

Chalfie and colleagues designed a genetic screen to isolate mutant *C. elegans* worms that were incapable of detecting a light brush stroke, a stimulus that normally activates one or more of six mechanoreceptive sensory neurons.[48] This screen led to the identification of 16 genes that are necessary for the proper function of this behavioral response.[13] Subsequent positional cloning of many of these genes has led to identification of several predicted proteins that together might make up a mechanotransduction complex at the sensory axon terminal (Fig. 7.3). The principal members of this hypothesized protein complex are MEC1, MEC5, and MEC9, which are all thought to be extracellular matrix components;[32,3] MEC4 and MEC10, which are known to be ion channel subunits;[49–51] MEC2, which is an integral membrane protein,[52] and MEC7 and MEC12, which are tubulin-like proteins inside the cell.[33,53] The model of a mechanotransducer that is based on these proteins is a speculative one since no direct evidence is available from *C. elegans* that these proteins do directly interact with each other in vivo to make up a mechanotransduction complex. However, an important point to make about this model is that it suggests that mechanotransduction has a much more complex molecular makeup

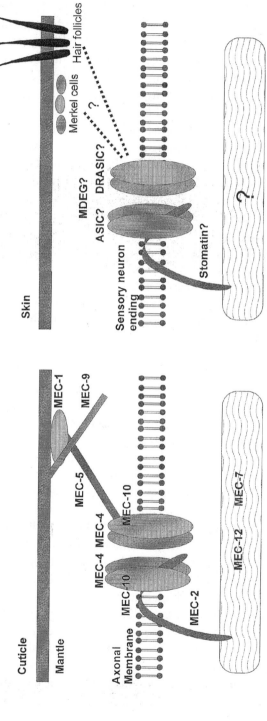

Figure 7.3 Model of mechanotransduction complex in sensory neurons of *C. elegans* and mammals. The mechanosensitive cation channel in *C. elegans* is thought to be composed of multiple copies of MEC4 and MEC10, and the channel is presumably linked to intracellular microtubules via MEC2. It is hypothesized that a mechanical stimulus at the mantle may gate the ion channel by creating tension between the extracellular proteins and the intracellular microtubules. In mammals, candidate mechanotransduction proteins are just now being identified, and so far, cation channels that have high homology to those in *C. elegans* include MDEG, ASIC, and DRASIC. Furthermore, a mammalian homolog of MEC2, stomatin, has been identified and may link the ion channel to the cytoskeletal network. So far it is only known that these candidate channels and stomatin are all expressed in DRG neurons. There is as yet no direct evidence to implicate them as playing a role in mechanotransduction in vertebrates.

than was assumed when stretch-activated ion channels were discovered.[54] Stretch-activated conductances have been detected in many cell types and it has been assumed that some of these channels might constitute a mechanotransducer in sensory neurons.[55] However, the model from *C. elegans*, a relatively simple organism, suggests that the molecular composition of a mammalian mechanotransducer may be much more complex than that in *C. elegans*. Indeed, the sequences of some of the genes which are particularly important for the touch response in *C. elegans* have not yet been identified (e.g., mec6) and the proteins encoded by these genes may very well radically change the model outlined in Figure 7.3. Another important point is that the Chalfie screen rejected mutants that resulted in lethal phenotypes. Thus it is possible that some genes may participate in making a mechanotransducer but have additional essential functions in the organism.[56] In mammals, the range of different mechanoreceptors is much more diverse than that in flies and worms, suggesting that the composition and regulation of the mechanotransduction complex in mammals is equivalently diverse. In mammals, different receptor types may have mechanotransduction complexes that have some common feature(s) as well some unique features that specify the nature of the mechanical response. This conceptual model of a mechanotransducer as a molecular complex whose detailed composition might determine receptor specificity is a compelling one. However, in mammals it is not clear what the individual components of such a complex might be.

7.5 MOLECULAR NATURE OF MECHANOTRANSDUCTION IN MAMMALS

The molecular nature of mammalian mechanotransduction is unequivocally not known. What, then, are the criteria for identifying such molecule(s) in mammals? One strategy that has been tested is to use expression cloning techniques to find candidate mechanotransduction genes. This strategy has recently paid off handsomely in the case of the capsaicin receptor.[57] Here, the ability of capsaicinlike agonists to induce calcium signals in cells expressing the capsaicin receptor was used to screen pools of cDNA clones expressed in human embryonic kidney (HEK) cells. The cloned capsaicin receptor, named vanilloid receptor-1, was shown further to confer a noxious heat-activated current to the cells that expressed it (see Chapter 9). The evidence indicates that this novel ion channel is an excellent candidate for the major component of the heat transduction apparatus in small sensory neurons.[58,59] In the case of mechanotransduction, the expression cloning approach has some drawbacks. Although one might expect to find a mechanically sensitive ion channel with this approach, it has been known for years that many channels (e.g., some chloride channels) are stretch sensitive and are not necessarily good candidates as sensory mechanotransduction ion channels. A more serious problem may be that as we have seen from work in *C. elegans* (Fig. 7.3), the mechanotransducer may be a complex of proteins that functions only as a mechanically activated cation conductance when all proteins of the complex are present. Indeed, the first attempt at expression cloning such a channel uncovered a candidate ion channel that has many attributes not expected of a mechanotransducing channel.[60] A cDNA from chicken was found, which when expressed in frog oocytes, induced a very large conductance following mechanical stimulation. This ion channel turned out to be a ligand-gated purinergic receptor, P2Y1, that was localized to small, presumably nociceptive sensory neurons. It is unlikely that a sensory mechanotransduction channel functions via a chemical intermediate because the process of mechanotransduction is simply too fast.[2,61] Furthermore, no evidence was presented in this first report that directly implicated this channel as part of the mechanotransducer in vivo.[60]

Another approach is to identify mammalian homologs of mechanotransduction genes that have previously been identified in lower organisms, since the capacity of sensory neurons to respond to mechanical stimuli is conserved from worms to humans. Even after mammalian homologs are identified, much work is needed to determine if they are expressed in appropriate tissues where they could feasibly contribute to a mechanotransducer (i.e., DRG neurons). Furthermore, the candidate proteins may have to be targeted to the mechanotransduction apparatus and, in some cases, be capable of interacting directly with other members of the complex. Finally, experiments must be designed to demonstrate conclusively that these proteins are necessary to transduce physiologically meaningful mechanical stimuli in mammalian sensory neurons. The last requirement is naturally the most difficult to demonstrate, but recent advances in mouse molecular genetics, such as gene targeting, together with physiological techniques allow one to test directly the involvement of candidate genes in mechanotransduction. Thus, by using homologous recombination techniques in mouse embryonic stem cells, it is possible to knock out the function of a given gene (loss of function). Conversely, it is also possible to ask whether the overexpression of a given gene is capable of modulating the function of a mechanotransducer. Recently developed electrophysiological preparations can then be used to measure quantitative aspects of single-mechanoreceptor function in genetically altered mice.[7,15]

Naturally, of central importance is the identity of the actual ion channel component of the mechanotransducer. The genes encoding the ion channel proteins in *C. elegans* genes have been known for some time, and up to a year ago, their closest known homologs in mammals were a family of amiloride-sensitive cation channels expressed predominantly in water-resorbing epithelia.[62] Recently, a new subfamily of these cation channels have been identified that are expressed not only in central neurons but also in many sensory neurons of the dorsal root ganglia. Three genes have so far been identified, including MDEG (mammalian degenerin), ASIC (acid-sensing ion channel), and DRASIC (dorsal root ganglion acid-sensing ion channel).[63-65] MDEG and ASIC were also cloned in humans by Corey and co-workers and were called BNAC1 and BNAC2, respectively.[66] When expressed in nonneuronal cell lines, each of these proteins is capable of forming a functional ion channel by itself.[64,65,67] In addition, stimulation with protons (acid) activates an inward current in cell lines expressing any one of these three channels alone.[64,65,67] However, the characteristics of the proton-gated current are dependent in some cases on the cell line used.[63,67] A new splice variant of MDEG called MDEG2 was also shown to modulate the kinetics and ion selectivity of the MDEG (now MDEG1) and DRASIC channels when coexpressed in COS cells.[67] These channels, with the exception of MDEG1, have all been reported to be expressed in small sensory neurons of the dorsal root ganglia in rat.[63,67] This suggests that they may form a heteromultimeric ion channel selectively in nociceptive neurons. It has been postulated that these channels function as pH sensors and are the molecular basis of the pH-activated current observed in nociceptors.[64] When ASIC and MDEG are expressed together in COS cells, they form a channel that has very similar activation properties to a channel found in small sensory neurons in culture.[68] It is clear that low pH can activate nociceptors in vivo and that the acidification of the extracellular space that occurs during inflammation may be the physiological stimulus that activates these neurons.[69,70] However, even if these channels were shown to be pH sensors, this would not rule out a role for these channels in mechanotransduction. The reported restricted expression of these channels to small-diameter DRG neurons might argue against a role in mechanotransduction since the large DRG neurons would then be devoid of a mechanosensitive channel, and large neurons are much more sensitive to mechanical stimuli than are nociceptive neurons (see above). However, in our laboratory we have found that these channels are expressed much more widely in the DRG than originally reported. With our in situ hybridization techniques, these channels are expressed equally by sensory neurons of all sizes (S.L. McIlwrath and G.R. Lewin, unpublished observations). These channels, or as yet unidentified mammalian homologs, remain good mechanotransducer candidates.

The *C. elegans* studies have taught us that the ion channel alone is probably insufficient to form a mechanotransducer. For this reason it is logical to look for genes encoding other nonchannel proteins that may associate with a mechanotransduction complex. One such candidate that seems to have a central role in the nematode mechanotransducer is the integral membrane protein MEC2.[52,71] In humans, this protein was first isolated from erythrocytes using biochemical techniques and was called erythrocyte band 7.2 kb because it is one of a group of major integral membrane proteins in these cells.[72,73] The protein was also named stomatin after the hereditary disease stomatocytosis, which is associated with a reduction in the stomatin protein in erythrocytes.[72] Based on its distribution in mouse and human tissues, stomatin appears to be a poor candidate as part of a mechanotransducer (e.g., Ref. 73). However, the MEC2 protein in *C. elegans* shows remarkable homology to the human and mouse stomatin proteins in that it is 65% identical in amino acids in a long segment of the C terminus. Based on the fact that the mec-2 gene is necessary for mechanotransduction in *C. elegans,* we have gone on to examine whether the mammalian homolog is expressed in sensory neurons in the DRG. To do this, we raised antibodies against the mouse protein and used these in combination with in situ hybridization techniques to show that indeed, this protein is expressed abundantly by all sensory neurons.[74] Thus stomatin is at least expressed appropriately for playing a functional role as part of a mechanotransduction complex in mammals. Since BDNF can regulate mechanosensitivity in some sensory neurons, we have looked to see if stomatin expression can be regulated by BDNF. At the level of mRNA, there appears to be no strong regulation by BDNF, but it is still possible that BDNF can regulate other mechanotransduction genes at the level of transcription. It is also possible that the targeting or function of mechanotransduction proteins can be modulated after activation of neurotrophin tyrosine kinases receptors. We are currently beginning experiments with transgenic mice to determine whether the stomatin protein is involved directly in the process of mechanotransduction.

7.6   CONCLUSIONS

Detection and transmission of mechanical stimuli are the major functions of somatic sensory neurons. Despite this, the molecular and biochemical mechanisms that underlie mechanotransduction were, until several years ago, completely unknown. However, very recent studies of mechanotransduction in the worm *C. elegans* have opened up new possibilities for an understanding of mechanotransduction at the molecular level. In comparison to a simple worm, the process of mechanotransduction in mammals is likely to be far more complex and diverse given the great diversity of mammalian mechanoreceptors as well as the many ways in which their sensitivity can be regulated. Nevertheless, the studies in *C. elegans* have laid the foundation and provided tools for understanding mechanotransduction in mammals. The nature of the vertebrate mechanoreceptive apparatus is likely to be of key importance for an understanding of peripheral sensory processes in both normal and disease states. A more molecular understanding may also provide genetic explanations and therapies for sensory disorders.

REFERENCES

1. Perl, E. R. (1992). Function of dorsal root ganglion neurons. In: Sensory neurons diversity, development, and plasticity, ed. Scott, S. A., Oxford University Press, New York, pp. 3–27.

2. French, A. S. (1992). Mechanotransduction. Annu. Rev. Physiol. 54:135–152.

3. Lewin, G. R. (1996). Neurotrophins and the specification of neuronal phenotype. Philos. Trans. R. Soc. Lond. B Biol. Sci. 351:405–411.

4. Lewin, G. R., and Barde, Y.-A. (1996). Physiology of the neurotrophins. Annu. Rev. Neurosci. 19:289–317.

5. Lewin, G. R., and Mendell, L. M. (1993). Nerve growth factor and nociception. Trends Neurosci. 16:353–359.

6. Lewin, G. R., and Mendell, L. M. (1994). Regulation of cutaneous C-fiber heat nociceptors by nerve growth factor in the developing rat. J. Neurophysiol. 71:941–949.

7. Airaksinen, M. S., Koltzenburg, M., Lewin, G. R., Masu, Y., Helbig, C., Wolf, E., Brem, G., Toyka, K. V., Thoenen, H., and Meyer, M. (1996). Specific subtypes of cutaneous mechanoreceptors require neurotrophin-3 following peripheral target innervation. Neuron 16:287–295.

8. Stucky, C. L., Koltzenburg, M., DeChiara, T., Lindsay, R. M., and Yancopoulos, G. D. (1998). Neurotrophin 4 (NT-4) is required for the survival of a subclass of hair follicle receptors. J. Neurosci. 18:7040–7046.

9. Lewin, G. R., Ritter, A. M., and Mendell, L. M. (1993). Nerve growth factor–induced hyperalgesia in the neonatal and adult rat. J. Neurosci. 13(5):2136–2148.

10. Lewin, G. R., Rueff, A., and Mendell, L. M. (1994). Peripheral and central mechanisms of NGF-induced hyperalgesia. Eur. J. Neurosci. 6:1903–1912.

11. McMahon, S. B., Bennett, D. L., Priestley, J. V., and Shelton, D. L. (1995). The biological effects of endogenous nerve growth factor on adult sensory neurons revealed by a trkA–IgG fusion molecule. Nature Med. 1:774–780.

12. Carroll, P., Lewin, G. R., Koltzenburg, M., Toyka, K. V., and Thoenen, H. (1998). A role for BDNF in mechanosensation. Nature Neurosci. 1:42–46.

13. Tavernarakis, N., and Driscoll, M. (1997). Molecular modeling of mechanotransduction in the nematode *Caenorhabditis elegans*. Annu. Rev. Physiol. 59:659–689.

14. Garcia Anoveras, J., and Corey, D. P. (1997). The molecules of mechanosensation. Annu. Rev. Neurosci. 20:567–594.

15. Koltzenburg, M., Stucky, C. L., and Lewin, G. R. (1997). Receptive properties of mouse sensory neurons innervating hairy skin. J. Neurophysiol. 78:1841–1850.

16. Catton, W. T. (1970). Mechanoreceptor function. Physiol. Rev. 50:297–318.

17. Katz, B. (1950). Depolarisation of sensory terminals and the inititation of impulses in the muscle spindle. J. Physiol. 111:261–282.

18. Loewenstein, W. R., and Skalak, R. (1966). Mechanical transmission in a Pacinian corpuscle: an analysis and a theory. J. Physiol. (Lond.) 182:346–378.

19. Iggo, A., and Muir, A. R. (1969). The structure and function of a slowly adapting touch corpuscle in hairy skin. J. Physiol. (Lond.) 200:763–796.

20. Ikeda, I., Yamashita, Y., Ono, T., and Ogawa, H. (1994). Selective phototoxic destruction of rat Merkel cells abolishes responses of slowly adapting type I mechanoreceptor units. J. Physiol. (Lond.) 479:247–256.

21. Senok, S. S., Baumann, K. I., and Halata, Z. (1996). Selective phototoxic destruction of quinacrine-loaded Merkel cells is neither selective nor complete. Exp. Brain Res. 110:325–334.

22. Mearow, K. M., and Diamond, J. (1988). Merkel cells and the mechanosensitivity of normal and regenerating nerves in *Xenopus* skin. Neuroscience 26:695–708.

23. Diamond, J., Mills, L. R., and Mearow, K. M. (1988). Evidence that the Merkel cell is not the transducer in the mechanosensory Merkel cell–neurite complex. Prog. Brain Res. 74:51–56.

24. Mills, L. R., and Diamond, J. (1995). Merkel cells are not the mechanosensory transducers in the touch dome of the rat. J. Neurocytol. 24:117–134.

25. English, K. B., Harper, S., Stayner, N., Wang, Z. M., and Davies, A. M. (1994). Localization of nerve growth factor (NGF) and low-affinity NGF receptors in touch domes and quantification of NGF mRNA in keratinocytes of adult rats. J. Comp. Neurol. 344:470–480.

26. Kinkelin, I., Stucky, C. L., Toyka, K. V., and Koltzenburg, M. (1999). Post-natal loss of marked cells, but not slowly-adapting mechanoreceptors in mice lacking the neutotrophin receptor p. 75. Eur. J. NeuroSci. 11.

27. Koschorke, G. M., Meyer, R. A., and Campbell, J. N. (1994). Cellular components necessary for mechanoelectrical transduction are conveyed to primary afferent terminals by fast axonal transport. Brain Res. 641:99–104.

28. Sharma, R. V., Chapleau, M. W., Hajduczok, G., Wachtel, R. E., Waite, L. J., Bhalla, R. C., and Abboud, F. M. (1995). Mechanical stimulation increases intracellular calcium concentration in nodose sensory neurons. Neuroscience 66:433–441.

29. Sullivan, M. J., Sharma, R. V., Wachtel, R. E., Chapleau, M. W., Waite, L. J., Bhalla, R. C., and Abboud, F. M. (1997). Non-voltage-gated Ca^{2+} influx through mechanosensitive ion channels in aortic baroreceptor neurons. Circ. Res. 80:861–867.

30. Cunningham, T. J., Wachtel, R. E., and Abboud, F. M. (1997). Mechanical stimulation of neurites generates an inward current in putative aortic baroreceptors in vitro. Brain Res. 757:149–154.

31. Garcia Anoveros, J., Ma, C., and Chalfie, M. (1995). Regulation of *Caenorhabditis elegans* degenerin proteins by a putative extracellular domain. Curr. Biol. 5:441–448.

32. Du, H., Gu, G., William, C. M., and Chalfie, M. (1996). Extracellular proteins needed for *C. elegans* mechanosensation. Neuron 16:183–194.

33. Gu, G., Caldwell, G. A., and Chalfie, M. (1996). Genetic interactions affecting touch sensitivity in *Caenorhabditis elegans*. Proc. Natl. Acad. Sci. USA 93:6577–6582.

34. Koltzenburg, M. (1995). Stability and plasticity of nociceptor function and their relationship to provoked and ongoing pain. Semin. Neurosci. 7:199–210.

35. McMahon, S. B., Lewin, G. R., and Wall, P. D. (1993). Central hyperexcitability triggered by noxious inputs. Curr. Opin. Neurobiol. 3:602–610.

36. Treede, R. D., Meyer, R. A., Raja, S. N., and Campbell, J. N. (1992). Peripheral and central mechanisms of cutaneous hyperalgesia. Prog. Neurobiol. 38:397–421.

37. Schmelz, M., Schmidt, R., Bickel, A., Handwerker, H. O., and Torebjork, H. E. (1997). Specific C-receptors for itch in human skin. J. Neurosci. 17:8003–8008.

38. Habler, H. J., Janig, W., and Koltzenburg, M. (1988). A novel type of unmyelinated chemosensitive nociceptor in the acutely inflamed urinary bladder. Agents Actions 25:219–221.

39. Habler, H. J., Janig, W., and Koltzenburg, M. (1990). Activation of unmyelinated afferent fibres by mechanical stimuli and inflammation of the urinary bladder in the cat. J. Physiol. (Lond.) 425:545–562.

40. Dmitrieva, N., and McMahon, S. B. (1996). Sensitisation of visceral afferents by nerve growth factor in the adult rat. Pain 66:87–97.

41. Berninger, B., and Poo, M. (1996). Fast actions of neurotrophic factors. Curr. Opin. Neurobiol. 6:324–330.

42. McMahon, S. B., Armanini, M. P., Ling, L. H., and Phillips, H. S. (1994). Expression and coexpression of Trk receptors in subpopulations of adult primary sensory neurons projecting to identified peripheral targets. Neuron 12:1161–1171.

43. Diamond, J., Coughlin, M., Macintyre, L., Holmes, M., and Visheau, B. (1987). Evidence that endogenous beta nerve growth factor is responsible for the collateral sprouting, but not the regeneration, of nociceptive axons in adult rats. Proc. Natl. Acad. Sci. USA 84:6596–6600.

44. Ernfors, P., Lee, K. F., and Jaenisch, R. (1994). Mice lacking brain-derived neurotrophic factor develop with sensory deficits. Nature 368:147–150.

45. Jones, K. R., Farinas, I., Backus, C., and Reichardt, L. F. (1994). Targeted disruption of the BDNF gene perturbs brain and sensory neuron development but not motor neuron development. Cell 76:989–999.

46. Minichiello, L., Casagranda, F., Tatche, R. S., Stucky, C. L., Postigo, A., Lewin, G. R., Davies, A. M., and Klein, R. (1998). Point mutation in trkβ causes loss of NT-4-dependent neurons without major effects on diverse BDNF responses. Nueron 21(2):335–345.

47. McAllister, A. K., Katz, L. C., and Lo, D. C. (1997). Opposing roles for endogenous BDNF and NT-3 in regulating cortical dendritic growth. Neuron 18:767–778.

48. Chalfie, M. (1993). Touch receptor development and function in *Caenorhabditis elegans*. J. Neurobiol. 24:1433–1441.

49. Driscoll, M., and Chalfie, M. (1991). The mec-4 gene is a member of a family of *Caenorhabditis elegans* genes that can mutate to induce neuronal degeneration. Nature 349:588–593.

50. Hong, K., and Driscoll, M. (1994). A transmembrane domain of the putative channel subunit MEC-4 influences mechanotransduction and neurodegeneration in *C. elegans.* Nature 367:470–473.

51. Lai, C. C., Hong, K., Kinnell, M., Chalfie, M., and Driscoll, M. (1996). Sequence and transmembrane topology of MEC-4, an ion channel subunit required for mechanotransduction in *Caenorhabditis elegans.* J. Cell Biol. 133:1071–1081.

52. Huang, M., Gu, G., Ferguson, E. L., and Chalfie, M. (1995). A stomatin-like protein necessary for mechanosensation in *C. elegans.* Nature 378:292–295.

53. Hamelin, M., Scott, I. M., Way, J. C., and Culotti, J. G. (1992). The mec-7 beta-tubulin gene of *Caenorhabditis elegans* is expressed primarily in the touch receptor neurons. EMBO J. 11:2885–2893.

54. Hamill, O. P., and McBride, D. W. Jr. (1996). The pharmacology of mechanogated membrane ion channels. Pharmacol. Rev. 48:231–252.

55. Erxleben, C. (1989). Stretch-activated current through single ion channels in the abdominal stretch receptor organ of the crayfish. J. Gen. Physiol. 94:1071–1083.

56. Kernan, M., Cowan, D., and Zuker, C. (1994). Genetic dissection of mechanosensory transduction: mechanoreception-defective mutations of *Drosophila.* Neuron 12:1195–1206.

57. Caterina, M. J., Schumacher, M. A., Tominaga, M., Rosen, T. A., Levine, J. D., and Julius, D. (1997). The capsaicin receptor: a heat-activated ion channel in the pain pathway. Nature 389:816–824.

58. Cesare, P., and McNaughton, P. (1996). A novel heat-activated current in nociceptive neurons and its sensitization by bradykinin. Proc. Natl. Acad. Sci. USA 93:15435–15439.

59. Reichling, D. B., and Levine, J. D. (1997). Heat transduction in rat sensory neurons by calcium-dependent activation of a cation channel. Proc. Natl. Acad. Sci. USA 94:7006–7011.

60. Nakamura, F., and Strittmatter, S. M. (1996). P2Y1 purinergic receptors in sensory neurons: contribution to touch-induced impulse generation. Proc. Natl. Acad. Sci. USA 93:10465–10470.

61. Gottschaldt, K. M., and Vahle-Hinz, C. (1981). Merkel cell receptors: structure and transducer function. Science 214:183–186.

62. Voilley, N., Galibert, A., Bassilana, F., Renard, S., Lingueglia, E., Coscoy, S., Champigny, G., Hofman, P., Lazdunski, M., and Barbry, P. (1997). The amiloride-sensitive Na$^+$ channel: from primary structure to function. Comp. Biochem. Physiol. A. Physiol. 118:193–200.

63. Waldmann, R., Champigny, G., Voilley, N., Lauritzen, I., and Lazdunski, M. (1996). The mammalian degenerin MDEG, an amiloride-sensitive cation channel activated by mutations causing neurodegeneration in *Caenorhabditis elegans.* J. Biol. Chem. 271:10433–10436.

64. Waldmann, R., Champigny, G., Bassilana, F., Heurteaux, C., and Lazdunski, M. (1997). A proton-gated cation channel involved in acid-sensing. Nature 386:173–177.

65. Waldmann, R., Bassilana, F., de Weille, J., Champigny, G., Heurteaux, C., and Lazdunski, M. (1997). Molecular cloning of a non-inactivating proton-gated Na^+ channel specific for sensory neurons. J. Biol. Chem. 272:20975–20978.

66. Garcia-Anoveros, J., Derfler, B., Neville-Golden, J., Hyman, B. T., and Corey, D. P. (1997). BNaC1 and BNaC2 constitute a new family of human neuronal sodium channels related to degenerins and epithelial sodium channels. Proc. Natl. Acad. Sci. USA 94:1459–1464.

67. Lingueglia, E., de Weille, J., Bassilana, F., Heurteaux, C., Sakai, H., Waldmann, R., and Lazdunski, M. (1997). A modulatory subunit of acid sensing ion channels in brain and dorsal root ganglion cells. J. Biol. Chem. 272:29778–29783.

68. Bassilana, F., Champigny, G., Waldmann, R., de-Weille, J. R., Heurteaux, C., and Lazdunski, M. (1997). The acid-sensitive ionic channel subunit ASIC and the mammalian degenerin MDEG form a heteromultimeric H^+-gated Na^+ channel with novel properties. J. Biol. Chem. 272:28819–28822.

69. Steen, K. H., Reeh, P. W., Anton, F., and Handwerker, H. O. (1992). Protons selectively induce lasting excitation and sensitization to mechanical stimulation of nociceptors in rat skin, in vitro. J. Neurosci. 12:86–95.

70. Steen, K. H., Steen, A. E., Kreysel, H. W., and Reeh, P. W. (1996). Inflammatory mediators potentiate pain induced by experimental tissue acidosis. Pain 66:163–170.

71. Huang, M., and Chalfie, M. (1994). Gene interactions affecting mechanosensory transduction in *Caenorhabditis elegans.* Nature 367:467–470.

72. Stewart, G. W., Hepworth-Jones, B. E., Keen, J. N., Dash, B. C., Argent, A. C., and Casimir, C. M. (1992). Isolation of cDNA coding for an ubiquitous membrane protein deficient in high Na^+, low K^+ stomatocytic erythrocytes. Blood 79:1593–1601.

73. Gallagher, P. G., and Forget, B. G. (1995). Structure, organization, and expression of the human band 7. 2b gene, a candidate gene for hereditary hydrocytosis. J. Biol. Chem. 270:26358–26363.

74. Mannsfeldt, A. G., Carroll, P., Stock, C. C., Lewin, G. R. (1999). Stomatin, a Mec-Z like protein, is expressed by mammalian sensory neurons. Mol Cell NeuroSci 13(6):391–404.

CHAPTER 8

Role of Bradykinin B_1 and B_2 Receptors in Nociception and Inflammation

NADIA M. J. RUPNIAK, JEANETTE LONGMORE, AND RAYMOND G. HILL

Merck Sharp and Dohme Research Laboratories, Neuroscience Research Centre
Terlings Park, Harlow, Essex

8.1 INTRODUCTION

Kinins are believed to be primary mediators of pain and inflammation, acting both to activate nociceptors directly and to induce prolonged inflammatory hyperalgesia. Kinins are released in damaged tissues from bloodborne kininogen precursors by the action of kallikreins. In addition to their algogenic and vasodilator properties,[1,2] kinins trigger an inflammatory positive feedback cycle, stimulating the release of prostaglandins and cytokines, which in turn amplify the responsiveness of inflamed tissue to kinins.[3,4] Elevated levels of circulating bradykinin have been demonstrated in patients with rheumatoid arthritis, confirming the involvement of bradykinin in pathophysiological processes of inflammatory disease.[5] Kinins are also believed to mediate the bone resorption seen in chronic inflammatory conditions such as periodontitis, osteomyelitis, and rheumatoid arthritis.[6] These observations provide a compelling rationale for the development of kinin antagonists as analgesic and anti-inflammatory drugs.

The actions of bradykinin are mediated by means of two distinct receptors designated B_1 and B_2. Both receptors were cloned by Hess and colleagues.[7,8] Bradykinin itself is thought to act mainly through B_2 receptors that are widely and constitutively expressed, for example on immune cells and on neuronal and vascular tissues.[9] The direct activation of B_2 receptors on nociceptors[10] probably explains why intradermal injection of bradykinin is extremely painful in humans.[2,11] Although B_2 receptor antagonists might therefore be

Molecular Basis of Pain Induction, Edited by John N. Wood
ISBN 0-471-34607-1   Copyright © 2000 by Wiley-Liss, Inc. All rights reserved.

expected to possess analgesic activity, concerns over the safety implications of blocking a putative cardioprotective function of bradykinin[12] has dampened enthusiasm to develop such compounds. The B$_1$ receptor shows 10- to 50-fold higher affinity for des-Arg[10][kallidin] and for the metabolite des-[Arg^9]bradykinin than for bradykinin and is expressed in low abundance in normal tissues; the de novo synthesis of B$_1$ receptors is increased over time following tissue damage and exposure to inflammatory agents.[3,13]

Unlike the B$_2$ receptor, the ability of B$_1$ receptor stimulation to activate nociceptors directly has not been firmly established. However, the inducible nature of B$_1$ receptors at the site of injury may make this a more attractive target for drug development since selective antagonists might be expected to cause minimal disruption of normal physiology in noninflamed tissues and so cause few unwanted side effects. The decision about which bradykinin receptor to target for drug development therefore depends on a careful evaluation of their contributions to painful inflammatory disease and whether their blockade can be achieved without compromising clinical safety.

8.2 PRODUCTION OF KININS IN RESPONSE TO TISSUE INJURY

Kinins are produced in the blood and tissues in response to tissue damage. These include bradykinin, which acts at the B$_2$ receptor subtype, and des-[Arg^9]bradykinin and des-[Arg[10]]kallidin, which are B$_1$ receptor–preferring peptides[5,14,15] (Fig. 8.1). Although the details of the enzymic biosynthesis of bradykinin were known in considerable detail from the work of Rocha e Silva and his colleagues, it was not until 1959 that the identity of bradykinin as a nine-amino acid peptide was revealed.[16] The production of bradykinin from inactive precursors and its rapid degradation in tissues has complicated the study of its pharmacology in vivo.

The production of bradykinin and cognate peptides from their precursor molecules following tissue damage involves serine protease enzymes known generically as kallikreins. Tissue kallikrein and plasma kallikrein are members of different enzyme families,[17,18] but both lead to production of bradykinin. In plasma, activated factor XII cleaves prekallikrein to give active plasma kallikrein, which in turn cleaves high-molecular-weight kininogen to give bradykinin. In the tissues, damage or inflammation leads to release of proteases that cleave prekallikrein to give tissue kallikrein, which then cleaves low-molecular-weight kininogen to give bradykinin and Lys-bradykinin.[17] Production of kinins is stimulated by a variety of inflammatory stimuli and can be evoked by bacterial endotoxins, local irritation (e.g., with uric acid crystals), or antigen/antibody reactions, and degranulating mast cells release proteases that have kallikrein-like activity.[19] It is also significant that the ac-

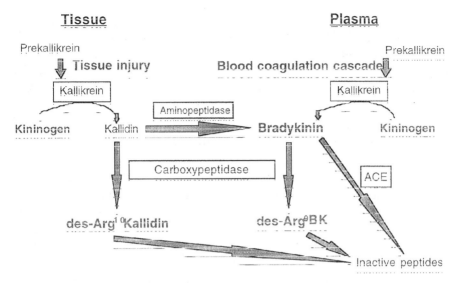

Figure 8.1   Production of kinins in response to tissue injury.

tivity of kininases, which normally limit the lifetime of kinins in the biophase, is inhibited by the acid environment of inflamed tissues, thus increasing effective kinin levels. It has also been reported that levels of the B_1 receptor–preferring peptide des-[Arg^9]bradykinin are elevated more than those than those of bradykinin itself during inflammation produced by intradermal carageenan injection.[20]

8.3   ROLE OF BRADYKININ AND OTHER KININS IN PAIN AND INFLAMMATION

Armstrong and his colleagues[21] were the first to show that kinins were produced in an experimental blister on human skin and could cause pain when applied to a blister base. Since pure synthetic bradykinin has been available, it has become readily apparent that this peptide can directly activate nociceptor fibers, innervating many tissues, including skin, joint, muscle, and internal viscera.[19,22–24] Bradykinin is the most potent algogen known and one of the few that stimulates nociceptors in the absence of other chemical agents. Physiologically, it is probably more significant that bradykinin powerfully potentiates the actions of other substances released by tissue inflammation and damage, such as prostaglandins, serotonin, and cytokines[25] (see Ref. 26 for a review). More recently it has been shown that bradykinin is degraded to des-[Arg^9]-bradykinin, which is also an important activator of kinin receptors.

Interestingly, there are tissue-specific differences in the sensitivity of nociceptors to bradykinin. It has been estimated that about half of all unmyelinated and small myelinated afferent fibers in skin are sensitive to excitation by bradykinin (as defined by a 1-min exposure to 10^{-5} M bradykinin), while in deeper tissues over 90% of C fibers may be bradykinin sensitive.[27] It has also been suggested that units that are not overtly sensitive to bradykinin can, nevertheless, show sensitisation of their responses to thermal noxia in the presence of bradykinin.[28] After inflammation with carageenan, more than 80% of cutaneous nociceptors were found to be bradykinin sensitive.[29]

Bradykinin can be shown to produce its excitatory effects on nociceptors by direct depolarization, and recordings from anatomically identified dorsal root ganglion neurones reveals that it is only a proportion of the smaller neurones that are sensitive to bradykinin. Intracellular recordings have shown that the response to bradykinin is through the activation of phospholipase C (PLC). This leads to elevation in intracellular Ca^{2+} and activation of protein kinase C (PKC), and it has been shown that inhibitors of PKC may reduce responses to bradykinin.[30] As the actions of prostaglandins and bradykinin on sensory neurones are additive, the stimulation of prostaglandin production by PLC activation is also relevant.[30] Production of prostaglandins can also be stimulated by bradykinin-induced activation of phospholipase A$_2$ in non-neuronal cells.[26] The dual action of prostaglandins and bradykinin on nociceptors increases intracellular cyclic AMP levels, which inhibits the slow after-hyperpolarization, thereby increasing the effective burst duration following stimulation.[26] Interaction between kinins and cytokines are also important, in part because of the up-regulation of kinin receptor expression by cytokines[31] (see below).

Indirect effects of bradykinin are important determinants of the effect of tissue inflammation on nociceptor activity (Fig. 8.2). The activation of primary afferent nociceptors and sympathetic neurones leads to release of transmitters contained in the peripheral terminals of these neurones. Neuropeptides released from sensory neurones include substance P, which produces profound neurogenic extravasation plus a smaller amount of vasodilation by activation of NK$_1$ receptors.[32,33] It is interesting to note that bradykinin-induced bronchoconstriction in asthmatics was reduced by aerosol administration of the NK$_1$ receptor antagonist FK-224.[34] Release of calcitonin gene–related peptide (CGRP) from the same population of sensory neurones causes vasodilatation and also potentiates the extravasation action of substance P.[32,35] The influence of sympathetic neurone activation and the release of monoamines on inflammation is somewhat controversial. Levine and his colleagues[36,37] have argued for an important role of the sympathetic postganglionic nerve in the production of inflammation and hyperalgesia by bradykinin. In their experiments, activation of the sympathetic nerves, either indirectly by mast cell degranulation or more directly by injection of bradykinin, produced an extravasation response that was decreased by chem-

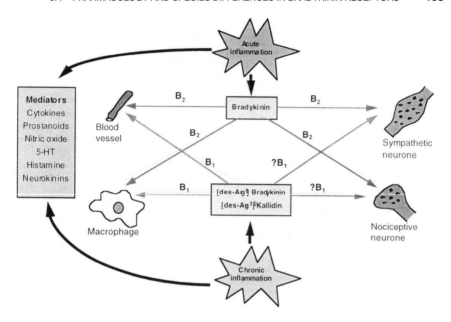

Figure 8.2 Roles of kinins in pain and inflammation. (Modified from Ref. 94.)

ical or surgical sympathectomy.[37,38] Others have conversely found that although peptide depletion with capsaicin or blockade of prostaglandin synthesis with indomethacin would reduce bradykinin-induced hyperalgesia, chemical sympathectomy had no effect.[39,40] Kinins release histamine and serotonin from mast cells and may also be chemotactic and attract immune competent cells to the site of inflammation.[26] It is clear that sensory ganglia are well innervated by postganglionic sympathetic and parasympathetic nerve fibers, however,[41] recent work suggests that there is a direct action of bradykinin that is independent of the sympathetic nerves and a negative feedback operating through the nociceptive afferents and the hypothalomopituitary adrenal axis, which depends on an intact sympathetic system.[42] Bradykinin excites sympathetic ganglion neurones by inhibition of an M-type K^+ current by means of $G_{\alpha q/11}$.[43] Paradoxically, bradykinin can also *inhibit* voltage-dependent N-type Ca^{2+} currents in some cells by a mechanism involving the protein kinase p38-2.[44]

8.4 MOLECULAR PHARMACOLOGY AND SPECIES DIFFERENCES IN BRADYKININ RECEPTORS

The cloning of B_1 and B_2 receptors from human, rat, mouse and rabbit has helped to interpret some of the differences in the pharmacological profiles of B_1 and B_2 receptors across species. For B_1 receptors there are striking species differences in the affinity of the des-[Arg] metabolites of kallidin and bradykinin, the endogenous ligands for B$_1$ receptors (and also differences in the affinity of synthetic Leu-substituted analogs of these metabolites). Des-[Arg^{10}]kallidin has much higher affinity than des-[Arg^9]bradykinin for the human B$_1$ receptor; this difference is less for the rabbit receptor, while the rat and mouse receptors have higher affinity for des-[Arg^9]bradykinin.[45] Furthermore, des-[Arg^{10}Leu^9]kallidin and des-[Arg^{9}Leu^8]bradykinin are partial agonists at the mouse B$_1$-receptor, but antagonists at the human receptor.[45,46] The affinity and selectivity of ligands for B$_1$ receptors can also vary across species. For example, B9858, a designer peptide B$_1$ receptor–selective antagonist, has greater than 1000-fold selectivity for human B$_2$ over B$_2$ receptors (0.04 nM compared to 146 nM), whereas affinity for the mouse B$_1$ receptor is much lower (5.4 nM), and selectively over mouse B$_2$ receptors is reduced to approximately 30-fold.[45] Overall, the pharmacological profile of human and rabbit B$_1$ receptors is similar (although there are some minor differences) and contrast to the profiles of rat and mouse receptor.[47–50]

The peptide-binding domains for the B$_1$ receptor are uncharacterized, although it is known that for peptides the presence of lysl or D-Arg groups at the N terminal are important for affinity, and amino acids at positions 7 and 8 seem to be important for receptor activation and for selectivity over the B$_2$ receptor, respectively.[51–53] The human B$_1$ receptor gene is regulated by two promoters and it is tempting to speculate that expression, either constitutive or inducible, is regulated by one or the other of these promoters.[54]

In most species bradykinin is the endogenous ligand for B$_2$ receptors. Good pharmacological tools are available, including peptide antagonists (e.g., HOE 140) and non-peptide B$_2$ receptor selective agonists (FR190097) and antagonists (FR167344, FR173657, WIN 64338).[55–57] Species differences exist in the affinity of both peptide and nonpeptide B$_2$ receptor antagonists. For example, binding studies have shown that FR167344 and FR173657 show higher affinity (subnanomolar) for rat and guinea pig B$_2$ receptors compared to human B$_2$ receptors (65 nM).[56,58,59] Unlike the B$_1$ receptor, the overall pharmacological profile of B$_2$ receptors across species does not fall conveniently into clear-cut divisions.[60] The peptide-binding domains to the B$_2$ receptor have been partially characterized using anti-iodiotypic antibodies and site-directed mutagenesis. Extracellular domains 3 and 4 (Fig. 8.3) and the upper regions of transmembrane domains 4 and 7 are important for bradykinin and HOE 140 binding and for receptor activation.[61] Transmembrane 3 (particularly ^{118}Lys) is important for determining peptide selectivity between bradykinin receptor subtypes.[62] Interestingly, sequence alignment of the human, rat, mouse, and rabbit B$_2$ receptors shows most diversity in the fourth extracellular domain and the upper regions of transmembrane 7, both of which are important for peptide binding. Several polymorphisms of the

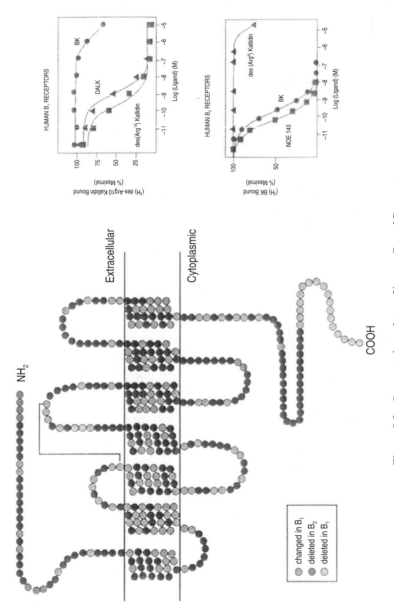

Figure 8.3 Sequence homology of human B₁ and B₂ receptors.

155

human B$_2$ receptor gene have been identified, including changes to the promotor region and a change resulting in a switch from a tyrosine to a cysteine residue at position 14. The impact of these changes or the involvment of B$_2$ receptors in hereditary disease is unknown.[63]

The sequence homology between B$_1$ and B$_2$ receptors is low (35% at the amino acid level for human B$_1$ and B$_2$ receptors[50,60] (Fig. 8.3). Although it has been possible to make peptide dimers with dual affinity for both B$_1$ and B$_2$ receptors,[51] it would be challenging to design small synthetic molecules with dual affinity for both B$_1$ and B$_2$ receptors. In addition, since bradykinin receptors show similar levels of homology to other G-protein-coupled receptors (e.g., 30% homology to the angiotensin AT$_2$ receptor), this may limit the level of attainable specificity.

8.5 TISSUE DISTRIBUTION AND EXPRESSION OF BRADYKININ RECEPTORS

The distribution and expression of B$_1$ and B$_2$ receptors has recently been reviewed extensively (see Refs. 64 to 66 for detailed descriptions). This review will focus on recent discoveries, particularly those dealing with the distribution of bradykinin receptors in human tissues.

B$_1$ receptors are often regarded as atypical in that they are not always expressed on the cell surface, and their expression is inducible.[64,66] The induction of B$_1$ receptors is generally believed to involve de novo synthesis of B$_1$ receptor protein since it can be inhibited by mRNA and protein synthesis inhibitors such as actinomycin D and cyclohexamide.[64] This is supported by the observation that B$_1$ receptor induction can lead to an increase in receptor density or number of binding studies, or in an increase in the magnitude of the functional response, but is not always associated with changes in the affinity or potency of B$_1$ receptor ligands.[8,67]

It is generally assumed that under normal conditions B$_1$ receptors are not constitutively expressed in tissues, but that expression can be induced or upregulated. In some studies, upregulation is measured by the appearance of specific B$_1$ receptor sites determined using radioligands or antibodies, and in other studies by development of a functional response to selective B$_1$ receptor agonists or antagonists. It should be remembered that the appearance of binding sites does not imply that these "receptors" are functional proteins, and on the other hand, the development of a functional response does not exclude the existence of a preformed, nonfunctional receptor protein. Tissue injury can evoke the expression of B$_1$ receptors and/or functional response. This can be seen in some animal assays, such as persistent hyperalgesia.[26] Importantly, B$_1$ receptor expression has been detected in inflamed tissues in humans, specifically in human stomach obtained as biopsy material from patients with gastritis, but not in the same tissue from control patients.[68] Other inducing factors are pharmacological agents including inflammatory mediators such as interleukins, cytokines, or bacterial toxins lipopolysaccharide (LPS) and growth factors.[60,64] The presence of an inflammatory stimulus is not a prerequisite and the induction of a B_1 receptor–mediated responses in isolated tissue preparations can be evoked by incubation in physiological salt solutions (at 37°C).[64,65] The length of the induction period can vary depending on the species; in vivo experiments have shown that induction of B_1 receptor expression evoked by LPS injection takes 2 h in rabbits compared to 12 to 24 h in rats.[13,69] For human isolated tissues (e.g., coronary artery, umbilical vein, and ileum), the length of the induction time varies from 3 h to overnight incubation.[70–72] The up-regulation of B_1 receptor expression is important since it results in amplification of tissue responses to kinins and increased responsiveness to the long-lived des[Arg] metabolites of native kinins.

There are exceptions to the general assumption that in native tissues B_1 receptor–mediated responses cannot be detected except following tissue injury or disease. These exceptions may be species-dependent phenomena. B_1 receptor expression (either inducible or constitutive) has not been reported in guinea pig tissues[60]; no B_1 receptor–mediated responses have been detected in normal tissues from rabbit, rat, pig, or cow.[64–66] In contrast, responses to B_1 receptor agonists have been reported in hemodynamic studies using normal dogs and cats.[64,66,73] Human tissues may also express constitutive B_1 receptors. In human isolated ileum (a tissue that under normal conditions is unresponsiveness to B_1 receptor agonists), protein synthesis inhibitors reduced but did not completely abolish B_1 receptor induction, suggesting the existence of preformed, nonfunctional receptor protein.[70] B_1 receptor immunostaining is present on vascular smooth and endothelial cells in normal human blood vessels and also in vessels with atherosclerotic lesions,[74] although no pharmacological studies were conducted with these vessels to determine receptor functionality. The existence of preformed, nonfunctional receptor protein may explain the apparent short time course for B_1 receptor induction (2 to 3 h for some tissues).[65] This issue should be addressed using a combination of selective B_1 receptor radioligands or antibodies and determination of the absence or presence of a functional B_1 receptor response.

B_2 receptors are regarded as the constitutive bradykinin receptor in that they are expressed in tissues under normal conditions.[60] However, there is some evidence that B_2 receptor expression can also be up-regulated. In dog, cultured tracheal smooth muscle cells incubation (24 h) with forskolin leads to an increase in the number of B_2 receptor binding sites, an effect that can be blocked by protein synthesis inhibitors.[54] Up-regulation of B_2 receptors by interluekin-1 has also been reported for cultured human synovial cells.[75]

B$_1$ and B$_2$ receptors are expressed on a wide variety of cell types from different species and these summarized in Table 8.1. Of particular relevance to the role of bradykinin receptors in inflammation and nociception is the presence of both B$_1$ and B$_2$ receptors in blood vessels (vascular smooth muscle and endothelial cells) and blood cells (including macrophages). These receptors are involved in the regulation of blood flow and microvascular permeability[64,66] and mediate the extravasation of plasma proteins in response to some inflammatory agents.[65,66] Activation of B$_1$ and B$_2$ receptors on macrophages promotes the release of inflammatory mediators (see Fig. 8.2) and at least part of the anti-inflammatory and antinociceptive effects of bradykinin receptor antagonists could be mediated through blockade of receptors on macrophages that have infiltrated the tissue injury or inflammation site. In humans, the recent development of receptor subtype-specific antibodies has allowed the demonstration of B$_2$ receptors on endothelial and synovial cells and on fibroblasts in synovial membranes from patients with inflammatory joint disease.[76] Surprisingly, no B$_1$ receptor immunoreactivity was detected in these tissues despite the presence of a chronic inflammatory disease.

TABLE 8.1   Cell Types Expressing B$_1$ Receptors and B$_2$ Receptors[a]

B$_1$ Receptor Sites/Responses	B$_2$ Receptor Sites/Responses
Smooth muscle	Smooth Muscle
*Gastrointestinal tract[66,70]	Gastrointestinal tract[66]
*Vascular[66,74,76,77]	*Vascular[66,71,74,76]
Genitourinary tract[66]	*Genitourinary[66]
Airway[66]	Airway[66]
Blood cells	Ocular[66]
*Neutrophils[66,78]	Blood cells
*Macrophages[66,74,76]	*Macrophages[74,76]
Lymphocytes[66]	Neutrophils[78]
*Endothelial cells[66,76,77]	*Endothelial cells[66,76,77]
*Fibroblasts[8,66,74]	*Fibroblasts[8,76]
Neuronal	Neuronal
Superior cervical ganglia[31,79]	Superior cervical ganglia[79]
CNS (human thalamus, hypothalamus)[10]	*Sensory neurons[26,66,79,80]
Spinal cord (human substantia gelatinosa	CNS (cortex, hypothalamus,
and interneurons)[77]	*caudate, pons, medulla)[77,81]
Bone	Skeletal muscle[82]
Osteoclasts[66]	*Kidney[66,83]
Osteoblasts[66]	*Skin[84]
	*Epithelial cells[85]
	*Synovial cells[66,75,76]
	*Cancer cells[86]

[a] Data were determined either phamacologically using functional assays or by radioligand binding and immunocytochemistry with receptor specific antibodies. An asterisk denotes receptors found in human tissues.

It is generally accepted that B_2 receptors are present on nociceptive C and Aδ fibers innervating skin, joint, muscle, tooth pulp, and viscera[26,80] and on postganglionic sympathetic fibers.[26,31,79] Bradykinin activates nociceptors and sensitizes them to other physical and chemical stimuli[26] and activation of B_2 receptors on sympathetic fibers results in blood flow changes and the release of secondary mediators which in turn promote extravasation and/or sensitize nociceptors[26] (see Fig. 8.2). The expression of B_1 receptors on sensory and sympathetic neurones is less clear cut. B_1 receptor agonist des-[Arg^9]bradykinin or des-[Arg^{10}]kallidin failed to activate primary afferents in a spinal nociceptive reflex preparation[30] or cultured rats dorsal root ganglion.[87] No B_1 receptor–mediated responses were detected in dorsal root sensory ganglia (IL1β treated) obtained from either wild-type or B_2 receptor knockout mice, despite the presence of B_1 receptor mRNA.[79] In mouse and rat superior cervical ganglia (sympathetic) B_1 receptor–mediated responses can only be detected following induction with IL1β *and* in the presence of captopril, a peptidase inhibitor.[31,88] These findings suggest that the B_1 receptors that contribute to inflammatory hyperalgesia may not be located on sensory neurones but may be expressed by other cells that release mediators that sensitize or directly activate nociceptors.

There is evidence for a role of central B_2 receptors in blood pressure control and, more relevant to this review, in the processing of nociceptive information. Injection of bradykinin into the brain either intracerebroventricularly or intrathecally increases nociceptive behaviors and blood pressure.[26,80] B_2 receptor binding sites (determined using radioligand binding or immunohistochemistry) are present in cerebral cortex, hypothalamus, caudate, subfornical organ, red nucleus, pons, and some nuclei in the medulla (e.g., solitary tract nucleus[26,76,80,81]). Most relevant to nociception are the B_2 receptor sites present in the spinal cord (superficial layers of the dorsal horn and descending noradrenergic bulbospinal neurones[76,80]). Until recently, no B_1 receptor sites were reported in the central nervous system. However, Cassim et al.[76] used immunocytochemical techniques to show B_1 receptors in human brain (hypothalamus and thalamus) and spinal cord (substantia gelatinosa and some interneurones). The role of these B_1 receptors is unknown. The development of improved pharmacological tools for the B_1 receptor, with greater selectivity and metabolic stability, will help to clarify this issue.

8.6 ANTINOCICEPTIVE ACTIVITY OF PEPTIDE BRADYKININ RECEPTOR ANTAGONISTS

Until recently, the only pharmacological tools that were available to explore the roles of different kinin receptors in pain and inflammation were peptide antagonists, such as the selective bradykinin B_1 receptor antagonist des[Arg^9-

Leu^8]bradykinin, and the B$_2$ antagonist HOE 140. As will be discussed, there are a number of problems associated with the use of peptide antagonists to elucidate the function of bradykinin receptors in vivo. However, studies using des-Arg^9[Leu^8]bradykinin are consistent with the proposal of an important role of B$_1$ receptors in inflammatory hyperalgesia. Of particular interest is the ability of des-Arg^9[Leu^8]bradykinin to reverse or prevent the persistent ($\geq$ 24 h) mechanical and thermal hyperalgesia caused by intra-articular injection of Freund's adjuvant, or by ultraviolet irradiation of the skin in rats; in contrast, the B$_2$ antagonist HOE 140 was ineffective or only weakly active in these assays.[89–91] Moreover, intra-articular injection of the B$_1$ agonist des-[Arg^9]bradykinin exacerbated hyperalgesia caused by Freund's adjuvant, indicating local induction of B$_1$ receptors at the site of inflammation.[89,92] Studies of intraarticular plasma extravasation in antigen-induced arthritis also reveal an evolving role for B$_1$ receptors in the maintenance of chronic inflammation.[93] In other studies examining the effects of ultraviolet irradiation of the paws, thermal hyperalgesia in rats was further increased by intravenous injection of des-[Arg^9]bradykinin and to a lesser extent by bradykinin; this effect of both agonists was reversed by des-Arg^9[Leu^8]bradykinin but not by HOE 140, implicating B$_1$ rather than B$_2$ receptors in persistent hyperalgesia.[91] These findings have led to the proposal that stimulation of the B$_2$ receptor initiates the acute nociceptive and inflammatory response to bradykinin and that the inducible B$_1$ receptor may play an important role in the development and maintenance of chronic inflammatory hyperalgesia.[94] Consistent with this view is the more restricted activity of peptide B$_2$ receptor antagonists such as HOE 140 and NPC 567 in acute nociception tests, such as inhibition of acetic acid–induced abdominal constriction[95,96] and tests of carrageenan or urate-induced hyperalgesia.[95,97]

Unfortunately, discrimination of the potentially different roles of B$_1$ and B$_2$ receptors from such in vivo studies is compromised by several difficulties. The use of peptide receptor antagonists is problematic because of their metabolic lability and evidence for partial agonist activity. Thus, carboxypeptidases are able to convert certain peptide B$_2$ receptor antagonists into *B$_1$* receptor blockers,[98] and the B$_1$ receptor specificity of the antinociceptive effects of des-Arg^9[Leu^8]bradykinin is similarly complicated by its degradation by peptidases in vivo.[99] Peptide antagonists may also behave as partial agonists, as has been reported using in vitro functional assays for des-Arg^9[Leu^8]bradykinin.[45,46,100] An unexplained anomaly is that the dose-response curves for both peptide B$_1$ and B$_2$ antagonsits in in vivo assays are typically bell shaped with narrow active dose windows, such that antinociceptive efficacy is lost as the dose is increased[92,101] (Fig. 8.4). This narrow active dose window makes it difficult to be sure that appropriate doses of the antagonists were evaluated in attempting to determine the relative contributions of B$_1$ or B$_2$ receptors in assays of acute or chronic hyperalgesia. Finally,

Carrageenan induced hyperalgesia (rat)   Formalin paw late phase (mouse)

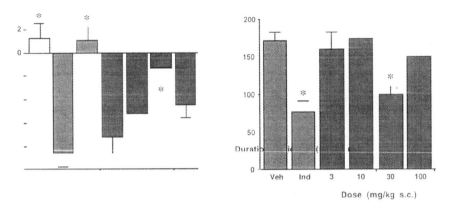

Figure 8.4 Narrow dose window for antinociceptive activity of des-Arg^9[Leu^8]bradykinin in the formalin and carrageenan paw tests in mice and rats. Mice received an intraplantar injection of formalin (20 µL of 2.5% solution) 10 min after the test compounds; the duration of licking was recorded throughout the period 10 to 20 min thereafter. In rats, test compounds were administered 2 h after intraplantar injection of carrageenan (4.5 mg) and the change in paw pressure thresholds was determined 1 h later. (From Ref. 92.)

the proposed distinction between B$_2$ receptor activation in *acute* nociception, compared with the inducible B$_1$ receptor appearing relatively more important in *chronic* inflammatory hyperalgesia, does not readily account for the antinociceptive and anti-inflammatory activity of des-Arg^9[Leu^8]bradykinin in several acute assays, including formalin paw,[92,101,102] capsaicin-induced dermal inflammation,[103] and carrageenan-induced hyperalgesia.[92] In these assays, nociception or inflammation is assessed ≤ 30 min after injection of the inflammatory agent, an observation that is not easily reconciled with the low levels of constitutive expression of the B$_1$ receptor.

To attempt to overcome the limitations associated with des-Arg^9[Leu^8]-bradykinin, we assessed the antinociceptive activity of B9858 (Lys-Lys^0, Hyp^3, Igl^5, D-Igl^7, Oic^8, des-Arg^{9}bradykinin), which has recently been described as a potent, stable peptide B$_1$ receptor antagonist.[52] Unlike Arg^9[Leu^8]bradykinin, B9858 behaved as a full antagonist at cloned human and murine B$_1$ receptors using an in vitro aequorin bioluminescence assay.[45] However, the expectation that B9858 might exhibit a wider antinociceptive dose range compared with des-Arg^9[Leu^8]bradykinin in vivo was not borne out in either the carrageenan or formalin paw assays (unpublished observations).

The difficulties associated with the use of peptide antagonists for in vivo functional pharmacology studies underlines the need to develop selective, metabolically stable, nonpeptide B$_1$ and B$_2$ receptor antagonists. Recently, the first orally active nonpeptide B$_2$ antagonist, FR173657, was described.[104] This compound was found to inhibit bradykinin-induced bronchoconstriction and carrageenan-induced paw edema in rodents but has not yet been evaluated for its effects on nociception. Progress is also being made to develop nonpeptide B$_1$ antagonists such as the compounds exemplified in a patent filed by Sanofi.

8.7   PHENOTYPE OF *BKr*$^{-/-}$ MICE

The ability to produce knockout mice with targeted disruption of genes encoding specific proteins has become a popular alternative approach to evaluate the function of neurotransmitter receptors in vivo, particularly where suitable pharmacological antagonists are not yet available. Mice in which the bradykinin B$_2$ receptor was knocked out (*Bk2r*$^{-/-}$) have been available for several years, so these have been characterized in most detail. Unlike tissues from wild-type animals, membrane preparations from the ileum or uterus of *Bk2r*$^{-/-}$ mice provided no detectable binding of [^{3}H]bradykinin, and there were no functional responses to bradykinin in uterine or neuronal tissues.[106]

Recently, we described the behavior of *Bk2r*$^{-/-}$ mice in a range of conscious animal nociception assays. In view of the known algogenic effects of bradykinin that are believed to be mediated by means of B$_2$ receptor activation, we observed surprisingly subtle changes in nociception in *Bk2r*$^{-/-}$ mice.[92] As would be expected following deletion of this gene, *Bk2r*$^{-/-}$ mice failed to exhibit a nociceptive behavioral response to intraplantar injection of bradykinin (Fig. 8.5), confirming that the direct activation of nociceptors by bradykinin agonists involves the B$_2$ rather than the B$_1$ receptor, at least in non-inflamed tissues. These findings are consistent with the ability of HOE 140 and other peptide B$_2$ receptor antagonists to inhibit nociception elicited by bradykinin in animals and humans.[2,95,96] The *Bk2r*$^{-/-}$ mice also failed to develop paw edema or thermal hyperalgesia in response to intraplantar injection of carrageenan, indicating that the action of bradykinin at B$_2$ receptors is an essential initial step in the inflammatory response to this polysaccharide. This observation is consistent with the inhibition of carrageenan-induced edema and thermal hyperalgesia by peptide B$_2$ antagonists such as NPC 567.[97]

In contrast to their abnormal response to bradykinin and to carrageenan, *Bk2r*$^{-/-}$ mice exhibited intact nociceptive responses in a number of other tests. Their spinal nociceptive reflexes, assessed using a paw flick test, appeared normal, suggesting that bradykinin is not involved in the activation of thermal nociceptors in the absence of inflammation or tissue damage. Moreover, nociception and inflammatory hyperalgesia elicited by intraplantar injection of formalin or complete Freund's adjuvant were indistinguishable in *Bk2r*$^{-/-}$ and wild-type mice (Fig. 8.5). This finding was unexpected in view of reports that

Intraplantar injection of bradykinin   Late phase response to formalin

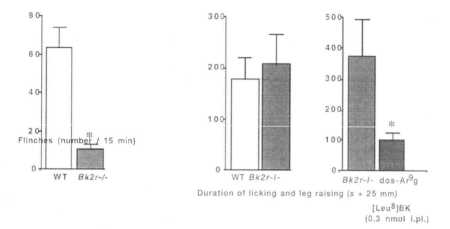

Figure 8.5 Response of *Bk2r⁻/⁻* mice to intraplantar injection of bradykinin or formalin. Aversive behaviors elicited by intraplantar injection of bradykinin (10 nmol) or formalin (2.5%) were recorded by direct observation for up to 35 min. Also shown is the inhibition of the late-phase response to formlin by intraplantar injection of des-Arg^9[Leu^8]bradykinin (0.3 nmol) in *Bk2r⁻/⁻* mice. (From Ref. 92.)

peptide B$_2$ receptor antagonists such as HOE 140 and NPC 567 could attenuate nociceptive responses evoked by formalin[101] and increase the load tolerated by the arthritic joints of experimental rats.[107] Interestingly, the antinociceptive effect of the B$_1$ receptor antagonist des-Arg^9[Leu^8]bradykinin against the late-phase response to formalin was still demonstrable in *Bk2r⁻/⁻* mice (Fig. 8.5), indicating that induction of B$_1$ receptors is not dependent on B$_2$ receptor stimulation. The findings from phenotypic characterization of *Bk2r⁻/⁻* mice suggests that B$_2$ receptor activation is required for some, but not all, responses to noxious stimuli and that the clinical potential of B$_2$ receptor antagonists to treat chronic pain and inflammation may therefore be limited.

The first bradykinin B$_1$ receptor knockout mice (*Bk1r⁻/⁻*) have been generated only recently; unlike wild-type animals, administration of bacterial lipopolysaccharide to *Bk1r⁻/⁻* mice failed to increase B$_1$ receptor mRNA in peripheral tissues (heart, lungs, kidney, liver, ileum, and stomach). In isolated tissue preparations (stomach and ileum) the contractile response to the B$_1$ receptor agonist des-[Arg^9]bradykinin was absent in *Bk1r⁻/⁻* mice.[108] Such animals provide a means to circumvent the limitations of currently available peptide bradykinin antagonists to clarify the relative contributions of the B$_1$ and B$_2$ receptors to acute and chronic noxious and inflammatory responses. The phenotype of *Bk1r⁻/⁻* mice in assays of acute and chronic inflammatory hyperalgesia has not yet been characterized; this remains an important objective for future investigations.

8.8 B₁ OR B₂ RECEPTORS AS DRUG DEVELOPMENT TARGETS

The existence of two bradykinin receptors begs the question of which is the better target for drug development. The low (35%) sequence homology between the B₁ and B₂ receptors suggests that it would be difficult to design a pharmacological antagonist that would block both of these and still retain adequate selectivity over other G protein–coupled receptors. Faced with the need to choose one receptor as a target for development, it is important to assess which of these is the most compelling.

The evidence summarized in Table 8.2 indicates that at present the B₁ receptor remains an attractive target because it is induced locally at the site of tissue injury, so that blocking this receptor should cause minimal disturbance of physiology in normal tissues, and because studies using peptide B₁ receptor antagonists indicate that these are active in a wide range of nociception assays involving both acute and chronic inflammation. Although the response of *Bk1r⁻/⁻* mice to noxious stimulation has not yet been assessed, these animals appear healthy, and no adverse consequence of blocking or deleting the B₁ receptor is known at present. In contrast to this are a number of emerging reservations about the B₂ receptor as an analgesic drug target. Pharmacological blockade of the B₂ receptor results in antinociception in only a narrow range of animal assays compared with B₁ antagonists. While recognizing the limitations of studies using peptide antagonists, it is clear that the subtle changes in response to noxious stimuli seen in *Bk2r⁻/⁻* mice are broadly consistent with this conclusion.

A second important area of concern regarding the development of B₂ receptor antagonists involves the ubiquitous and constitutive expression of these receptors that may give rise to adverse effects, particularly involving the

TABLE 8.2   B₁ or B₂ Receptor: Which Is the Best Drug Target?

	B₁	B₂
Antinociceptive activity of peptide antagonists	Wide range of acute and chronic assays	Limited activity in acute assays
Phenotype of *Bkr⁻/⁻* mice	Not known	Respond to most noxious stimuli
Expression	Inducible	Constitutive
Potential harmful effects	None known	Cardioprotection? Hypertension?

cardiovascular system. A major issue surrounds the potential for provoking or exacerbating hypertension by blocking B_2 receptors. The kallikrein-kinin system regulates water and sodium excretion and so participates in blood pressure homeostasis. Although $Bk2r^{-/-}$ mice exhibit normal resting blood pressure, recent studies have demonstrated that the hypertensive response to a high-salt diet was almost doubled in $Bk2r^{-/-}$ mice compared with wild-type controls.[109,110] These observations suggest that drugs blocking the B_2 receptor might predispose individuals to develop salt-sensitive hypertension and may counteract the beneficial effects of antihypertensive therapies. The contribution of B_1 receptor–mediated events to blood pressure homeostasis has not yet been investigated under these conditions. Another major clinical safety concern is that the B_2 receptor antagonist HOE 140 has been shown to attenuate the antiarrhythmic (cardioprotective) effects of ischemic preconditioning in anesthetized dogs.[12] Again, the consequences of blocking the B_1 receptor have not been established under these conditions.

8.9   CONCLUSIONS AND FUTURE DIRECTIONS

There is a strong preclinical rationale for the development of bradykinin antagonists to treat pain and inflammation. Both B_1 and B_2 receptors represent potential analgesic drug targets, although the B_1 receptor is currently of most interest because it may provide greater clinical efficacy in chronic pain states and a more favorable clinical safety profile. The question of whether bradykinin antagonists can be developed successfully into safe and effective anti-inflammatory analgesic drugs awaits the identification of nonpeptide antagonists that have high affinity for the human receptor and careful preclinical safety and efficacy studies in appropriate species. Studies to characterize the expression and localization of bradykinin in normal and pathological tissues will also make an important contribution to our understanding of their role in health and disease.

REFERENCES

1. Coffman, J. (1966). The effect of aspirin on pain and hand blood flow responses to intra-arterial injection of bradykinin. Clin. Pharmacol. Ther. 7:26–37.

2. Whalley, E. T., Clegg, S., Stewart, J. M., and Vavrek, R. J. (1987). The effect of kinin agonists and antagonists on the pain response of the human blister base. Arch. Pharmacol. 336:652–655.

3. Regoli D., and Barabe, J. (1980). Pharmacology of bradykinin and related kinins. Pharmacol. Rev. 32:1–46.

4. Burch, R. M., Connor, J. R., and Tiffany, C. W. (1989). The kallikrein–kinino-gen–kinin system in chronic inflammation. Agents Actions 27:258–260.

5. Hargreaves, K. M., Troullos, E., Dionne, R. A., Schmidt, E. A., Schafer, S., and Joris, J. L. (1988). Bradykinin is increased during acute and chronic inflammation: therapeutic implications. Clin. Pharmacol. Ther. 6:613–621.

6. Ljunggren, O., and Lerner, U. H. (1990). Evidence for BK$_1$ bradykinin receptor-mediated prostaglandin formation in osteoblasts and subsequent enhancement of bone resorption. Br. J. Pharmacol. 101:382–386.

7. Hess, J. F., Borkowski, J. A., Young, G. S., Strader, C. D., and Ransom, R. W. (1992). Cloning and pharmacological characterisation of a human bradykinin (BK-2) receptor. Biochem. Biophys. Res. Commun. 184:260–268.

8. Menke, J. G., Borkowski, J. A., Bierilo, K. K., MacNeil, T., Derrick, A. W., Schneck, K. A., Ransom, R. W., Strader, C. D., Linemeyer, D. L., and Hess, J. F. (1994). Expression cloning of a human B$_1$ bradykinin receptor. J. Biol. Chem. 269:21583–21586.

9. Sharif, N. A., and Whiting, R. L. (1991). Identification of B$_2$-bradykinin receptors in guinea-pig brain regions, spinal cord and peripheral tissues. Neurochem. Int. 18:89–96.

10. Steranka, L. R., Manning, D. C., de Haas, C. J., Ferkany, J. W., Borosky, S. A., Connor, J. R., Vavrek, R. J., and Stewart, J. M. (1988). Bradykinin as a pain mediator: receptors are localized to sensory neurons, and antagonists have analgesic actions. Proc. Natl. Acad. Sci. USA 85:3245–3249.

11. Manning, D. C., Srinivasa, N. R., Meyer, R. A., and Campbell, J. N. (1991). Pain and hyperalgesia after intradermal injection of bradykinin in humans. Clin. Pharmacol. Ther. 50:721–729.

12. Vegh, A., Papp, J. G., and Parratt, J. (1994). Attenuation of the antiarrhythmic effect of ischaemic preconditioning by blockade of bradykinin B$_2$ receptors. Br. J. Pharmacol. 113:1167–1172.

13. Regoli, D. C., Marceau, F., and Lavigne, J. (1981). Induction of B$_1$ receptors for kinins in the rabbit by a bacterial lipopolysaccharide. Eur. J. Pharmacol. 71:105–115.

14. Barlas, A., Sugio, K., and Greenbaum, L. A. (1985). Release of T-kinin and bradykinin in carageenin induced inflammation in the rat. FEBS Lett. 190:268–270.

15. Farmer, S. G. (1997). The handbook of immunopharmacology: the kinin system, Academic Press, San Diego, Calif.

16. Boissonas, R. A., Guttman, S. T., and Jaquenoud, P. A. (1960). Synthèse de la L-arginyl-L-prolyl-L-prolyl-glycyl-L-phenylanalyly-L-seryl-L-phenylalanyl-L-arginine: distinction entre cet octapeptide et la bradykinine. Helv. Chim. Acta. 43:1481–1487.

17. Bhoola, K. D., Figueroa, C. D., and Worthy, K. (1992). Bioregulation of kinins: kallikreins, kininogens and kininases. Pharmacol. Rev. 44:1–80.

18. Clements, J. A. (1997). The molecular biology of the kallikreins and their roles in inflammation. In: The handbook of immunopharmacology: the kinin system, ed. Farmer, S. G., Academic Press, San Diego, Calif., pp. 72–97.

19. Kress, M., and Reeh, P. W. (1996). Chemical excitation and sensitization in nociceptors. In: Neurobiology of nociceptors, ed. Belmonte, C., and Cervero, F., Oxford University Press, Oxford, pp. 258–297.

20. Burch, R. M., and DeHaas, C. (1990). A bradykinin antagonist inhibits carrageenan edema in rats. Naunyn Schmiedebergs Arch. Pharmacol. 342: 189–193.

21. Armstrong, D., Dry, R. M. L., Keele, C. A., and Markham, J. M. (1952). Pain-producing substances in blister fluid and serum. J. Physiol. 117:4P.

22. Handwerker, H. O. (1976). Influence of algogenic substances and prostaglandins on discharges of unmyelinated cutaneous nerve fibres identified as nociceptors. In: Advances in pain research and therapy, ed. Bonica, J. J., and Albe-Fessard, D. G., Raven Press, New York, pp. 41–51.

23. Kumazawa, T., and Mizumura, K. (1980). Chemical responses of polymodal receptors of the scrotal contents in dogs. J. Physiol. 299:219–231.

24. Schaible, H.-G., and Grubb, B. D. (1993). Afferent and spinal mechanisms of joint pain. Pain 55:5–54.

25. Dray, A. (1994). Tasting the inflammatory soup: role of peripheral neurones. Pain Rev. 1:153–171.

26. Dray, A., and Perkins, M. (1997). Kinins and pain. In: The handbook of immunopharmacology: the kinin system, ed. Farmer, S. G., Academic Press, San Diego, Calif., pp. 157–172.

27. Lang, E., Novak, A., Reeh, P. W., and Handwerker, H. O. (1990). Chemosensitivity of fine afferents from rat skin in vitro. J. Neurophysiol. 63:887–901.

28. Beck, P. W., and Handwerker, H. O. (1974). Bradykinin and serotonin effects on various types of cutaneous nerve fibres. Pflugers Arch. 347:209–222.

29. Kirchoff, C. G., Jung, S., Reeh, P. W., and Handwerker, H. O. (1990). Carrageenan inflammation increases bradykinin sensitivity of rat cutaneous nociceptors. Neurosci. Lett. 111:206–210.

30. Dray, A., Patel, I. A., Perkins, M. N., and Rueff, A. (1992). Bradykinin-induced activation of nociceptors: receptor and mechanistic studies on the neonatal rat spinal cord-tail preparation in vitro. Br. J. Pharmacol. 107:1129–1134.

31. Seabrook, G. R., Bowery, B. J., and Hill, R. G. (1995). Bradykinin receptors in mouse and rat isolated superior cervical ganglion. Br. J. Pharmacol. 115:368–372.

32. Brain, S. D., and Williams, T. J. (1985). Inflammatory oedema induced by synergism between calcitonin gene related peptide and mediators of increased vascular permeability. Br. J. Pharmacol 86:855–860.

33. Shepheard, S. L., Williamson, D. J., Williams, J., Hill, R. G., and Hargreaves, R. J. (1995). Comparison of the effects of sumatriptan and the NK$_1$ antagonist

CP-99,994 on plasma extravasation in dura mater and c-fos mRNA expression in trigeminal nucleus caudalis of rats. Neuropharmacology 34:255–261.

34. Ichinose, M., Nakajima, N., Takahashi, T., Yamauchi, H., Inoue, H., and Takishima, T. (1992). Protection against bradykinin-induced bronchoconstriction in asthmatic patients by neurokinin receptor antagonist. Lancet 340: 1248–1251.

35. Williamson, D. J., Hargreaves, R. J., Hill, R. G., and Shepheard, S. L. (1997). Sumatriptan inhibits neurogenic vasodilation of dural blood vessels in the anaesthetized rat: intravital microscope studies. Cephalalgia 17:525–531.

36. Taiwo, Y. O., Heller, P. H., and Levine, J. D. (1990). Characterisation of distinct phospholipases mediating bradykinin and noradrenaline hyperalgesia. Neuroscience 39:523–531.

37. Basbaum, A. I., and Levine, J. D. (1991). The contribution of the nervous system to inflammation and inflammatory disease. Can. J. Physiol. Pharmacol. 69:647–651.

38. Coderre, T. J., Chan, A. K., Helms, C., Basbaum, A. I., and Levine, J. D. (1991). Increasing sympathetic nerve terminal-dependent plasma extravasation correlates with decreased arthritic joint injury in rats. Neuroscience 40:185–189.

39. Koltzenburg, M., Kress, M., and Reeh, P. W. (1992). The nociceptor sensitisation by bradykinin does not depend on sympathetic neurons. Neuroscience 46:465–473.

40. Schuligoi, R., Donnerer, J., and Amann, R. (1994). Bradykinin-induced sensitization of afferent neurons in the rat paw. Neuroscience 59:211–215.

41. Kummer, W. (1994). Sensory ganglia as a target of autonomic and sensory nerve fibres in the guinea pig. Neuroscience 59:739–754.

42. Green, P. G., Janig, W., and Levine, J. D. (1997). Negative feedback neuroendocrine control of inflammatory response in the rat is dependent on the sympathetic postganglionic neuron. J. Neurosci. 17:3234–3238.

43. Jones, S., Brown, D. A., Milligan, G., Willer, E., Buckley, N. J., and Caulfield, M. P. (1995). Bradykinin excites rat sympathetic neurons by inhibition of M currents through a mechanism involving B_2 receptors and $G_{\alpha q/11}$. Neuron, 64:394–405.

44. Wilk-Blaszczak, M. A., Stein, B., Xu, S., Barbosa, M. S., Cobb, M. H., and Belardetti, F. (1998). The mitogen-activated protein kinase p38-2 is necessary for the inhibition of N-type calcium current by bradykinin. J. Neurosci. 18:112–118.

45. MacNeil, T., Feighner, S., Hreniuk, D. L., Hess, J. F., and Van der Ploeg, L. H. T. (1997). Partial agonists and full antagonists at the human and murine bradykinin B_1 receptors. Can. J. Physiol. Pharmacol. 75:735–740.

46. Allogho, S. N., Gobell, F., Pheng, L. H., Nguyen-Le, X. K., Neugebauer, W., and Regoli, D. (1995). Kinin B_1 and B_2 receptors in mouse. Can. J. Physiol. Pharmacol. 73:1759–1764.

47. Gobeil, F., Neugebauer, W., Nguyen-Le, X. K., et al. (1997). Pharmacological profiles of the human and rabbit B_1 receptors. Can. J. Physiol. Pharmacol. 75:591–595.

48. Brown, M., Weeb, M., Phillips, E., Skidmore, E., and McIntyre, P. (1995). Molecular studies on kinin receptors. Can. J. Physiol. Pharmacol. 73:780–786.

49. Hess, J. F., Borkowski, J. A., MacNeil, T., et al. (1994). Differential pharmacology of cloned human and mouse B_2 bradykinin receptors. Mol. Pharmacol. 45:1–8.

50. Hess, J. F. (1997). Molecular pharmacology of kinin receptors. In: The handbook of immunopharmacology: the kinin system, ed. Farmer, S. G., Academic Press, San Diego, Calif., pp. 45–56.

51. Gera, L., Stewart, J. M., Whalley, E. T., Burkard, M., and Zuzack, J. S. (1996). A new class of potent bradykinin antagonist dimers. Immunopharmacol 33:178–182.

52. Stewart, J. M., Gera, L., Hanson, W., Zuzack, J. S., Burkard, M., McCullough, R., and Whalley, E. T. (1996). A new generation of bradykinin antagonists. Immunopharmacol 33:51–60.

53. Reissmann, S., Schwuchow, C., Seyfarth, L., et al. (1996). Highly selective bradykinin agonists and antagonists with replacement of proline residues by *N*-methyl-D- and L-phenylalanine. J. Med. Chem. 39:929–936.

54. Yang, X., and Polgar, P. (1996). Genomic structure of the human bradykinin B_1 receptor gene preliminary characterisation of its regulatory regions. Biochem. Biophys. Res. Commun. 222:718–725.

55. Aramori, I., Zenhok, J., Morikawa, N., et al. (1997). Nonpeptide mimic of bradykinin with long-acting properties at the bradykinin B_2 receptor. Mol. Pharmacol. 52:16–20.

56. Aramori, I., Zenhok, J., Morikawa, N., et al. (1997). Novel subtype-selective nonpeptide bradykinin receptor antagonists FR16344 and FR173657. Mol. Pharmacol. 51:171–176.

57. Scherrer, D., Daeffler, L., Trifilieff, A., and Gies, J.-P. (1995). Effects of WIN64338, a nonpeptide bradykinin B_2 receptor antagonist, on guinea-pig trachea. Br. J. Pharmacol. 11:1127–1128.

58. Inamura, N., Asano, M., Hatori, C., et al. (1997). Pharmacological characterisation of a novel, orally active, nonpeptide bradykinin B_2 receptor antagonist, FR 167344. Eur. J. Pharmacol. 333:79–86.

59. Griesbacher, T., Sametz, W., Legat, F. J., et al. (1997). Effects of a non-peptide B_2 antagonist FR173657 on kinin-induced smooth muscle contraction and relaxation, vasoconstriction and prostaglandin release. Br. J. Pharmacol. 121:469–476.

60. Regoli, D., Rizzi, A., Calo, G., Nsa Allogho, S., and Gobeil, F. (1997). B1 and B2 kinin receptors in various species. Immunopharmacol. 36:143–147.

61. Abd Alla, S., Quitterer, U., Grigoriev, S., et al. (1997). Extracellular domains of the bradykinin B_2 receptor involved in ligand binding and agonist sensing defined by antipeptide antibodies. J. Biol. Chem. 271:1748–1755.

62. Fathy, D. B., Mathis, S. A., Leeb, T., and Leeb-Lundberg, L. M. F. (1998). The third transmembrane domains of the human B1 and B2 bradykinin receptors subtypes are involved in discriminating between subtype-selective ligands. J. Biol. Chem. 273: 12210–12218.

63. Braun, A., Kammerer, S., Bohme, E., Muller, B., and Roscher, A. A. (1995). Identificantion of polymorphic sites of the human bradykinin B$_2$ receptor gene. Biochem. Biophys. Res. Commun. 211:234–240.

64. Marceau, F. (1995). Kinin B$_1$ receptors: a review. Immunopharmacol 30:1–26.

65. Marceau, F. (1997). Kinin B$_1$ receptor induction and inflammation. In: The handbook of immunopharmacology: the kinin system, ed. Farmer, S. G., Academic Press, San, Diego, Calif., pp. 143–156.

66. Hall, J. M., and Morton, I. K. M. (1997). The pharmacology and immunopharmacology of kinin receptors. In: The handbook of immunopharmacology: the kinin system, ed. Farmer, S. G., Academic Press, San Diego, Calif., pp. 9–44.

67. Drummond, G. R., and Cocks, T. M. (1995). Endothelium-dependent relaxations mediated by inducible B$_1$ and constitutive B$_2$ kinin receptors in the bovine isolated coronary artery. Br. J. Pharmacol. 116:2473–2481.

68. Bhoola, R., Ramsaroop, R., Naidoo, S., Muller-Esterl, W., and Bhoola, K. D. (1997). Kinin receptor status in normal and inflamed gastric mucosa. Immunopharmacol 36:161–166.

69. Tokumasu, T., Veno, A., and Oh-ishi, S. (1995). A hypotensive response induced by des-Arg^9-bradykinin in young brown/Norway rats pretreated with endotoxin. Eur. J. Pharmacol. 274:225–228.

70. Zuzack, J. S., Burkard, M. R., Cuadrado, D. K., Greer, R. A., Selig, W. M., and Whalley, E. T. (1996). Evidence of a bradykinin B1 receptor in human ileum: pharmacological comparison to the rabbit aorta B1 receptor. J. Pharmacol. Exp. Ther. 227:1337–1343.

71. Gobeil, F., Pheng, L. H., Badini, I., et al. (1996). Receptors for kinins in the human isolated umbilical vein. Br. J. Pharmacol. 118:289–294.

72. Drummonds, G. R., and Cocks, T. M. (1995). Endothelium-dependent relaxation to the B$_1$ kinin receptor agonist des-Arg^9-bradykinin in human coronary arteries. Br. J. Pharmacol. 116:3083–3085.

73. Santiago, J. A., Garrison, E. A., Champion, H. C., et al. (1995). Analysis of responses to kallidin, DABK, and DAK in feline hindlimb vascular bed. Am. J. Physiol. 269:H2057–H2064.

74. Raidoo, D. M., Ramsaroop, R., Naidoo, S., Muller-Esterl, W., and Bhoola, K. D. (1997). Kinin receptors in human vascular tissue: their role in atheromatous disease. Immunopharmacol 36:153–160.

75. Bathon, J. M., Manning, D. C., Goldman, D. W., Towns, M. C., and Proud, D. (1992). Characterisation of kinin receptors on human synovial cells and upregulation of receptor number by interleukin-1. J. Pharmacol. Exp. Ther. 260: 384–392.

76. Cassim, B., Naidoo, S., Ramsaroop, R., and Bhoola, K. D. (1997). Immunolocalisation of bradykinin receptors on human synovial tissue. Immunopharmacol 36:121–126.

77. Raidoo, D. M., and Bhoola, K. D. (1997). Kinin receptors on human neurones. J. Neuroimmunol. 77:39–44.

78. Carl, V. S., Moore, E. E., Moore, F. A., and Whalley, E. T. (1996). Involvement of bradykinin B1 and B2 receptors in human PMN elastase release. Immunopharmacol, 33:325–329.

79. Seabrook, G. R., Bowery, B. J., Heavens, R., et al. (1997). Expression of B_1 and B_2 bradykinin receptors mRNA and their functional role in sympathetic gnaglia and dorsal root sensory ganglia neurones from wild-type and B_2 receptor knockout mice. Neuropharmacol 36:1009–1017.

80. Lopes, P., Kar, S., Chretien, L., Regoli, D., Quirion, R., and Couture, R. (1995). Quantitative autoradiographic localization of [^{125}I-Tyr^8]bradykinin receptor binding sites in the rat spinal cord: effects of neonatal capsaicin, noradrenergic deafferentation, dorsal rhizotomy and peripheral axotomy. Neuroscience 68:867–881.

81. Caligiorne, S. M., Santos, R. A. S., and Campagnole-Santos, M. J. (1996). Cardiovascular effects produced by bradykinin microinjection into the nucleus tractus solitarii of anaesthetized rats. Brain Res., 720:183–190.

82. Figueroa, C. D., Dietze, G., and Muller-Esterl, W. (1996). Immunolocalization of bradykinin B2 receptors on skeletal muscle cells. Diabetes 45 Suppl. 1:S24–S28.

83. Song, Q., Wang, D. Z., Harley, R. A., Chao, L., and Chao, J. (1996). Cellular localization of low-molecular-weight kininogen and bradykinin B2 receptor mRNAs in human kidney. Am. J. Physiol. 270:F919–F926.

84. Schremmer-Danninger, E., Heinz-Erian, P., Topfer-Petersen, E., and Roscher, A. A. (1995). Autoradiographic localisation and characterisation of bradykinin receptors in human skin. Eur. J. Pharmacol. 283:207–216.

85. Wiernas, T. K., Griffin, B. W., and Sharif, N. A. (1997). The expression of functionally-coupled B_2-bradykinin receptors in human corneal epithelial cells and their pharmacological characterization with agonists and antagonists. Br. J. Pharmacol. 121:649–656.

86. Chan, D., Gera, L., Helfrich, B., Helm, K., Stewart, J., Whalley, E., and Bunn, P. (1996). Novel bradykinin antagonist dimers for the treatment of human lung cancers. Immunopharmacol 33(1–3):201–204.

87. Nagy, I., Matesz, K., Woolf, C. J., and Urnan, L. (1993). Cobalt uptake enables identification of capsaicin and bradykinin sensitive sub-populations of rat dorsal root gangion cells in vitro. Neuroscience 56:167–172.

88. Babbedge, R., Dray, A., and Urban, L. (1995). Bradykinin depolarises the rat isolated superior cervical ganglion via B_2 receptor activation. Neurosci. Lett. 193:161–164.

89. Davis, A. J., and Perkins, M. N. (1994). Induction of B_1 receptors in vivo in a model of persistent inflammatory mechanical hyperalgesia in the rat. Neuropharmacol 33:127–133.

90. Perkins, M. N., Campbell, E., and Dray, A. (1993). Antinociceptive activity of the bradykinin B$_1$ and B$_2$ receptor antagonists, des-Arg^9[Leu^8]-BK and HOE 140, in two models of persistent hyperalgesia in the rat. Pain 53:191–197.

91. Perkins, M. N., and Kelly, D. (1993). Induction of bradykinin B$_1$ receptors in vivo in a model of ultra-violet irradiation-induced thermal hyperalgesia in the rat. Br. J. Pharmacol. 110:1441–1444.

92. Rupniak, N. M. J., Boyce, S., Webb, J. K., Williams, A. R., Carlson, E., Borkowski, J. A., Hess, J. F., and Hill, R. G. (1997). Effects of the bradykinin B$_1$ receptor antagonist des-Arg^9[Leu^8]bradykinin and genetic disruption of the B$_1$ receptor on nociception in rats and mice. Pain 71:89–97.

93. Cruwys, S. C., Garrett, N. E., Perkins, M. N., Blake, D. R., and Kidd, B. L. (1994). The role of bradykinin B$_1$ receptors in the maintenance of intra-articular plasma extravasation in chronic antigen-induced arthritis. Br. J. Pharmacol. 113:940–944.

94. Dray, A., and Perkins, M. N. (1993). Bradykinin and inflammatory pain. Trends Neurosci. 16:99–104.

95. Steranka, L. R., DeHaas, C. J., Vavrek, R. J., Stewart, J. M., Enna, S. J., and Snyder, S. H. (1987). Antinociceptive effects of bradykinin antagonists. Eur. J. Pharmacol. 136:261–262.

96. Heapy, C. G., Shaw, J. S., and Farmer, S. C. (1993). Differential sensitivity of antinociceptive assays to the bradykinin antagonist HOE 140. Br. J. Pharmacol. 108:209–213.

97. Costello, A. H., and Hargreaves, K. M. (1989). Suppression of carrageenan-induced hyperalgesia, hyperthermia and edema by a bradykinin antagonist. Eur. J. Pharmacol. 171:259–263.

98. Regoli D., Drapeau, G., Rovero, P., Dion, S., Rhaleb, N. E., Barabe, J., D'Orleans-Juste, P., and Ward, P. (1986). Conversion of kinins and their antagonists into B$_1$ receptor activators and blockers in isolated vessels. Eur. J. Pharmacol. 127:219–224.

99. Erdos, E. G. (1990). Some old and some new ideas on kinin metabolism. J. Cardiovasc. Pharmacol. 15:S20–S24.

100. Meini, S., Lecci, A., and Maggi, C. A. (1996). The longitudinal muscle of rat ileum as a sensitive monoreceptor assay for bradykinin B1 receptors. Br. J. Pharmacol. 117:1619–1624.

101. Correa, C. R., and Calixto, J. B. (1993). Evidence for participation of B$_1$ and B$_2$ kinin receptors in formalin-induced nociceptive response in the mouse. Br. J. Pharmacol. 110:193–198.

102. Shibata, M., Ohkubo, T., Takahashi, H., and Inoki, R. (1989). Modified formalin test: characteristic biphasic pain response. Pain 38:347–352.

103. Mantione, C. R., and Rodriguez, R. (1990). A bradykinin (BK)$_1$ receptor antagonist blocks capsaicin-induced ear inflammation in mice. Br. J. Pharmacol. 99:516–518.

104. Asano, M., Inamura, N., Hatori, C., Sawai, H., Kujiwara, T., Katayama, A., Kayakiri, H., Satoh, S., Abe, Y., Inoue, T., Sawada, Y., Nakahara, K., Oku, T., and Okuhara, M. (1997). The identifaction of an orally active, nonpeptide bradykinin B_2 receptor anatgonist, FR173657. Br. J. Pharmacol. 120:617–624.

105. Borkowski, J. A., Ransom, R. W., Seabrook, G. R., Trumbauer, M., Chen, H., Hill, R. G., Strader, C. D., and Hess, J. F. (1995). Targeted disruption of a B2 bradykinin receptor gene in mice eliminates bradykinin action in smooth muscle and neurons. J. Biol. Chem. 270(23):13706–13710.

106. Davis, A., and Perkins, M. N. (1993). The effect of capsaicin and conventional analgesics in two models of monoarthritis in the rat. Agents Actions 38 Spec. No:C10–C12.

107. Pesquero, J. B. (1997). Molecular characterisation and targeted disruption of the mouse B_1 receptor gene. Presented at Gordon Research Conference on Kallikreins and Kinins, Italy.

108. Alfie, M. E., Sigmon, D. H., Pomposiello, S. I., and Carretero, O. A. (1997). Effect of high salt intake in mutant mice lacking bradykinin B_2 receptors. Hypertension 29:483–487.

109. Alfie, M. E., Yang, X. P., Hess, F., and Carretero, O. A. (1996). Salt-sensitive hypertension in bradykinin B_2 receptor knockout mice. Biochem. Biophys. Res. Commun. 224:625–630.

CHAPTER 9

Capsaicin and Vanilloid Receptors

IAIN F. JAMES

Novartis Institute for Medical Sciences
London

REY GARCIA, ANASTASIA LIAPI, AND JOHN N. WOOD

University College London
London

9.1   INTRODUCTION

Capsaicin is the hot component of chili peppers and has proved an invaluable pharmacological tool over recent years, because of its selective excitatory and toxic effects on damage-sensing peripheral neurons. Thanks to molecular cloning studies,[1,2] we now know that these effects are mediated through a specific receptor named VR1 (vanilloid receptor-1), which is also activated by noxious heat as well as by the low pH often associated with tissue damage. In this chapter we review early studies on capsaicin, attempts to exploit its specific actions to develop new analgesic drugs, and recent progress in understanding the mechanism of capsaicin action through activation of specific receptors.

9.2   EARLY STUDIES ON CAPSAICIN

Capsaicin has been a part of the human diet for thousands of years. It has also been used in folk medicine for a variety of conditions, from the treatment of rheumatism and gastric ulcers to appetite stimulation and hair restoration. Capsaicin was first isolated in 1876[3] and the structure (Fig. 9.1) was determined in 1919.[4] The current interest in the biological effects of capsaicin

Molecular Basis of Pain Induction, Edited by John N. Wood
ISBN 0-471-34607-1   Copyright © 2000 by Wiley-Liss, Inc. All rights reserved.

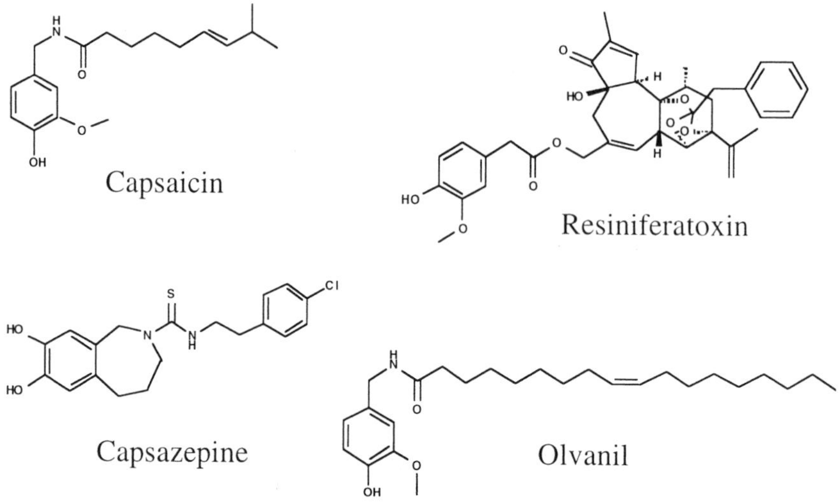

Capsaicin

Resiniferatoxin

Capsazepine

Olvanil

Figure 9.1 Structures of capsaicin analogs.

dates from the work of Jancso and his colleagues in Hungary in the late 1960s and early 1970s (for a review of this period, see Szolcsanyi[5]), who showed specific structural requirements for the induction of pain by capsaicin through its action on nociceptive sensory neurons. More recent work has concentrated on the molecular mechanisms underlying the actions of capsaicin culminating in the recent cloning of a capsaicin receptor.[1]

The pharmacological effects of capsaicin include induction of pain, plasma extravasation, decrease in body temperature, decrease in blood pressure, and changes in heart rate. All these actions are mediated by selective activation of a subset of sensory neurons, the polymodal nociceptors. Capsaicin causes depolarization of sensory neurons, increases in intracellular calcium, and release of neuropeptides such as calcitonin gene–related peptide (CGRP). Capsaicin is also a selective neurotoxin. Long-term treatment can cause selective loss of unmyelinated sensory fibers (C fibers) in newborn and adult rats. Rapid desensitization is a characteristic of capsaicin action. The initial excitatory response is often followed by insensitivity to subsequent applications of capsaicin and inactivation to other noxious stimuli. In rats, mice, and humans, capsaicin causes an increase in nociceptive thresholds probably mediated by this type of inactivation. The excitatory, desensitizing, and toxic effects of capsaicin are selective for sensory C fibers and a population of Aδ fibers. Hence capsaicin has been a useful tool to study the functions and properties of sensory neurons. These aspects of capsaicin biology have been reviewed comprehensively elsewhere.[6] In this chapter we concentrate on the cellular and molecular aspects of capsaicin action and discuss the current major issues concerning the actions of capsaicin. We concentrate on capsaicin receptors and the molecular mechanisms of neuronal activation and desensitization.

9.3   EFFECTS OF CAPSAICIN ON SENSORY NEURONS

The effects of capsaicin on sensory neuron activity have been reviewed extensively by Szolcsanyi[7] and Bevan and Docherty.[8] There is little to add to these reviews except for the discussion of multiple types of capsaicin-evoked inward currents (see Section 9.4.2) and the properties of the cloned channel (Section 9.4.3). In summary, capsaicin causes depolarization and firing of sensory C fibers. The depolarization is caused by capsaicin-induced inward currents carried mainly by Ca^{2+} and Na^+ ions mediated by opening of a nonspecific cation channel. The ion permeability sequence for the channel is $Ca^{2+} > Mg^{2+} > K^+ > Na^+$. It is possible to monitor activation of sensory neurons by capsaicin by following uptake of radioactive $^{45}Ca^{2+}$.[9] This assay has been used to study the structure–activity requirements for capsaicin analogs[10] and to characterize properties of capsaicin receptors (Section 9.4).

Opening of capsaicin-sensitive channels is mediated by binding to a site on the channel molecule (see below). There are two widely used antagonists of capsaicin. Capsazepine is a close analog of capsaicin and is a competitive antagonist.[11] Ruthenium red is a noncompetitive antagonist.[11-13]

Capsaicin-induced excitation of sensory neurons is followed by desensitization to subsequent applications of capsaicin. Receptor desensitization is calcium dependent[14,15] and probably involves calcium-dependent dephosphorylation of the receptor.[14] At higher concentrations, in addition to causing receptor desensitization, capsaicin also causes inactivation of neurons to other noxious stimuli, such as heat and bradykinin.[16,17] The mechanism of inactivation is not well understood.

9.4   CAPSAICIN RECEPTORS

There are four indirect lines of evidence supporting the existence of a specific receptor for capsaicin: (1) There are strict structural requirements for capsaicinlike activity[10]; (2) capsaicin acts on mammalian sensory neurons and not on other cell types[9]; capsaicin sensitivity is regulated by nerve growth factor (NGF) in these cells[18]; (3) photoaffinity probes based on capsaicin cause long-lasting agonist effects on sensory neurones[19]; and (4) there is a competitive antagonist (capsazepine) of capsaicin action.[11] Taken together, these four observations provide strong support for the view that capsaicin interacts with a receptor to excite sensory neurones. This has been confirmed by the development of binding assays and by the recent cloning of the VR1 ion channel that is activated by capsaicin.

9.4.1   Resiniferatoxin Binding

Capsaicin and its close analogs are not suitable ligands for measuring binding because of their relatively low potencies and lipophilicity. The discovery that the plant toxin resiniferatoxin (RTX; Fig. 9.1) has similar actions to capsaicin, but is much more potent, allowed the development of binding assays with [³H]RTX. Initial reports suggested that the affinity of RTX for sites on sensory neurones in the rat was 0.27 nM and that the Hill slope was close to 1, suggesting a single class of noninteracting sites.[20] Binding was inhibited by capsaicin but not phorbol esters (which have some structural similarity to RTX). Similar results were reported by Winter et al.,[21] who found a K_d value of 0.66 nM and a Hill slope of 0.99. In these experiments, RTX binding was inhibited by a series of capsaicin analogs. RTX sites were found in DRG and spinal cord, but not liver, heart, skeletal muscle, cerebellum, or cerebral cortex. Both capsaicin sensitivity and RTX binding were regulated by NGF. Irradiation inactivation experiments suggested a molecular weight of around 270 kD for the binding protein.[22]

In a series of later experiments, Szallasi et al.[23] changed the protocol for the binding assay and now reported that binding of RTX to membranes from rat DRG showed positive cooperativity with an apparent K_d value of 0.024 nM and a Hill slope of 1.7. Furthermore, analogs of RTX apparently showed different degrees of cooperativity,[24] and one analog abolished the cooperative nature of RTX binding.[25] The physical basis and functional consequences of these properties is unclear.

From here the binding experiments became more confusing. Table 9.1 is an attempt to summarize some of the published data. In peripheral tissues (e.g., rat urinary bladder) binding of RTX is noncooperative[27] but has the same affinity as in DRG. In other species the apparent affinity of RTX for its binding sites differs considerably from the rat sites. For example, in pig DRG and in guinea pig spinal cord the values of K_d were reported as 2.2 and 5 nM, compared to about 0.02 nM for the rat (reviewed by Szallasi[26]). Even in the same species, affinity varied from tissue to tissue. In the pig the K_d value was 2.2 nM in DRG and 0.27 nM in spinal cord. In the rat the values were 0.02 nM in DRG, 0.03 nM in urinary bladder, 0.25 nM in airways, and 3 nM in colon.[26] These differences have been used as part of the argument for multiple receptors (see Section 9.4.2). In our current model capsaicin receptors are expressed selectively on sensory neurons. We would therefore expect binding in the spinal cord to represent receptors on the central terminals of sensory neu-

TABLE 9.1   Properties of RTX Binding Sites Vary Between Tissue, Species, and Research Groups

Species	Tissue	K_d (nM)	Positive Cooperativity	Reference
Pig	DRG	2.2		Szallasi[26]
Rat	DRG	0.27	No	Szallasi and Blumberg[20]
	DRG	0.66	No	Winter et al.[21]
	DRG	0.024	Yes	Szallasi et al.[23]
	Urinary bladder	0.03	No	Szallasi et al.[27]
	Urinary bladder	0.06	Yes	Acs et al.[28]
	Colon	3	No	Szallasi[26]
	Airways	0.25	No	Szallasi[26]
	Spinal cord			Szallasi[26]
Guinea pig	Spinal cord			Szallasi[26]
Human	Spinal cord			Szallasi[26]

rons and binding in bladder, airways, and colon to represent receptors on the peripheral terminals. If the affinities are genuinely different in these tissues, either there are different receptors that are transported to central and peripheral terminals differentially with different peripheral receptors in different tissues, or there are high densities of receptor subtypes that are expressed on cells other than sensory neurons. Acs et al.[28] showed that the properties of RTX binding sites were the same in the cell bodies, central terminals, peripheral terminals, and axons of rat sensory neurones.

In general, data from binding assays are confusing. Different groups have reported different binding properties. For example, Acs et al.[28] found cooperative binding for RTX in rat urinary bladder. As mentioned above, Szallasi et al.[27] reported noncooperative binding. Estimates of affinity vary widely between tissues and between species, and there are hints of different activities in functional and binding assays (see below). The inconsistencies in binding data are likely to be resolved as cloned vanilloid receptor subtypes are identified.

9.4.2   Multiple Receptors

Evidence for Multiple Receptors from Binding Assays.   The evidence for multiple receptors from binding assays can be divided into three categories, none of which is definitive. First, there are the reports of different binding properties in different tissues discussed above. Since the only three groups to have published on RTX binding disagree on many details of binding data (see Section 9.4.1 and Table 9.1), this work needs clarification before any final interpretations are made.

Second, for a few compounds there are differences in potencies between binding and calcium uptake assays. For example, Winter et al.[21] found that although the absolute potencies differed, in general the rank order of potencies for a series of capsaicin and RTX analogs were the same in binding and calcium uptake assays. There were two exceptions: capsazepine, which had lower activity in the binding assay than predicted from its activity as an antagonist in the calcium uptake assay, and VOS (*N*-vanillyloctylsulfonamide), which had an EC_{50} value of 2.5 μM in the uptake assay but was inactive up to 100 μM in the binding assay. Acs et al.[29] found a similarly low activity in the binding assay compared to calcium uptake for capsazepine, and saw differences in rank orders of potencies in the two assays for a series of RTX analogs. Classically, differences in rank potencies are taken as indicative of multiple receptors.

Third, there is an argument for receptor subtypes based on differences between activation and desensitization in the calcium uptake assay,[30] which may be summarized as follows. Treatment of DRG neurons with low concentrations of RTX for 6 h leads to inactivation of subsequent responses to RTX and capsaicin in the calcium uptake assay. Under these conditions the concentration response curve for RTX-induced desensitization was similar to the RTX binding curve. In the calcium uptake assay the potency of RTX was much less than in the assay of desensitization. Potency for desensitization with capsaicin was the same as potency in the calcium uptake assay and correlated with affinity of capsaicin in the binding assay. Desensitization to RTX was supposedly not caused by neurotoxicity, because RTX binding sites were still detectable after the pretreatment. These results were interpreted to mean that there must be two receptors. One (called the R-type) controls desensitization but not uptake and is measured in the RTX binding assay. The other (C-type) controls uptake and is not measured in the RTX binding assay.[30] Furthermore, mast cell lines also take up calcium in response to capsaicin and RTX.[31] Pretreatment of mast cells with RTX also causes desensitization, but in this case the potency for desensitization corresponds to the potency in the uptake assay. Vanilloids were not toxic in mast cells and RTX binding was undetectable. The conclusion drawn was that mast cells express only the C-type receptor.

The finding that bone marrow–derived mast cells respond to capsaicin is very important. It is the first demonstration of capsaicin receptors on cells other than sensory neurons and opens up the possibility that endogenous ligands involved in activating sensory neurons through the capsaicin receptor may also have actions on cells of the immune system. Mast cells are present within DRG as well as being associated with the peripheral terminal of C fibers. The argument that these data support the existence of C and R types of receptor, however, is not compelling. It depends entirely on the separation of desensitization from calcium uptake in DRG neurons, but not in mast cells. The fact that no high-affinity binding sites were detected on mast cells probably reflects much lower levels of expression than in neurons. Biro et al. demonstrate that mast cells express only 10% of the receptor levels found in the DRG neurons.

To induce desensitization in the calcium uptake assay, neurons were treated with RTX for 6 h. In our hands, desensitization in the calcium uptake assay with capsaicin is complete within 10 min and with RTX within 20 min (Fig. 9.2). Desensitization of the capsaicin-induced currents also occurs within minutes.[14,15] The 6-hour time course suggests toxicity rather than desensitization. The only evidence against toxicity is that RTX binding sites were still detectable. RTX sites can be measured in membrane preparations, and clearly they could still be present on dead cells. Lack of toxicity (desensitization) at low concentrations of RTX in mast cells could reflect the low level of receptor expression or could reflect differences between the two cell types in mechanisms for handling intracellular calcium.

Evidence for Multiple Receptors from Heterogeneity of Ion Currents.   In single neurons from DRG or trigeminal ganglia under voltage clamp, there are different patterns of current in response to capsaicin and some of its

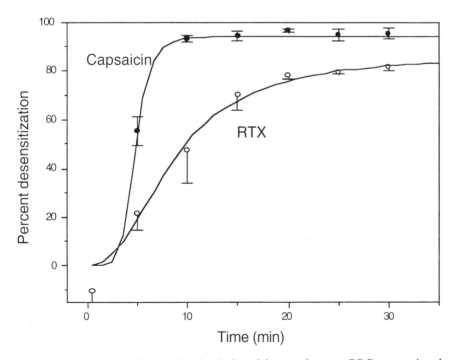

Figure 9.2   Time course of desensitization in the calcium uptake assay. DRG neurons in culture were pretreated with capsaicin or RTX for the times shown. Capsaicin-induced calcium uptake was measured. Data are shown as percent desensitization compared to untreated cells.

analogs. Liu and Simon[32] saw two inward currents evoked by capsaicin. One was rapidly activating, and another was much slower. Similarly, Petersen et al.[33] saw at least two currents in response to capsaicin, which in addition to having different kinetics, had different concentration–response relationships. The slower current was activated at lower concentrations of capsaicin than the fast current. The currents were apparently independent because they could be induced separately. Other compounds, piperine and zingerone, acting by binding to vanilloid receptors, could induce the different currents selectively. Zingerone activated only fast currents; piperine activated only slow currents.[34] The nonpungent capsaicin analogs, olvanil and glyceryl nonivamide (GLNVA), also activated two currents in trigeminal ganglion neurons. The activation kinetics for these currents were considerably slower than those activated by capsaicin.[35] In some cases the two currents showed different rates of desensitization. For example, tachyphylaxis of the rapidly activating current was induced more readily than the slowly activating current after treatment with the RTX analog PPAHV.[36] The heterogeneity of currents and the different desensitization properties have been used as evidence for multiple receptors.

In general, evidence for heterogeneity of binding sites is not strong, and heterogeneity of current activation does not inevitably lead to the conclusion that there is more than one vanilloid receptor. Experience with other systems tells us that there are more than likely multiple vanilloid receptors. Expression of recombinant receptors will tell us if different receptors, or different combinations of receptor subunits, have the properties predicted from measurements of binding, desensitization, and ion currents.

9.4.3   Cloned Receptors

A functional vanilloid (capsaicin) receptor (VR1) activated both by capsaicin and noxious heat (48°C) has been cloned by the Julius laboratory.[1] Pools of clones that conferred capsaicin sensitivity were isolated from a rat DRG cDNA library in the shuttle vector pcDNA3. Increases in intracellular calcium in HEK293 cells transfected with defined pools of cDNA clones were measured using the calcium-sensitive dye Fura-2. The sequence and proposed topology of rat VR1 are shown in Figure 9.3. The functional receptor resembles members of the trp family of proteins in terms of topological organization. Trp proteins are 6-transmembrane monomers first identified in *Drosophila* in the transient receptor potential (trp) mutants, which show deficits in photoreception. VR1 has the characteristic N-terminal ankyrin repeats, and considerable sequence similarity is also apparent in, but is limited to, the sixth transmembrane domain, its flanking sequences, and the loop between transmembrane domains 5 and 6 believed to form part of the presumptive pore region.

AMINO ACID SEQUENCE OF VR1

ⓄⓊⓉⓁⒾⓃⒺⒹ ⒷⓄⓁⒹ: predicted protein kinase A phosphorylation sites
Bold: ankyrin repeats
<u>UNDERLINED:</u> transmembrane regions
SHADOWED ITALICS : pore loop between transmembrane regions five and six

MEQRASLDSEESESPPQENSCLDPPDRDPNCKPPPVKPHIFTTRSR

TRLFGKGDSEEASPLDCPYEEGGLASCPIITVSSVLTIQRPGDGPAS

VRPSSQDSVSAGEKPPRLYDRRSIFDAVAQSNCQELESLLPFLQRSK

KRL<u>T</u>DSEFKDPETGKTCLLKAMLNLHNGQNDTIALLLDVARKTDS

LKQFVNASYTDSYY**KGQTALHIAIERRNMTLVTLLVENGADV**

QAAANGDFFKKTKGRPGFY**FGELPLSLAACTNQLAIVKFLLQ**

NSWQPADISARDSVGNTVLHALVEVADNTVDNTKFVTSMYNEILIL

GAKLHPTLKLEEITNR**KGLTPLALAASSGKIGVLAYILQREIHE**

PECRHLSRKF<u>TEWAYGPVHSSLYDLSCIDTCEKNSVLEVIAYSSSET</u>

PNRHDMLLVEPLNRLLQDKWDRFVKR<u>IFYFNFFVYCLYMIIFTAAAYY</u>

RPVEGLPPYKLKNTVGDYFRVTGEIL<u>SVSGGVYFFFRGIQY</u>FLQRRP<u>S</u>

LKSLFVD<u>SYSEILFFVQSLFMLVSVVLYF</u>SQRKEYVASMV<u>FSLAMGW</u>

<u>TNMLYYTRGFQQMGIYAVMIE</u>KMILRD<u>LCRFMFVYLVFLFGFSTAVV</u>

TLIEDGKNNSLPMESTPHKCRGSACKP*GNSYNSLYSTCLELFKF*

*TIGMG*DLEFTENYD<u>FKAVFIILLLAYVILTYILLLNMLIALMGE</u>TVNKI

AQESKNIWKLQRAITILDTEKSFLKCMRKAFRSGKLLQVGFTPDGKD

DYRWCFRVDEVNWTTWNTNVGIINEDPGNCEGVKRTLSFSLRSGRV

SGRNWKNFALVPLLRDASTRDRHATQQEEVQLKHYTGSLKPEDAEVF

KDSMVPGEK

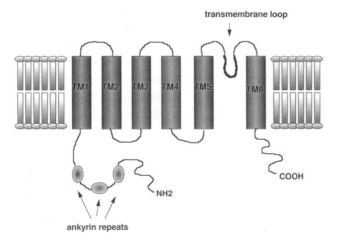

Figure 9.3 Amino acid sequence and proposed membrane spanning regions of VR1.

The fact that the first cloned capsaicin receptor is a member of a known channel family has provided some insights into its properties. Several lines of evidence have suggested that some trp channels may provide the molecular basis for the phenomenon known as capacitative calcium entry (CCE). CCE is loosely defined as the influx of Ca^{2+} from the extracellular space following inositol 1,4,5-triphosphate–induced depletion of internal calcium stores.[37] As such, it has also been referred to as store-operated calcium entry, which appears to be ubiquitous, having been observed in most cells examined for this particular mode of calcium influx. Expression of *Drosophila* trp (Dtrp) in Sf9[38] and 293T cells[39] causes the appearance of novel membrane currents that show modest selectivity for Ca^{2+} and are sensitive to store depletion. In contrast, *Drosophila* trp-like (Dtrpl) forms a rather nonselective, constitutively active cation channel when expressed heterologously.[40] To date, six mammalian trp genes have been cloned and sequenced, either through initial searches of expressed sequence tag databases using the *Drosophila* trp amino acid sequence as the query sequence, or through degenerate reverse transcription-polymerase chain reaction (RT-PCR) using primers designed from the highly conserved regions (transmembrane domains 5 and 6) of *Drosophila* trp and trpl. Trp(s) 1,[41,42] 3,[43] 4,[44] and 6[45] have been sequenced in full, and partial sequences have also been reported for trp(s) 2 and 5,[43] the former of which may be a pseudogene. Functional expression of the available full-length clones in mammalian cells enhances CCE,[43–47] whereas expression of trp cDNA fragments in antisense orientation interfered with endogenous CCE,[43,46] providing a direct connection between trp(s) and store-operated calcium entry. Like *Drosophila* trp, bovine trp 4 appears to be fairly selective for Ca^{2+} and sensitive to store depletion when expressed in HEK293 cells.[44] When expressed in CHO cells, human trp 1 is also activated by store depletion, but the channel formed is fairly nonselective.[47] Trp(s) 3 and 6 have also been functionally expressed and form nonselective cation channels insensitive to store depletion.[45,48] Homomeric and/or heteromultimeric interactions between the different trp proteins may help explain the functional heterogeneity of store-operated conductances observed in various cell types.

The capsaicin vanilloid receptor VR1 also probably exists in a multimeric form as a cation-selection ion channel with a preference for calcium, but does not appear to play any role in capacitative calcium entry. Whether VR1 can heteromultimerize with other trp's or further VR1-like receptors is as yet unknown, but there is certainly strong evidence for an additional capsaicin-activated VR1-like receptor present in mast cells. Biro et al. have characterized a calcium uptake response in these cells, as discussed above.

There are already a large number of trp family members, and there is evidence for other VR1-like receptors. It is likely that these related channels will be gated by a variety of signals. For example, the VR-L gene (vanilloid receptor-like) was cloned by homology to VR1. It is expressed in sensory neurones and lymphocytes but is not activated by capsaicin, moderate heat, or low pH.[49,60] The endogenous activator of this channel is not yet known although high temperatures may activate the channel.[60] The human trp family members trpC6 and trpC3 are activated by diacylglycerol (DAG), which in turn is produced by activation of phospholipase C (PLC).[50] Membrane-impermeable analogs of DAG were active on inside-out patches containing the trp channels, but not on whole cells. Hence the DAG binding site is probably on the intracellular domain of the channel. Similarly, the light-sensitive channels from *Drosophila* trp and trpl are activated by polyunsaturated fatty acids (e.g., arachidonic acid and linolenic acid), which could be generated from DAG.[51] These examples represent a mechanism linking activation of membrane-associated phospholipases, possible after G protein–coupled receptor occupation, to activation of trp channels via an endogenous lipophilic ligand binding to the intracellular surface of the channel.

The VR1 channel may also fall into the same category. Capsaicin can activate VR1 when applied from either the extracellular or cytosolic side of the membrane, but the impermeant capsaicin analog DA5018 is effective only if applied on the cytosolic side.[52] DAG is inactive at VR1 channels.[50] It is feasible that there is another endogenous lipophilic activator of VR1 that normally binds to this site. Other members of the trp family not activated by DAG (e.g., trpC 1, 4, and 5)[50] may also turn out to be activated by other lipophilic mediators.

Noxious heat and lipid mediators are not the only potential activators of VR1. Bevan and Gepetti[53] suggested that proton- and capsaicin-gated currents in DRG represent activation of the same ion channels. More recently, Tominaga et al.[2] have shown that in excised patches, single VR1 channels are activated directly by heat. In addition, protons decreased the temperature threshold for VR1 activation so that at room temperature a moderate reduction in pH caused activation. They concluded that VR1 acts as an integrator of the various pain-producing stimuli and that the effect of any one stimulus cannot be considered in isolation. These observations are particularly intriguing in the context of studies on soups of inflammatory mediators carried out by the Reeh laboratory. They have found that an inward current is evoked by bradykinin, prostaglandin E2, and 5-hydroxytryptamine (5-HT) in sensory neurons at low pH but not at physiological pH.[54] As the current is blocked by 10 μM capsazepine, it is possible that the vanilloid receptor/ion channel is responsible for the inward current. In addition, the same group have provided evidence that a variety of nonsteroidal anti-inflammatory aspirinlike drugs are capsaicin channel blockers on sensory neurons in culture. These observations have yet to be confirmed with expressed VR1 receptors, but they provide one possible mechanism for the analgesic actions of capsaicinlike drugs that desensitize the receptor. Intriguingly, anandamide, an endogenous canna-binoid has also been shown to activate VR1. It is possible that G-proteins link occupation of various receptors to activation of the channel.[61]

9.5   CAPSAICIN AS AN ANALGESIC

Capsaicin causes excitation of polymodal nociceptors and hence is pungent and painful. There is also a paradoxical antinociceptive activity (reviewed by Dray and Dickenson[55]). Some analogs of capsaicin [e.g., olvanil (Fig. 9.1)] have antinociceptive activity in vivo without any overt excitatory side effects (reviewed by Campbell et al.[56]). The mechanistic basis for capsaicin-induced antinociception is not well understood, nor is the separation of excitation from antinociception in olvanil-like compounds. Certainly, olvanil binds to vanilloid receptors and activates the channel.[8] It is also an agonist with a similar potency to capsaicin in the calcium uptake assay.[21] However, it is a poor activator of C fibers.[57] The site of the antinociceptive effects of both capsaicin and olvanil seems to be central rather than peripheral.[57,58]

One plausible proposal for the analgesic mechanism of action of capsaicin was discussed above in relation to the action of inflammatory mediators. Another is that calcium entering the cell through vanilloid channels causes inactivation of voltage-activated calcium channels, resulting in depression of transmitter release from C-fiber terminals in the spinal cord. Capsaicin does cause inhibition of calcium currents in neurons that depolarize in response to capsaicin, and this effect is secondary to a rise in intracellular calcium.[59] Furthermore, both capsaicin and olvanil can inhibit KCl-stimulated release of neuropeptides from spinal cord.[57] If correct, this hypothesis provides only a partial explanation of capsaicin- and olvanil-induced antinociception. It depends entirely on activation of vanilloid channels by the antinociceptive agent and does not account for the lack of excitatory activity in compounds such as olvanil.

9.6   CONCLUSIONS

This is an active and stimulating period in capsaicin research. The cloning of VR1 and VR-L, the search for further subtypes of receptor, and the possible connection or interaction with trp channels will surely lead to more insights into the molecular mechanisms of capsaicin action and the physiological role of VR1, including how it is normally activated. Cloned receptors should also help us to understand how VR1 is regulated, as well as why capsaicin is analgesic and how olvanil and other compounds can work through vanilloid receptors to cause analgesia without the excitatory effects one might expect. Finally, the analysis of VR1 mouse null mutants and the molecular cloning of mast cell capsaicin-gated channels should provide further insights into the functional significance of vanilloid receptors and their role in pain and nociception.

REFERENCES

1. Caterina, M. J., Schumacher, M. A., Tominaga, M., Rosen, T. A., Line, J. D., and Julius, D. (1997). The capsaicin receptor: a heat-activated ion channel in the pain pathway. Nature 389:816–824.
2. Tominaga, M., Caterina, M. J., Malmberg, A. B., Rosen, T. A., Gilbert, H., Skinner, K., Raumann, B. E., Basbaum, A. I., and Julius, D. (1998). The cloned capsaicin receptor integrates multiple pain-producing stimuli. Neuron 21:531–543.
3. Thresh, M. (1876). Pharm. J. Trans. 7–15.
4. Nelson, E. K. (1919). J. Am. Chem. Soc. 127:1115–1472.
5. Szolcsanyi, J. (1984). In: Antidromic vasodilation and neurogenic inflammation, ed. Chahl, L. A., Szolcsanyi, J., and Lembeck, F., Academiai Kiado, Budapest, pp. 7–25.
6. Wood, J. N. (1993). Capsaicin in the study of pain, Academic Press, London.
7. Szolcsanyi, J. (1993). Actions of capsaicin on sensory receptors. In: Capsaicin in the study of pain, ed. Wood, J. N., Academic Press, London, pp. 1–26.
8. Bevan, S. J., and Docherty, R. J. (1993). Cellular mechanisms of the action of capsaicin. In: Capsaicin in the study of pain, ed. Wood, J. N., Academic Press, London, pp. 27–44.
9. Wood, J. N., Winter, J., James, I. F., Rang, H. P., Yeats, J., and Bevan, S. J. (1988). Capsaicin induced ion fluxes in dorsal root ganglion cells in culture. J. Neurosci. 8:3208–3220.
10. Walpole, C. S. J., and Wrigglesworth, R. (1993). Structural requirements for capsaicin agonists and antagonists. In: Capsaicin in the study of pain, ed. Wood, J. N., Academic Press, London, pp. 63–82.
11. Bevan, S., Hothi, S., Hughes, G., James, I. F., Rang, H. P., Shah, K., Walpole, C. S. J., and Yeats, J. (1992). Capsazepine: a competitive antagonist of the sensory neurone excitant capsaicin. Br. J. Pharmacol. 107:544–552.
12. Dray, A., Forbes, C. A., and Burgess, G. (1990). Ruthenium red blocks the capsaicin-induced increased in intracellular calcium and activation of membrane currents in sensory neurons as well as the activation of peripheral nociceptors in vitro. Neurosci. Lett. 110:52–59.
13. Amman, R., and Maggi, C. A. (1991). Ruthenium red as a capsaicin antagonist. Life Sci. 49:849–856.
14. Docherty, R. J., Yeats, J. C., and Boddeke, H. W. (1996). Inhibition of calcineurin inhibits the desensitization of capsaicin-evoked currents in cultured dorsal root ganglion neurones from adult rats. Pflugers Arch. 431:828–837.

15. Koplas, P. A., Rosenberg, R. L., and Oxford, G. S. (1997). The role of calcium in the desensitization of capsaicin response in rat dorsal root ganglion neurons. J. Neurosci. 17:3525–3537.

16. Marsh, S. J., Stansfeld, C. E., Brown, D. A., Davey, R., and McCarthy, D. (1987). The mechanism of action of capsaicin on C-type neurons and their axons in vitro. Neuroscience 23:275–289.

17. Dray, A., Bettaney, J., and Forster, P. (1990). Actions of capsaicin on peripheral nociceptors. Br. J. Pharmacol. 101:727–733.

18. Winter, J., Forbes, C. A., Sterberg, J., and Lindsay, R. M. (1988). Nerve growth factor (NGF) regulates adult rat cultured dorsal root ganglion neuron responses to capsaicin. Neuron 1:973–981.

19. James, I. F., Walpole, C. S. J., Hixon, J., Wood, J. N., and Wrigglesworth, R. (1988). Long lasting agonist activity produced by capsaicin-like photoaffinity probe. Mol. Pharmacol. 33:643–649.

20. Szallasi, A., and Blumberg, P. M. (1990). Specific binding of resiniferatoxin, an ultrapotent capsaicin analog, by dorsal root ganglion membranes. Brain Res. 524:106–111.

21. Winter, J., Walpole, C. S. J., Bevan, S., and James, I. F. (1993). Characterization of resiniferatoxin binding sites on sensory neurons: co-regulation of resinifera-toxin binding and capsaicin sensitivity in adult dorsal root ganglia. Neuroscience 57:747–757.

22. Szallasi, A., and Blumberg, P. M. (1991). Molecular target size of the vanilloid (capsaicin) receptor in pig dorsal root ganglia. Life Sci. 47:1399–1408.

23. Szallasi, A., Lewin, N. A., and Blumberg, P. M. (1993). Vanilloid (capsaicin) receptor in the rat: positive cooperativity of resiniferatoxin binding and its modulation by reduction and oxidation. J. Pharmacol. Exp. Ther. 266:678–683.

24. Appendino, G., Cravotto, G., Palmisano, G., Annunziata, R., and Szallasi, A. (1996). Synthesis and evaluation of phorboid 20-homovanillates: discovery of a class of ligands binding to the vanilloid (capsaicin) receptor with different degrees of cooperativity. J. Med. Chem. 39:3123–3131.

25. Szallasi, A., Acs, G., Cravatto, G., Blumberg, P. M., Lundberg, J. M., and Appendino, G. (1996). A novel agonist, phorbol 12-phenylacetate 13-acetate, 20-homovanillate, abolishes positive cooperativity of binding by the vanilloid receptor. Eur. J. Pharmacol. 299:221–228.

26. Szallasi, A. (1994). The vanilloid (capsaicin) receptor: receptor types and species differences. Gen. Pharmacol. 25:223–243.

27. Szallasi, A., Conte, B., Goso, C., Blumberg, P. M., and Manzini, S. (1993). Characterization of peripheral vanilloid (capsaicin) receptor in the urinary bladder of the rat. Life Sci. 52:PL221–PL226.

28. Acs, G., Palkovits, M., and Blumberg, P. M. (1994). Comparison of [^{3}H]resini-feratoxin binding by the vanilloid (capsaicin) receptor in dorsal root ganglia, spinal cord, dorsal vagal complex, sciatic and vagal nerves and urinary bladder. Life Sci. 55:1017–1026.

29. Acs, G., Lee, J., Marquez, V. E., and Blumberg, P. M. (1996). Distinct structure–activity relations for stimulation of 45Ca uptake and for high affinity binding in cultured dorsal root ganglion neurons and dorsal root ganglion membranes. Brain Res. Mol. Brain Res. 35:173–182.

30. Acs, G., Biro, T., Modarres, S., and Blumberg, P. M. (1997). Differential activation and desensitization of sensory neurons by resiniferatoxin. J. Neurosci. 17:5622–5628.

31. Biro, T., Maurer, M., Modarres, S., Lewin, N. E., Brodie, C., Acs, G., Acs, P., Paus, R., and Blumberg, P. M. (1998). Characterization of functional vanilloid receptors expressed by mast cells. Blood 91:1332–1340.

32. Liu, L., and Simon, S. A. (1996). Capsaicin-induced currents with distinct desensitization and Ca^{2+} dependence in rat trigeminal ganglion cells. J. Neurophysiol. 75:1503–1514.

33. Petersen, M., Lamotte, R. H., Klusch, A., and Kniffki, K.-D. (1996). Multiple capsaicin-evoked currents in isolated rat sensory neurons. Neuroscience 75:495–505.

34. Liu, L., and Simon, S. A. (1996). Similarities and differences in the currents activated by capsaicin, piperine, and zingerone in rat trigeminal ganglion cells. J. Neurophysiol. 76:1858–1869.

35. Liu, L., Lo, Y.-C., Chen, I.-J., and Simon, S. A. (1997). The responses of rat trigeminal ganglion neurons to capsaicin and two nonpungent vanilloid receptor agonists, olvanil and glyceryl nonamide. J. Neurosci. 17:4101–4111.

36. Liu, L., Szallasi, A., and Simon, S. A. (1998). A non-pungent resiniferatoxin analogue, phorbol 12-phenylacetate 13-acetate 20-homovanillate, reveals vanilloid receptor subtypes on rat trigeminal ganglion neurons. Neuroscience 84:569–581.

37. Putney, J. W., Jr. (1986). A model for receptor-regulated calcium entry. Cell Calcium 7:1–12.

38. Vaca, L., Sinkins, W. G., Hu, Y., Kunze, D. L., and Schilling, W. P. (1994). Activation of recombinant trp by thapsigargin in Sf9 insect cells. Am. J. Physiol. Nov.; 267(5 Pt. 1):C1501–C1505.

39. Xu, X.-Z. S., Li, H.-S., Guggino, W. B., and Montell, C. (1997). Coassembly of TRP and TRPL produces a distinct store-operated conductance. Cell 89:1155–1164.

40. Hu, Y., Vaca, L., Zhu, X., Birnbaumer, L., Kunze, D., and Schilling, W. P. (1994). Appearance of a novel Ca^{2+} influx pathway in Sf9 insect cells following expression of the transient receptor potential-like (trpl) protein of *Drosophila*. Biochem. Biophys. Res. Commun. 132:346–354.

41. Wes, P. D., Chevesich, J., Jeromin, A., Rosenberg, C., Stetten, G., and Montell, C. (1995). TRPC1, a human homolog of a *Drosophila* store-operated channel. Proc. Natl. Acad. Sci. USA 92:9652–9659.

42. Zhu, X., Chu, P. B., Peyton, M., and Birnbaumer, L. (1995). Molecular cloning of a widely expressed human homologue for the *Drosophila* trp gene. FEBS Lett. 373:193–198.

43. Zhu, X., Jiang, M., Peyton, M., Boulay, G., Hurst, R., Stefani, E., and Birnbaumer, L. (1996). Trp, a novel mammalian gene family essential for agonist-activated capacitative Ca^{2+} entry. Cell 85:661–671.

44. Philipp, S., Cacalie, A., Freichel, M., Wissenbach, U., Zimmer, S., Trost, C., Marquart, A., Murakami, M., and Flockerzi, V. (1996). A mammalian capacitative calcium entry channel homologous to *Drosophila* TRP and TRPL. EMBO J. 15:6166–6171.

45. Boulay, G., Zhu, X., Peyton, M., Jiang, M., Hurst, R., Stefani, E., and Birnbaumer, L. (1997). Cloning and expression of a novel mammalian homolog of *Drosophila* transient receptor potential (Trp) involved in calcium entry secondary to activation of receptors coupled by the Gq class of G protein. J. Biol. Chem. 272:29672–29680.

46. Birnbaumer, L., Zhu, X., Jiang, J., Boulay, G., Peyton, M., Vannier, B., Brown, D., Platano, D., Sadeghi, H., Stefani, E., and Birnbaumer, M. (1996). On the molecular basis and regulation of cellular capacitative calcium entry: roles for Trp proteins. Proc. Natl. Acad. Sci. USA 93:15195–15202.

47. Zitt, C., Zobel, A., Obukhov, A. G., Harteneck, C., Kalkbrenner, F., Luckhoff, A., and Schultz, G. (1996). Cloning and functional expression of a human Ca^{2+} permeable channel activated by calcium store depletion. Neuron 16:1189–1196.

48. Zhu, X., Jiang, M., and Birnbaumer, L. (1998). Receptor-activated Ca^{2+} influx via human trp3 stably expressed in human embryonic kidney (HEK) 293 cells. J. Biol. Chem. 273:133–142.

49. Garcia, R., Liapi, A., Cesare, T., Bonnert, T., Wafford, K., Clark, S., Young, J., Delmas, P., Whiting, P., McNaughton, P., and Wood, J. N. (1999). VR-L, a vanilloid-receptor-like orphan receptor, is expressed in T-cells and sensory neurons. J. Physiol. 518P:126P.

50. Hofmann, T., Obukov, A. G., Schaefer, M., Harteneck, C., Gudermann, T., and Schulz, G. (1999). Direct activation of human TRPC6 and TRPC3 channels by diacylglycerol. Nature 397:259–263.

51. Chyb, S., Raghu, P., and Hardie, R. C. (1999). Polyunsaturated fatty acids activate the *Drosophila* light-sensitive channels TRP and TRPL. Nature 397:255–259.

52. Jung, J., Hwang, S. W., Kwak, J., Lee, S.-Y., Kang, C.-J., Kim, W. B., Kim, D., and Oh, U. (1999). Capsaicin binds to the intracellular domain of the capsaicin-activated ion channel. J. Neurosci. 19:529–538.

53. Bevan, S., and Geppetti, P. (1994). Protons: small stimulants of capsaicin-sensitive sensory nerves. Trends Neurosci. 17:509–512.

54. Vyklicky, L., Knotkova-Urbancova, H., Vitaskova, Z., Vlachova, V., Kress, M., and Reeh, P. W. (1998). Inflammatory mediators at acidic pH activate capsaicin receptors in cultured sensory neurons from newborn rats. J. Neurophysiol. Feb.; 79(2):670–676.

55. Dray, A., and Dickenson, A. (1993). Capsaicin, nociception and pain. In: Capsaicin in the study of pain, ed. Wood, J. N., Academic Press, London, pp. 239–254.

56. Campbell, E., Bevan, S., and Dray, A. (1993). Clinical applications of capsaicin and its analogues. In: Capsaicin in the study of pain, ed. Wood, J. N., Academic Press, London, pp. 255–272.

57. Dickenson, A., Hughes, C., Rueff, A., and Dray, A. (1990). A spinal mechanism of action is involved in the antinociception produced by the capsaicin analogue NE 19550 (olvanil). Pain 43:353–362.

58. Dickenson, A., Ashwood, N., Sullivan, A. F., James, I. F., and Dray, A. (1990). Antinociception produced by capsaicin: spinal or peripheral mechanism? Eur. J. Pharmacol. 187:225–233.

59. Docherty, R. J., Robertson, B., and Bevan, S. (1991). Capsaicin causes prolonged inhibition of voltage-activated calcium currents in adult rat dorsal root ganglion neurones in culture. Neuroscience 40:513–521.

60. Caterina, M. J., Rosen, T. A., Tominaga, M., and Brake, A. J., Julius, D. (1999). A capsaicin-receptor homologue with a high threshold for noxious heat. Nature Apr. 1; 398(6726):436–441.

61. Zygmunt, P. M., Perersson, J., Andersson, D. A., Chuang, H., Sorgard, M., Di Marzo, V., Julius, D., and Hogetstatt, E. D. (1999). Vanilloid receptors on sensory nerves mediate the vasodilator action of anandemide. Nature 400:452–457.

CHAPTER 10

Examination of the Opioid System Using Targeted Gene Deletions

ANDREAS ZIMMER AND TED USDIN

National Institute of Mental Health
Bethesda, Maryland

10.1   INTRODUCTION

Opiates have been used for millennia to relieve pain. The identification of opiate receptors and endogenous opioid peptides, nearly 25 years ago, suggested that pharmaceutical opiates act on receptors that are part of a neuropeptide system.[1,2] They may mimic some of the functions of the endogenous system and also produce somewhat different net effects by flooding receptor sites. The anatomy of opiate systems was first defined using receptor autoradiography and peptide immunolocalization. This has been further refined by localization of cloned opiate receptors.[3] These data, in combination with extensive physiological studies, have provided considerable insight into where opiates act to modulate sensory information processing. Nonetheless, major questions about the normal physiological role(s) of opioid peptides and receptors remain: Are opioid peptides primary mediators for signaling pain, or any particular sensory modality, at any neuroanatomical level? What information do opioids modulate, and how? How do the different opiate systems interact with each other and with other neurotransmitter systems?

Mice with targeted mutations in the genes for opioid peptides or receptors provide a new set of tools that can be used to address these and other questions about the function and interaction of opiate systems. Several opioid knockout mice have recently been described. Initial studies have confirmed a number of ideas derived from previous anatomical, pharmacological, and physiological experiments, and they have presented some surprises as well. In this chapter

Molecular Basis of Pain Induction, Edited by John N. Wood
ISBN 0-471-34607-1   Copyright © 2000 by Wiley-Liss, Inc. All rights reserved.

we describe some of the results of this first generation of experiments and attempt to illuminate how knockout mice may be used in combination with other established techniques to provide more precise answers to questions about the mechanisms and circuitry underlying analgesia and reward.

Before discussing mouse mutants, a brief review of the molecular players may be helpful. More complete reviews can be found elsewhere.[2,4] Three genes each produce a protein precursor which through proteolytic processing gives rise to a number of opioid peptides. Proopiomelanocortin (POMC), also called the β-endorphin/adrenocorticotrophic hormone (ACTH) precursor, produces β-endorphin (β-END), a 31-residue opioid peptide, as well as adrenocorticotrophic hormone (ACTH) and three potential melanocyte stimulating hormone (MSH)-like peptides. Proenkephalin encodes four copies of [Met]enkephalin, one copy of [Leu]enkephalin, and two C-terminal extended [Met]enkephalins. Prodynorphin encodes α- and β-neoendorphin, as well as dynorphin A and dynorphin B. Processing and posttranslation modification of these peptides varies between tissues. All of the opioid peptides include the N-terminal sequence Tyr-Gly-Gly-Phe. [Met]enkephalin extends this with a methionine, and [Leu]enkephalin with a leucine. β-Endorphin is extended from the [Met]enkephalin sequence while the neo-endorphins and dynorphins are extended from the [Leu]enkephalin sequence. Three genes also encode the pharmacologically defined μ, δ, and κ opiate receptors (MOR, DOR, and KOR) which are members of the superfamily of seven transmembrane domain G-protein-coupled receptors. Following cloning of the delta opiate receptor, sequence homology-based techniques were used to clone the mu and kappa receptors, whose existence was established previously.

These experiments also lead to the identification of a receptor, ORL1, that was 50% identical to the known opioid receptors but did not bind to any of the opioid peptide ligands.[5,6] A search for its ligand resulted in identification of nociceptin, a heptade capeptide that closely resembles dynorphin A.[7–9] In contrast to opioid peptides, nociceptin causes allodynia or hyperalgesia upon intracerebroventricular or intrathecal injection.[7,10,11] Interestingly, the action of nociceptin can be blocked by nocistatin, another biologically active peptide derived from the same nociceptin precursor.[12]

10.2 GENERATING MUTANT MICE

Recently, several laboratories have used gene targeting to generate mouse strains with mutations in the MOR,[13–17] KOR,[18] and DOR[19] genes and in the preproenkephalin encoding gene Penk2,[20] the β-endorphin-encoding POMC genes[21] and in the nociceptin receptor ORL1.[22] These animals fail to produce the targeted components of the endogenous opioid system. This approach is now a standard technique in molecular genetics and has been described in several excellent reviews.[23–26] Inactivation of the genes encoding opioid receptors and endogenous peptide ligands was in most cases achieved through the homologous insertion of bacterial sequences into the target gene locus. These insertions, often accompanied by simultaneous deletion of target DNA sequences, all seemed to have resulted in the generation of null alleles (i.e., functionally inactive genes).

A notable exception was the targeted mutation of the β-endorphin-producing POMC gene. β-endorphin is generated, like other opioid peptides, through proteolytic cleavage of a polypeptide protein precursor, in this case proopiomelanocortin. Unlike other opioid precursors, proopiomelanocortin produces a variety of nonopioid peptides with different physiological activities, including adrenocorticotropic hormone (ACTH), melanocyte stimulating hormones (α-MSH, γ-MSH), and lipotropins, as well as β-endorphin. A POMC null allele may lead to severe developmental or physiological defects in homozygous animals, and thus it might have been difficult to determine the contribution of the β-endorphin deficiency to the overall phenotype. To overcome this potential problem, Rubenstein and co-workers (1993) devised a very elegant targeting strategy to introduce a point mutation into the POMC coding region. This specifically eliminated production of β-endorphin while leaving the rest of the gene essentially intact.[21,27]

All mice with mutations in the opioid system develop without any apparent anatomical defects, are fertile, and care for their offspring. A possible exception may be found in MOR knockout male mice, where a decrease in sperm count and motility was found.[16] Nevertheless, these mice were fertile. The absence of gross developmental defects was surprising, because a substantial body of evidence suggested that opioid peptides have developmental functions, in addition to their role as neurotransmitters. The preproenkephalin (Penk2) gene, for example, is widely expressed in many nonneuronal tissues during embryonic development and has been implicated in the development of mesodermal tissues.[28–30] In fact, the preproenkephalin cDNA was first isolated from a concavalin A–activated mouse T-helper cell line,[31] and it has been shown to be abundant in activated, but undetectable in resting, T cells. It is also well known that chronic morphine treatment of mice inhibits proliferation and differentiation of thymic lymphocytes and leads to apoptotic degeneration of the thymus.[32–34] Interestingly, Yu and co-workers showed that the proliferation of granulocyte-macrophage, erythroid, and multipotential progenitor cells was increased in MOR knockout mice.[16] These results may suggest that the endogenous opioid system plays an important role in the regulation of immune functions which are not easy to detect under standard laboratory conditions.

Nociceptin receptor knockouts displayed a temporary increase in the threshold of auditory brain stem responses after exposure to intense sound, indicating that the nociceptin system modulates auditory function.[22] Interestingly, nociceptin knockouts also showed improved performance in several tests of learning and memory.[35,36] Physiological analysis revealed that such animals had larger long-term potentiation in the hippocampal CA1 region.[36]

The absence of gross developmental defects does not exclude the possibility of a developmental role of opioid peptides, however, as other studies have demonstrated a remarkable redundancy of some signal-transduction pathways during embryonic development. Thus it may be necessary to generate double-mutant mice before developmental defects become apparent. In addition, subtle defects may have escaped detection.

10.3 EXPRESSION STUDIES

Expression of opioid receptors and their peptide ligands was studied in some knockout mice to verify the mutation and to determine whether regulation of the intact components of the opioid system was affected. In general, the mutated gene product was reduced in a gene dose-dependent manner.

Receptor binding studies were performed using radiolabeled ligands in MOR, DOR, KOR, and Penk2 knockout mice. Saturation analysis of ligand binding to total brain homogenates from heterozygous MOR, DOR, and KOR mutant animals revealed a 40 to 60% reduction of B_{max} values for the binding sites of the mutated receptors, while B_{max} and K_d values similar to those of wild-type mice were found for the binding sites of intact receptors.[13,14,17,18] Binding sites of mutant receptors were undetectable in homozygous mutants, whereas nonmutated receptors remained unchanged. Autoradiographic mapping confirmed these results and showed a similar spatial distribution of intact receptors throughout the brains of wild-type and knockout animals, as well as an equal reduction in mutant receptor binding sites in all areas where they are expressed in heterozygous animals.[13,18,37] Expression of opioid peptides in MOR and KOR knockouts was studied using in situ hybridization.[13,18] No differences in the levels and distribution of enkephalin, dynorphin, or proopiomelanocortin mRNAs were found.

Enkephalin knockout mice also exhibited a gene dosage-dependent reduction of Penk2 mRNA and enkephalin peptide levels (44% of wild-type levels in heterozygous mice, no detectable enkephalin immunoreactivity in homozygous mutants), while the expression of dynorphin and endorphin remained unchanged.[20] Interestingly, however, homozygous mutants exhibited a significant and regionally specific up-regulation of μ- and δ-receptor expression.[38] Together, these results may indicate that the expression of opioid receptors is regulated, in part, by ligand levels, while expression of the opioid peptides is not affected by the presence or absence of their receptor.

10.4 PAIN PERCEPTION AND STRESS-INDUCED ANALGESIA

The apparently good health of opioid knockout mice is important for the analysis of sensory mechanisms and animal behaviors. It is not uncommon for knockout mice to exhibit developmental defects and/or compromised health in addition to behavioral defects. In these instances it is often difficult to ascertain whether the behavioral abnormality is caused directly by the absence of the gene product or is due to pathological adaptations.

A number of tests have been developed to assess behavioral responses to nociceptive stimuli in mice.[39] The tail flick and hot plate tests measure response latencies to thermal nociceptive stimuli. It is generally assumed that behavioral responses in these assays involve different levels of information processing. The tail flick reaction is a spinal reflex; the hot plate assay also involves cerebral functions. Other commonly used assays include the application of chemical irritants, such as formalin injection under the skin of the hindpaw, or the intraperitoneal injection of a dilute solution of acetic acid or 2-phenyl-1,4-benzoquinone. In these tests, the number or frequency of particular nociceptive responses are quantitated.

Alterations in baseline nociceptive thresholds were seen in some opioid knockout mice. These nociceptive defects were dependent on the assay as well as the particular gene mutated. MOR knockout mice exhibited slight hyperalgesia in the tailflick test and the hot plate assay at high, but not low, stimulus temperatures (55 versus 52°C).[14] KOR knockouts exhibited normal nociceptive thresholds in all tests (tail immersion, hot plate, tail pressure, formalin), except for the acetic acid–induced writhing test, where they showed an increased number of nociceptive behaviors, indicating hyperalgesia.[18] Enkephalin knockout mice showed marked hyperalgesia in the hot plate test but reacted normally in the tail flick assay.[20] After injection of formalin, enkephalin-deficient mice failed to display normal recuperative behaviors, such as paw licking and paw lifting, but instead, became agitated and displayed periods of intense sniffing. Nociceptin receptor knockouts showed normal pain responses in the tail flick, hot plate, electric foot shock, and writhing tests.[22,35] No abnormalities in baseline nociceptive responses have been reported in DOR or endorphin knockout mice. Together, these results suggest that individual opioid receptors and opioid peptides have distinct roles in nociceptive signaling (Table 10.1).

These data strongly support the notion that genetic factors may contribute to the perception of pain. However, the perception of pain is also clearly dependent on situational factors. For example, stressful or dangerous situations can reduce the pain thresholds [stress-induced analgesia (SIA)], whereas anxiety or the expectation of pain can enhance the subjective experience of pain.[40] Several lines of evidence suggest that endogenous opioids play a major role in

TABLE 10.1   Major Phenotypes in Opioid Knockout Mice

Gene Product	Nociception and Analgesia	Other Phenotypes
MOR	• Hyperalgesia in tail flick test under some experimental conditions • Slight hyperalgesia in hot plate test at high temperatures • Insensitive to morphine • Normal heroin and M6G analgesia • Reduced responses to KOR agonists • Reduced responses to DOR agonists	• Absence of morphine withdrawal symptoms • Absence of morphine-induced conditioned place preference • Absence of morphine immunosuppression • Reduced fertility • Reduced sexual activity
DOR	• Normal morphine analgesia • Insensitive to DOR agonists	
KOR	• Increased visceral pain sensitivity • Normal morphine analgesia	• Attenuated morphine withdrawal symptoms
Nociceptin receptor	• Normal baseline nociceptive behaviors • Loss of nociceptin-induced hyperalgesia	• Loss of nociceptin-induced hypoactivity • Disregulation of hearing ability • Enhanced learning and memory • Larger long-term potentiation in CA1
Preproenkephalin	• Hyperalgesia in hot plate test • Abnormal responses in formalin test • Normal stress-induced analgesia	• Increased aggressive behaviors • Increased anxiety-related behaviors
Proopiomelanocortin	• Normal baseline nociceptive behaviors • Normal morphine analgesia • Reduced analgesia after warm water swim stress • Increased analgesia after cold water swim stress • Increased stress-induced analgesia after naloxone treatment	

an intrinsic pain modulatory system: electric stimulation of specific brain regions, such as the periaqueductal gray area, results in profound analgesia, which is reversed by opioid antagonists. On the other hand, microinjection of opioids into these brain regions can mimic the analgesic effect of the electrical stimulation. In rodents, several "natural" stimuli lead to stress-induced analgesia, which can often be abrogated with opioid antagonists.

Stress-induced analgesia was studied using various paradigms in mice that lacked β-endorphin[21] or enkephalin.[20] Enkephalin knockouts were subjected to repeated foot shocks, a procedure known to produce opioid-dependent analgesia. Analgesia was determined by measuring tail flick latencies before and after the foot shock stress. Wild type and knockout animals exhibited similar baseline tail flick latencies and a similar increase in the tail flick latency, indicating that similar levels of analgesia were induced. Analgesia was also produced in enkephalin deficient mice with a short swim stress and measured in the hot-plate assay. At high water temperatures (34°C), moderate analgesia was produced that seemed to be entirely dependent on the opioid system and was completely blocked with opioid antagonists. At low water temperatures (4°C), a very robust analgesia was induced that seemed to have an opioid-dependent and an opioid-independent component and it was only partially blocked with opioid antagonists. Enkephalin knockouts exhibited normal stress-induced analgesia at both temperatures, indicating that enkephalin is not essential for the responses measured in these paradigms.

β-Endorphin-deficient mice displayed significantly more analgesia than wild-type controls in the hot plate assay after a 3-min swim stress at low water temperature (10°C) but had normal analgesia at higher water temperatures (20°C). Stress-induced analgesia under these experimental conditions, however, was not blocked by naloxone and thus seemed to be predominantly nonopioid mediated. When analgesia was measured with the abdominal constriction assay, after a 45-s swim at 20°C, significant analgesia was found in wild-type mice that was partially blocked by naloxone. Paradoxically, β-endorphin mice exhibited significantly increased stress-induced analgesia after naloxone administration, while little or no analgesia was observed in knockout mice after saline injection. Together, these results suggest that nonopioid pain inhibitory mechanisms may be enhanced in β-endorphin deficient mice.

10.5 PHARMACOLOGICAL TESTING

It has been difficult to assess the role of individual opioid receptors in pharmacological responses to opioids. Although there is substantial evidence to suggest that morphine-induced analgesia is mediated primarily by MOR, DOR and KOR may also be involved.[41] MOR knockout mice were virtually resistant to the analgesic effects of morphine, as measured in the tail flick and hot plate tests, even at high cumulative doses (up to 56 mg/kg), whereas wild-type mice exhibited profound analgesia.[13,14,17] Heterozygous mice displayed an intermediate phenotype. This result was somewhat unexpected because morphine can bind and activate the DOR, and DOR-specific agonists can elicit analgesia in these nociceptive tests. Heroin and its major metabolite morphine-6β-glucuronide also failed to produce analgesia in MOR knockout animals.[42] However, preliminary reports suggest that animals with a partial deletion of the MOR gene (deleting only exon 1) still seem to display heroin and morphine-6β-glucuronide analgesia, while morphine has no effects in these mice.[15,43,44] These mice also show morphine-6β-glucuronide binding sites that are distinct from the traditional MOR binding site. Thus distinct receptors may be produced through differential splicing and/or promoter use at the MOR gene, and those receptors seem to mediate at least some of the effects of heroin.

The MOR also plays a predominant role in morphine reward and dependence. The rewarding effects of morphine, determined with the conditioned place preference test, were lost in MOR-deficient mice.[13] There were also no signs of physical morphine dependence in MOR knockout animals, as they lacked any naloxone-precipitated morphine withdrawal symptoms (jumping, sniffing, teeth chattering, ptosis, wet-dog shakes, paw tremor, tremor, diarrhea, weight loss, reduction in body temperature) and showed no chronic morphine-increased striatal adenylyl cyclase activity.[13] Finally, MOR knockout mice were resistant to morphine immunosuppression[45] and respiratory effects of morphine.[17,46]

Morphine analgesia was apparently unaffected in KOR[18] and DOR[19] knockout mice, providing further evidence that DOR and KOR have little, if any, contribution to morphine analgesia. On the other hand, the DOR- and KOR-specific agonists [D-Pen2,D-Pen5]enkephalin (DPDPE) and U-50,488H induced analgesia in wild-type but not in DOR and KOR knockout mice, respectively. Interestingly, KOR knockout mice also exhibited an attenuation of naloxone-precipitated morphine withdrawal symptoms. This result, together with the observation that κ-selective antagonists can precipitate withdrawal signs in morphine-dependent mice, suggests a modulatory role for the KOR in morphine dependence. On the other hand, the KOR does not appear to be involved in modulating the rewarding properties of morphine, as the morphine-conditioned place preference was not altered in KOR knockout mice.

Nociceptin receptor knockouts were resistant to the locomotor and hypoalgesic effects of nociceptin.[22,47] Analgesia, produced by a single injection of morphine, was normal in these animals. Nociceptin receptor-deficient mice did show a somewhat reduced tolerance to morphine analgesia following 5 days of its administration.[48]

The antinociceptive effect of morphine can be modulated by DOR agonists.[49–52] Coadministration of a subantinociceptive dose of the δ-selective agonist DPDPE increased the antinociceptive potency of morphine, whereas a subeffective dose of a different δ-selective agonist [D-Ala2,Met5]enkephalinamide (DAMA) decreased morphine antinociception. Similarly, subantinociceptive doses of [D-Ala2,Glu4]deltorphin resulted in a leftward displacement of the morphine dose–effect curve (i.e., positive modulation), whereas [Met5]enkephalin resulted in a rightward displacement of the morphine dose–effect curve (i.e., negative modulation). These studies suggested functional interactions between the μ- and δ-opioid receptors. Support for such an interaction was provided by the analysis of opioid receptor knockout mice. Although morphine analgesia was intact in DOR and KOR knockouts, MOR-deficient animals showed a marked reduction in analgesia and respiratory effects with δ-selective agonists DPDPE[14] and Tyr-D-Ser(O-*t*-Bu)-Gly-Phe- Leu-Thr(O-*t*-Bu) (7, BUBU),[13,53] but not with the κ-selective agonist U-50,488H.[46] These results indicate that MOR and DOR, but not MOR and KOR, cooperate in vivo to mediate opioid effects. It is not clear whether this receptor crosstalk occurs within the same cell or involves separate neurons. However, at the cellular level, DOR signaling appears to be intact, because the analysis of agonist-induced [^{35}S]GTPγS binding showed that DOR coupling to intracellular effectors is unchanged in MOR knockout animals. It therefore seems more likely that the MOR/DOR synergism involves functional interactions within a neuronal network.

10.6   SPONTANEOUS, EMOTIONAL, AGGRESSIVE, AND SEXUAL BEHAVIORS

Opioids are known to induce hyperactivity, whereas nociceptin administration leads to profound hypoactivity. If the opioid/nociceptin system were to play a dominant role in the regulation of activity states, it could be expected that opioid knockouts would be hypoactive, while nociceptin receptor knockouts could be expected to be hyperactive. Proenkephalin knockout mice showed a reduction in activity (approximately 20%) in the open field test.[20] The MOR knockouts also exhibited a slight hypolocomotion that was not changed after morphine treatment.[16] KOR-deficient mice behaved normally in the open field test.[18] Surprisingly, nociceptin receptor knockouts were also moderately hypoactive.[22] Locomotor activity was not changed by nociceptin administration in these animals, indicating that the nociceptin-induced hypoactivity is indeed mediated through the nociceptin receptor.

A more detailed analysis of exploratory behaviors in Penk2 knockout mice in the open field test reveled that these mice were also less likely than wild-type controls to enter the central area of the open field. This behavioral pattern is often considered an indication that emotional behaviors in these animals are affected. When these animals were tested for anxiety in another animal model, the O-maze test, they also exhibited signs of increased anxiety-like behaviors. Hence it is possible that the proenkephalin mutation affected emotional behaviors in these mice. Emotion-related responses were also analyzed in KOR knockout (open field, O-maze, elevated plus maze, Y-maze), but no significant differences between wild-type and mutant mice were found.

The response of enkephalin knockout mice to handling during animal husbandry and analgesia testing suggested that these animals may be more aggressive than wild-type littermates. Aggressive behaviors were therefore quantitated in the resident–intruder paradigm.[20] In this test the attack latency and attack intensity of an isolated male mouse toward another male introduced into its home cage is measured. Enkephalin knockout animal show less attack latency and more fighting activity than that shown by wild-type animals. However, the difference between knockout and wild-type mice became smaller when the experiment was repeated with the same animals: Wild-type mice became more aggressive with repeated violations of their territory, while responses of enkephalin knockouts remain unchanged. One interpretation is that enkephalin-deficient mice approach the maximum fighting response faster than do wild-type animals, but they do not appear to react more violently or viciously toward an intruder than do wild-type mice. In summary, the alterations in pain-, emotion-, and anxiety-related behaviors in Penk2 knockout mice have been interpreted as indicating that enkephalin is involved in the regulation of responses to painful or threatening environmental stimuli.

Although all mice with mutations in genes of the opioid system were fertile, Tian et al.[16] observed that it took male MOR knockout mice longer to impregnate a female compared to wild-type males and they produced somewhat smaller litters. The diminished reproductive behavior could in part be explained by a slightly reduced sperm count and diminished sperm motility in MOR mutant males. In addition, MOR knockout males produced significantly fewer seminal plugs after being left overnight in a cage with female mice. These findings prompted a more detailed analysis of sexual behavior, which was done by introducing an estrous-phase female wild-type mouse into the cage of mutant or wild-type males. Wild-type animals will first inspect the female and within a few minutes mount the female. Mutant males exhibited a significantly increased mounting latency, had fewer intromissions, and failed to ejaculate during the two hour test. These results show, that the endogenous opioid system plays an important role in murine sexual behavior and reproductive physiology.

10.7 CONCLUSIONS

The first round of experiments using mice with knockout mutations in opioid system genes is nearly complete (Table 1). These experiments have contributed to clarification of several questions about the functional role of different opiates (Fig. 10.1). In some cases they have provided strong support for an existing view of opiate function. For instance, they have confirmed that the MOR mediates morphine's effects in the tail flick, and hot plate tests and have demonstrated that it has a predominant role in mediating morphine's effects on reward and dependence. The initial observations of the responses of

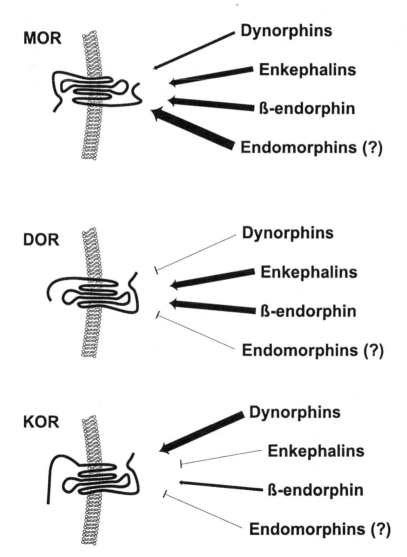

Figure 10.1 Binding potencies of endogenous ligands for the μ-, κ-, and δ-opioid receptors and the nociceptin receptor. The relative binding affinities are indicated by arrows. Note that the gene(s) that encode endorphins, two novel peptides with high affinity and specificity for the MOR isolated by Zadina et al.,[54] have not been cloned yet. Activation of the nociceptin receptor by nociceptin can be blocked with nocistatin, another biologically active peptide derived from the nociceptin precurser.

the different knockout mice in established pain measurement and behavioral paradigms emphasize that the different opioid receptors and peptides have different but not completely independent roles. Because these animals appear healthy and have no obvious developmental defects it should now be possible to use them to examine subtle behavioral and physiological phenomenon. The next generation of experiments with these animals should include fine dissection of which receptors and peptides are involved in different paradigms and should lead to insights into their roles in functional and anatomic pathways. Future experiments may use crosses between these and other knockout animals to examine redundancy and interplay between genes. It is quite reasonable to believe that they will contribute to mechanistic understanding of pain perception, tolerance, reward and the roles of opiates in a number of behaviors. These mice have demonstrated the great complexity in opioid physiology but have also provided tools for its examination.

REFERENCES

1. Brownstein, M. J. (1993). A brief history of opiates, opioid peptides, and opioid receptors. Proc. Natl. Acad. Sci. USA 90:5391–5393.
2. Kieffer, B. L. (1995). Recent advances in molecular recognition and signal transduction of active peptides: receptors for opioid peptides. Cell. Mol. Neurobiol. 15:615–635.
3. Mansour, A., Fox, C. A., Akil, H., and Watson, S. J. (1995). Opioid-receptor mRNA expression in the rat CNS: anatomical and functional implications. Trends Neurosci. 18:22–29.
4. Akil, H., Herz, A., and Simon, E. (1993). Opioids, Vol. 1, Springer-Verlag, New York.
5. Mollereau, C., et al. (1994). ORL1, a novel member of the opioid receptor family: cloning, functional expression and localization. FEBS Lett. 341:33–38.
6. Fukuda, K., et al. (1994). cDNA cloning and regional distribution of a novel member of the opioid receptor family. FEBS Lett. 343:42–46.
7. Meunier, J. C., et al. (1995). Isolation and structure of the endogenous agonist of opioid receptor-like ORL1 receptor [see comments]. Nature 377:532–535.
8. Mollereau, C., et al. (1996). Structure, tissue distribution, and chromosomal localization of the prepronociceptin gene. Proc. Natl. Acad. Sci. USA 93:8666–8670.
9. Reinscheid, R. K., et al. (1995). Orphanin FQ: a neuropeptide that activates an opioidlike G protein-coupled receptor. Science 270:792–794.
10. Mogil, J. S., et al. (1996). Orphanin FQ is a functional anti-opioid peptide. Neuroscience 75:333–337.
11. Okuda-Ashitaka, E., et al. (1996). Identification and characterization of an endogenous ligand for opioid receptor homologue ROR-C: its involvement in allodynic response to innocuous stimulus. Brain Res. Mol. Brain Res. 43:96–104.

12. Okuda-Ashitaka, E., et al. (1998). Nocistatin, a peptide that blocks nociceptin action in pain transmission. Nature 392:286–289.

13. Matthes, H. W., et al. (1996). Loss of morphine-induced analgesia, reward effect and withdrawal symptoms in mice lacking the μ-opioid-receptor gene. Nature 383:819–823.

14. Sora, I., et al. (1997). Opiate receptor knockout mice define μ receptor roles in endogenous nociceptive responses and morphine-induced analgesia. Proc. Natl. Acad. Sci. USA 94:1544–1549.

15. Schuller, A. G. P., et al. (1997). Heroin and M6G analgesia in μ opioid receptor deficient mice. Soc. Neurosci. Abst. 235:6.

16. Tian, M., et al. (1997). Altered hematopoiesis, behavior, and sexual function in μ opioid receptor-deficient mice. J. Exp. Med. 185:1517–1522.

17. Loh, H. H., et al. (1998). μ Opioid receptor knockout in mice: effects on ligand-induced analgesia and morphine lethality. Brain Res. Mol. Brain Res. 54:321–326.

18. Simonin, F., et al. (1998). Disruption of the kappa-opioid receptor gene in mice enhances sensitivity to chemical visceral pain, impairs pharmacological actions of the selective kappa-agonist U-50,488H and attenuates morphine withdrawal. EMBO J. 17:886–897.

19. Zhu, Y., et al. (1997). Genetic disruption of the mouse delta opioid gene. In: European Opioid Conference 6.

20. König, M., et al. (1996). Pain responses, anxiety, and aggression in mice deficient in pre-proenkephalin. Nature 383:535–538.

21. Rubinstein, M., et al. (1996). Absence of opioid stress-induced analgesia in mice lacking β-endorphin by site directed mutagenesis. Proc. Natl. Acad. Sci. USA 93:3995–4000.

22. Nishi, M., et al. (1997). Unrestrained nociceptive response and disregulation of hearing ability in mice lacking the nociceptin/orphanin FQ receptor. EMBO J. 16:1858–1864.

23. Zimmer, A. (1992). Manipulating the genome by homologous recombination in embryonic stem cells. Annu. Rev. Neurosci. 15:115–137.

24. Melton, D. W. (1994). Gene targeting in the mouse. Bioessays 16:633–638.

25. Bronson, S. K., and Smithies, O. (1994). Altering mice by homologous recombination using embryonic stem cells. J. Biol. Chem. 269:27155–27158.

26. Capecchi, M. R. (1994). Targeted gene replacement. Sci. Am. 270:52–59.

27. Rubenstein, M., Japon, M. A., and Low, M. J. (1993). Introduction of a point mutation into the mouse genome by homologous recombination in embryonic stem cells using a replacement type vector with a selectable marker. Nucleic Acids Res. 21:2613–2617.

28. Rosen, H., Polakiewicz, R. D., Benzakine, S., and Bar, S. Z. (1991). Proenkephalin A in bone-derived cells. Proc. Natl. Acad. Sci. USA 88:3705–3709.

29. Polakiewicz, R. D., and Rosen, H. (1990). Regulated expression of proenkephalin A during ontogenic development of mesenchymal derivative tissues. Mol. Cell. Biol. 10:736–742.

30. Polakiewicz, R. D., Behar, O. Z., Comb, M. J., and Rosen, H. (1992). Regulation of proenkephalin expression in cultured skin mesenchymal cells. Mol. Endocrinol. 6:399–408.

31. Zurawski, G., et al. (1986). Activation of mouse T-helper cells induces abundant pre-proenkephalin mRNA synthesis. Science 232:772–775.

32. Fuchs, B. A., and Pruett, S. B. (1993). Morphine induces apoptosis in murine thymocytes in vivo but not in vitro: involvement of both opiate and glucocorticoid receptors. J. Pharmacol. Exp. Ther. 266:417–423.

33. Freier, D. O., and Fuchs, B. A. (1993). Morphine-induced alterations in thymocyte subpopulations of B6C3F1 mice. J. Pharmacol. Exp. Ther. 265:81–88.

34. Sei, Y., Yoshimoto, K., McIntyre, T., Skolnick, P., and Arora, P. K. (1991). Morphine-induced thymic hypoplasia is glucocorticoid-dependent. J. Immunol. 146:194–198.

35. Mamiya, T., Noda, Y., Nishi, M., Takeshima, H., and Nabeshima, T. (1998). Enhancement of spatial attention in nociceptin/orphanin FQ receptor-knockout mice. Brain Res. 783:236–240.

36. Manabe, T., et al. (1998). Facilitation of long-term potentiation and memory in mice lacking nociceptin receptors. Nature 394:577–581.

37. Kitchen, I., Slowe, S. J., Matthes, H. W., and Kieffer, B. (1997). Quantitative autoradiographic mapping of mu-, delta- and kappa-opioid receptors in knockout mice lacking the mu-opioid receptor gene. Brain Res. 778:73–88.

38. Brady, L. S., et al. (1999). Region-specific up-regulation of opioid receptor binding in enkephalin knockout mice. Mol. Brain Res. 68:193–197.

39. Franklin, K. B. J., and Abbott, F. V. (1989). Techniques for assessing the effects of drugs on nociceptive responses. In: Psychopharmacology, Vol. 13, ed. Boulton, A. A., Baker, G. B., and Greenshaw, A. J., Humana Press, Totowa, N.J., pp. 145–216.

40. Craig, K. D. (1994). Emotional aspects of pain. In: Textbook of pain, 3rd ed., ed. Wall, P. D., and Melzack, R., Churchill Livingstone, Edinburgh, pp. 261–274.

41. Pasternak, G. W. (1993). Pharmacological mechanisms of opioid analgesics. Clin. Neuropharmacol. 16:1–18.

42. Kitanaka, N., Sora, I., Kinsey, S., Zeng, Z., and Uhl, G. R. (1998). No heroin or morphine 6-β-glucuronide analgesia in μ-opioid receptor knockout mice. Eur. J. Pharmacol. 355:R1–3.

43. Bolan, E. A., et al. (1998). Persistent high affinity 3H-Morphine-6-glucuronide binding in MOR-1 knockout mice. In: 29th International Narcotics Research Conference, Garmisch Partenkirchen, Germany.

44. Pintar, J. E., et al. (1998). Genetic analysis of opioid receptor function. In: 29th International Narcotics Research Conference, Garmisch Partenkirchen, Germany.

45. Gaveriaux-Ruff, C., Matthes, H. W., Peluso, J., and Kieffer, B. L. (1998). Abolition of morphine-immunosuppression in mice lacking the μ-opioid receptor gene. Proc. Natl. Acad. Sci. USA 95:6326–6330.

46. Matthes, H. W., et al. (1998). Activity of the delta-opioid receptor is partially reduced, whereas activity of the kappa-receptor is maintained in mice lacking the mu-receptor. J. Neurosci. 18:7285–7295.

47. Noda, Y., et al. (1998). Loss of antinociception induced by naloxone benzoylhydrazone in nociceptin receptor-knockout mice. J. Biol. Chem. 173:18047–18051.

48. Ueda, H., et al. (1997). Partial loss of tolerance liability to morphine analgesia in mice lacking the nociceptin receptor gene. Neurosci. Lett. 273:136–138.

49. Lee, N. M., Leybin, L., Chang, J. K., and Loh, H. H. (1980). Opiate and peptide interaction: effect of enkephalins on morphine analgesia. Eur. J. Pharmacol. 68:181–185.

50. Vaught, J. L., Rothman, R. B., and Westfall, T. C. (1982). Mu and delta receptors: their role in analgesia in the differential effects of opioid peptides on analgesia. Life Sci. 30:1443–1455.

51. Jiang, Q., Mosberg, H. I., and Porreca, F. (1990). Modulation of the analgesic efficacy and potency of morphine by [D-Pen2, D-Pen5]enkephalin in mice. Prog. Clin. Biol. Res. 328:449–452.

52. Heyman, J. S., Vaught, J. L., Mosberg, H. I., Haaseth, R. C., and Porreca, F. (1989). Modulation of mu-mediated antinociception by delta agonists in the mouse: selective potentiation of morphine and normorphine by [D-Pen2,D-Pen5]enkephalin. Eur. J. Pharmacol. 165:1–10.

53. Gacel, G., Dauge, V., Breuze, P., Delay-Goyet, P., and Roques, B. P. (1988). Development of conformationally constrained linear peptides exhibiting a high affinity and pronounced selectivity for delta opioid receptors. J. Med. Chem. 31:1891–1897.

54. Zadina, J. E., Hackler, L., Ge, L. J., and Kastin, A. J. (1997). A potent and selective endogenous agonist for the mu-opiate receptor. Nature 386:499–502.

CHAPTER 11

Role of Substance P in Nociception, Analgesia, and Aggression

STEPHEN P. HUNT, JOHN A. O'BRIEN, AND JAMES A. PALMER

MRC Laboratory of Molecular Biology
Cambridge, England

CHRISTOPHER A. DOYLE

University of Manchester
Manchester, England

CARMEN DE FELIPE

Universidad Miguel Hernandez
Alicante, Spain

11.1 INTRODUCTION

The peptide neurotransmitter substance P (SP) and its receptor (NK1) are widely distributed throughout the central nervous system (CNS). The actions of SP in the periphery and the brain have been reviewed extensively[1,2] and are not considered further here. In this review we focus on the roles of SP and NK1 receptors in nociception, thermoreception, and analgesia. Critical for these functions is the action of primary afferent SP on spinal cord NK1 receptors.

The release of SP into the spinal cord is triggered by noxious peripheral stimulation. Binding of SP to the NK1 receptor leads to depolarization and, via activation of protein kinase C, to an increased sensitivity of the NMDA receptor to glutamate (central hyperexcitability) and increased pain sensitivity (hyperalgesia). However, despite the introduction of specific NK1 antagonists, the function of SP in pain and nociception remains unclear. We have used two molecular approaches to increase our understanding of the role of

Molecular Basis of Pain Induction, Edited by John N. Wood

SP and NK1 receptors in nociception and cold thermoreception. In one series of experiments, we have used activation of the Fos transcription factor[3–5] to show that superficial and deep spinal NK1 neurons process nociceptive and thermoreceptive information in markedly different ways. Lamina I NK1 neurons appear to be involved in intensity discriminative aspects of pain and cooling, whereas deep NK1 cells are involved in spatial localization or the detection of particular nociceptive submodalities and do not seem to play an important role in cold thermoreception. In a second series of experiments we used homologous recombination in embryonic stem cells to disrupt the NK1 receptor gene in mice.[6] Analysis of NK1$^{-/-}$ mice revealed that there was a lack of encoding of the intensity of noxious stimuli and an absence of the characteristic amplification ("windup") of nociceptive reflexes. Furthermore, although SP was not involved in the signaling of acute pain, it was essential for the full development of analgesia and aggressive behavior, demonstrating important and unexpected roles for the peptide in the adaptive response to stress.

The chapter is therefore divided into three sections: (1) a general review of the anatomy and physiology of SP and NK1 receptors in the spinal cord, (2) an account of our current research showing that lamina I NK1 neurons encode the intensity of noxious and cold thermal stimuli, and (3) results from the NK1 gene knockout mouse revealing new and unexpected roles for the NK1 receptor.

11.2   SP AND ITS RECEPTOR (NK1) IN THE SPINAL CORD

11.2.1   Biosynthesis of Substance P

Substance P (SP) is a member of a family of related neuropeptides known as the tachykinins, which includes neurokinin A (NKA), neurokinin B (NKB), neuropeptide K (NPK), and neuropeptide γ (NPγ).[7] These peptides share a common C-terminal sequence, which is required for most of their biological activity.[8,9] The tachykinins are encoded by two distinct genes: preprotachykinin A (PPT-A) and preprotachykinin B (PPT-B). These genes were cloned in the 1980s, largely by Nakanishi's group.[10–17] SP, NKA, NPK, and NPγ are derived from the PPT-A gene and NKB is derived from the PPT-B gene.

11.2.2   SP in Primary Sensory Neurons and in the Spinal Cord

The distribution of SP within the brain has been reported extensively[18–32] and a summary of these results can be found in Ljungdahl et al.[33,34] In the spinal cord, large numbers of varicose axons immunoreactive for SP are present in lamina I and the outer (dorsal) region of lamina II in many species, including rat,[19,23,29,35,36] cat,[17] monkey,[37] and human,[38] although there is a moderate concentration in the inner (ventral) portion of lamina II and scattered fibers in the deeper layers of the cord. While a major proportion of the SP-positive axons in the superficial laminae (I and II) originate from SP-synthesizing primary afferent neurons in the dorsal root ganglia,[19,23,27,29,39] some axons also originate from local circuit neurons[35,39–41] and supraspinal sites.[42] These observations are consistent with data from radioimmunoassay, which showed that particularly high levels of SP are found in the dorsal root ganglia, the dorsal roots, and the dorsal horn, and that following section of the dorsal roots, SP levels in the dorsal horn are decreased markedly.[43] A similar depletion of SP occurs following axotomy.[27,44] The types of sensory neuron that express SP have small cell bodies and small unmyelinated or thinly myelinated axons.[20] This observation was confirmed in electrophysiological experiments, where SP-containing primary sensory neurons were shown to have conduction velocities in the Aδ- and C-fiber ranges.[45] Aδ- and C fibers conduct nociceptive and thermoreceptive information.[46–48] Additional evidence for the presence of SP in unmyelinated primary afferent C fibers comes from the use of capsaicin in neonatal animals. Capsaicin, which selectively destroys C fibers, produces an irreversible loss of SP from the superficial dorsal horn.[49–52]

For many years SP was assumed to be the only mammalian tachykinin. However, in the 1980s, several new members of the tachykinin family were discovered.[12,53–57] Due to the route of biosynthesis of tachykinins (see above), SP and NKA colocalize throughout the mammalian central nervous system (CNS)[58–60] and the two tachykinins are coreleased into the superficial laminae of the spinal cord following noxious peripheral stimulation.[58,61–65] The CNS distribution of NKB does not overlap with that of other tachykinins[43,66–68] and the PPT-B gene is not expressed by sensory neurons and is absent from primary afferent terminals.[7] Some investigators have reported the presence of NKB in the dorsal root ganglia, the dorsal roots, or in the spinal dorsal horn,[43] but the levels were negligible compared to SP and NKA.

11.2.3   Release of SP into the Spinal Cord

The release of SP from primary afferent terminals was first shown by electrical or chemical (55 mM K$^+$) stimulation of the dorsal roots and inspection of the perfusate for SP by radioimmunoassay and high-pressure liquid chromatography (HPLC).[69,70] This release of SP is also evoked by capsaicin or by sciatic nerve stimulation at intensities sufficient to activate C fibers.[62,71–74] SP release from dorsal root ganglion neurons grown in culture has also been reported.[75] More recent studies using push-pull cannulae[76] or antibody-coated microelectrode probes[63-65] have shown that SP is released into the spinal cord only by noxious stimuli. Innocuous stimuli (e.g., gentle brushing) are ineffective.

11.2.4   Spinal Distribution of the SP Receptor (NK1 Receptor)

Tachkinins exert their actions via one or more of the three neurokinin (NK) receptors (designated NK1, NK2 and NK3), which preferentially bind the peptides SP, NKA, and NKB, respectively.[7,77] Autoradiographic studies using ^{125}I- or ^{3}H-SP or SP analogs[78-88] have shown that SP binding sites (NK1 receptors) are widely distributed throughout the CNS. For reviews discussing the distribution of SP binding sites in the mammalian brain, see Refs. 89 to 91. In the spinal cord, the heaviest concentrations of SP binding sites are found in lamina I, the medial third of laminae III to VII, and in lamina X.[78-81,85]

Recent elucidation of the NK1 receptor structure[92] has enabled antisera to be raised against unique sequences of the protein.[93-96] NK1 immunoreactivity has now been studied extensively in many regions of the CNS,[94,96-100] and data obtained with these antibodies have confirmed that, in the spinal cord, lamina I contains the greatest number of NK1 receptor-bearing neurons and dendrites.[99,101-104] The deeper laminae contain only a moderate number of NK1 cells, most of which are located throughout III and in the medial third of IV, V, and VI. Lamina II is almost devoid of NK1 cells. Most spinal NK1-immunoreactive neurons (over 90%), including all of those in lamina I, do not contain γ-aminobutyric acid (GABA) or glycine[102] and are therefore excitatory in nature. Most, if not all, lamina I neurons which receive synaptic input from SP-positive axons are noci-specific and co-contain enkephalin.[147] Physiological[104,148] and morphological[103,118] studies have shown close synaptic coupling of SP-containing axons and NK1 receptor–bearing structures in the superficial dorsal horn, and it seems reasonable to assume that these enkephalinergic cells would express NK1 receptors. Less than 50% of neurons in the deep dorsal horn that receive contacts from SP-containing terminals co-contain enkephalin.[147] Double-labeling studies in which NK1 immunocytochemistry was combined with retrograde axonal tracing have shown that a large proportion of NK1 neurons in lamina I project to the thalamus[105] and to the parabrachial nuclei,[106] with many neurons sending axon collaterals to both.[106] A few NK1-positive cells in the deep laminae also ascend to the brain.

Cloning of the NK1 receptor cDNA[77,107] has allowed the distribution of NK1 mRNA expressing cell bodies to be located using in situ hybridization.[108-113] In the spinal cord, most labeled neurons occur in lamina I.[114]

There is no molecular[115] or morphological[78] evidence for the presence of the NK2 receptor in the CNS. This is curious, since large amounts of the endogenous ligand NKA are found in the CNS (see above). The NK3 receptor is, however, found differentially distributed within the CNS, with high levels being found in the spinal dorsal horn.[78]

11.2.5   Ligand–Receptor Mismatch

The distribution patterns of SP and NK1 receptors do not necessarily correlate, and considerable mismatch has been reported in the CNS.[82,84,116,117,242] However, since all three mammalian tachykinins can act as full agonists at each of the tachkinin receptors,[7] it is possible that NKA or NKB act as NK1 agonists in regions where SP is not present and that SP binds to NK2 and NK3 receptors when NKA and NKB are absent. In the spinal cord, the only notable ligand-receptor mismatch occurs in lamina II (the substantia gelatinosa), which receives a dense innervation from axons containing SP but contains very few NK1 receptor–bearing structures (see above). However, the few NK1-positive dendrites that are present receive a direct synaptic input from primary afferent SP-containing terminals.[118]

11.2.6   Coexistence of SP with Other Neurotransmitters

The following transmitters are colocalized with SP in primary sensory neurons and will be coreleased with SP into the superficial dorsal horn of the spinal cord following high-threshold peripheral stimulation.[62,71–74]

1. *NKA.* This is discussed above.

2. *Glutamate.* SP has been shown to be colocalized with glutamate in a subpopulation of sensory neurons within the dorsal root ganglia[123] and, accordingly, the two transmitters are co-stored in the terminals of primary sensory neurons[124–126] and co-released upon stimulation. SP mediates a slow EPSP in postsynaptic neurons of the spinal cord (see below), whereas glutamate produces a fast response.[127] There is evidence of interaction between SP and glutamate in the spinal cord, with SP enhancing NMDA receptor responses.[128] This is an important event in the generation of central hyperexcitability and and is discussed further below.

3. *Calcitonin gene–related peptide (CGRP).* Although nearly all SP-immunoreactive neurons in the sensory ganglia also contain CGRP, there are many neurons that contain CGRP alone.[119–122] As one would predict, capsaicin treatment depletes not only SP but also CGRP.[121] The functional consequences of SP/CGRP cotransmission are described below.

4. Bombesin[143]

The following transmitters are colocalized with SP in the brain.

1. *5-Hydroxytryptamine (5-HT).* The first example of SP coexisting with another transmitter was the colocalization with 5-HT in nuclei of the rat medulla oblongata.[24,30,129] Many neurons in this region project to the spinal cord,[42,130,131] and later studies showed that SP immunoreactive spinal projection neurons from the raphe nuclei are also positive for 5-HT,[132,133] although many contain 5-HT only. Destruction of the serotoninergic neurons in the raphe by neurotoxins results in an almost complete loss of 5-HT in both the ventral and dorsal horns of the spinal cord.[24] It was also seen that SP immunoreactivity in the ventral horn was virtually abolished.[134,135] The functional significance of this coexistence is poorly understood but appears at first glance to be paradoxical. It is known that this serotonergic pathway provides descending inhibition to the spinal cord.[136] However, if SP is coreleased, this would lead to excitation of the postsynaptic cell.

2. *Other transmitters.* SP is colocalized with GABA in the olfactory bulb, entopeduncular nucleus, neocortex, and striatum[137–140]; with acetylcholine (choline acetyltransferase) in the reticular system[141]; with dopamine (tyrosine hydroxylase) in the olfactory bulb[137]; with somatostatin in the entopeduncular nucleus[142]; with dynorphin in striatal projection neurons[144]; and with cholecystokinin in neurons of the mesencephalic periaqueductal central gray matter.[145] The latter neurons project to the spinal cord.[146]

11.2.7   Actions of SP in the Spinal Cord

Much of the attention that SP has received in spinal cord physiology is due to its suggested role as a nociceptive neurotransmitter, and there is now considerable biochemical evidence to support this claim. For example, SP is found selectively within nociceptive primary sensory neurons,[45,195] and noxious stimulation of the skin[63–65,76] and joint[149] triggers the release of immunoreactive SP into the superficial dorsal horn. Innocuous stimuli are ineffective. SP release into the dorsal horn can also be achieved by electrical stimulation of the nociceptive C fibers.[62] These findings support a role for SP in the transmission of nociceptive information from the periphery to the neurons of the spinal cord.

Similar conclusions have been drawn from electrophysiological experiments. When applied to the spinal cord by perfusion or ionophoresis, NK1 agonists consistently excite subpopulations of neurons.[101,149–152,193] The excitatory response, which is selective for nociceptive neurons,[150,151,193] is characteristically delayed in onset and prolonged[151,194] and mimics the slow, sustained depolarization evoked in spinal cord neurons by electrical activation of C fibers[153] or intraplantar injection of formalin.[154,155] Studies using NK1 receptor antagonists[154,156] have shown that it is the long-lasting component of C-fiber slow synaptic potentials which is mediated, at least partly, by the action of SP at the NK1 receptor. The early component, which is resistant to NK1 antagonists, is sensitive to NMDA antagonism.[156] Electrophysiological studies have also shown that NK1 and NMDA receptors are important mediators of the central hyperexcitability (or sensitization) that follows sustained activity in nociceptive afferents. Evidence that SP and glutamate coexist in nociceptive primary afferent terminals[123,125,126] and that NMDA receptor activity is enhanced by NK1 receptor activation[157–161] implies that an interaction between the two receptors may account for the increased neuronal excitability. These data are supported by the fact that SP also enhances neuronal responses to cutaneous mechanical stimulation,[150,157] an effect that is further amplified if SP is coadministered with glutamate or NMDA.[158] This SP-induced hyperexcitability is long lasting and affects responses to both innocuous and noxious mechanical stimulation, and this has led to the suggestion that it is important to the generation of hyperalgesia.[158,162] A number of potential means exist whereby NK1 receptor–mediated effects might facilitate NMDA receptor function and lead to central sensitization and hyperalgesia. One suggestion is that NK1 activation leads to release of intracellular calcium,[163] which, in turn, produces a protein kinase C–dependent phosphorylation of the NMDA receptor. This partially removes its voltage-dependent Mg^{2+} blockade,[164,165] increases glutamate sensitivity, and leads to the recruitment of subthreshold inputs.[166] Additional action on the glycine binding site of the NMDA receptor may also be involved.[159] Following chronic peripheral inflammation[167] or nerve transection[168,169] there is an up-regulation of SP in a subpopulation of large-diameter nonnociceptive ($A\beta$) primary afferents (see also Refs. 170 and 171) and a large increase in NK1 mRNA[114,170] and protein[172] expression in many laminae I and II spinal cord neurons. The primary afferent phenotypic switch, to one resembling C fibers, would increase SP release into the dorsal horn (and the dorsal column nuclei), which in view of the concomitantly elevated levels of NK1 would be predicted to powerfully potentiate central excitability and inflammatory hyperalgesia. The up-regulation of SP in certain spinal cord neurons following various types of peripheral inflammation[173,174] might have an additional effect.

Behavioral studies also support the idea of a role for SP in the transmission of nociceptive information to the spinal cord. For example, intrathecal (IT) SP increases the gain of the nociceptive flexion reflex for prolonged periods,[175,176] an action that parallels the long-term increase in central hyperexcitability[150,157,158] and which is prevented by pretreatment with NK1 antagonists.[175,177] Furthermore, IT injection of SP produces biting and scratching behavior similar to that elicited by intradermal injection of acetic acid or hypertonic saline[178,179] and shortens the latency of paw withdrawal following a noxious thermal stmulus.[180] These effects can also be prevented by prior or coadministration of NK1 antagonists.[180,181] NK1 antagonists are also effective in preventing writhing responses associated with activation of visceral nociceptors following intraperitoneal injection of phenylbenzoquinone[182] or acetic acid.[183] Since NK1 antagonists are effective in these nociceptive behavioral assays only when given before or at the same time as the stimulus, the activation of NK1 receptors by SP seems to contribute to the generation, but not the maintainance, of hyperalgesia. SP has received most attention with regard to its role in the generation of formalin-induced inflammatory hyperalgesia. Subcutaneous formalin injection results in a biphasic exciation of dorsal horn nociceptive neurons[154] and a sterotypical two-phase behavior of biting, licking, and flicking the paw.[182–185] The first phase, 0 to 10 min, is due to a primary afferent discharge (C fibers) produced by the stimulus. The second phase, lasting from 10 to 60 min, is due partially to sensitization (hyperexcitability) of spinal neurons resulting from the first-phase afferent discharge and partially to a second period of afferent discharges produced by a local inflammatory reaction in the paw. While the first phase is sensitive to NMDA but not NK1 antagonists,[186] a large body of evidence has shown that the second phase is powerfully reduced, or abolished, by preemptive NK1 antagonism[154,182–185] and is therefore mediated, at least in part, by SP. The inflammatory hyperalgesia produced by subcutaneous carrageenan[185] and complete Freund's adjuvant[187] is, similarly, reduced by pretreatment with NK1 antagonists. Tail flick and hot plate latencies are unchanged.[188]

11.2.8   Calcitonin Gene–Related Peptide and SP Actions

Most SP-immunoreactive neurons in the sensory ganglia also contain CGRP[119–122] and the two peptides will be released together from the terminals of primary sensory neurons. Behaviorally, intrathecal CGRP potentiates SP-induced scratching and biting behavior,[122] and SP and CGRP have been shown to synergistically modulate the nociceptive flexor reflex.[176] CGRP also inhibits the enzyme that hydrolyzes SP[189] and potentiates the release of SP[190] and glutamate[191] into the dorsal horn. CGRP has also be shown to potentiate the actions of SP in the periphery, such as increasing the SP-induced plasma extravasation from the skin of rats.[192]

11.2.9   SP Inactivation

The actions of substance P are rapidly terminated by specific peptidases. At present no reuptake mechanism has been found for intact SP,[196,197] but reuptake has been shown to occur for one of the products of proteolytic breakdown.[198] The enzyme responsible for the majority of the termination of the actions of SP is neutral endopeptidase-24.11 (NEP; enkephalinase; EC 3.4.24.11), and this enzyme is present in large quantities in the CNS.[199–201] Other enzymes found in the CNS are also known to hydrolyze SP; acetylcholine esterase (AChE) degrades SP and has an overlapping distribution with SP in the dorsal horn of chick spinal cord[202]; cathepsin D is found in high quantities in calf brain and hydrolyzes SP.[203] An enzyme with very high specificity for SP found in human and rat brain[204,205] was termed *substance P–degrading enzyme.* Its distribution in the rat spinal cord matches that of SP, suggesting that it may be an important enzyme in the metabolism of SP.[206] An inhibition of petidase activity in the spinal cord results in a remarkable diffusion of SP throughout the entire dorsal horn.[62]

11.2.10   Second Messenger Coupling of the NK1 Receptor

Activation of the NK1 receptor causes an increase in phospholipid turnover at sites that correlate with SP binding in the CNS.[212,213] The NK1 receptor is linked to a G-protein that activates the enzyme phospholipase C (PLC).[207] This specific isoform of PLC hydrolyzes phosphatidylinositol bisphosphate (PIP_2),[208,209] a phospholipid found on the inner face of the plasma membrane, and results in the formation of inositol trisphosphate (IP_3) and diacylglycerol.[210,211] IP_3 activates an IP_3 receptor that also acts as a calcium channel on the endoplasmic reticulum[214] to cause an increase in intracellular free Ca^{2+} from intracellular stores, which can then regulate calcium-calmodulin kinases (CAM kinases). Increases in intracellular Ca^{2+} therefore occur in a subpopulation of spinal dorsal horn neurons following the application of SP.[215]

11.2.11   Specific NK1 Receptor Agonists and Antagonists

Once the sequence of SP was elucidated, amino acid substitutions were made to determine the residues important for activity and selectivity. It was found that the C-terminal pentapeptide (SP_{7-11}) confers the biological activity of SP.[216] Other substitutions, particularly at position Gly^9, were performed to produce selective SP agonists such as septide[217] and $[Sar^9, Met(O_2)^{11}]SP$,[218] which are selective for the NK1 receptor and still maintain high activity.

   The first antagonists to be developed were peptides, but these often displayed low potency and selectivity[219] and were sometimes neurotoxic.[220] Recently, highly selective and potent nonpeptide antagonists have been developed. CP-96,345 is an extremely potent antagonist at the NK1 receptor at concentrations of less than 1 nM and is inactive at the NK2 and NK3 receptors.[221] However, it may have nonspecific actions on Ca^{2+} channels.[222,223] Following the discovery of the Ca^{2+} channel action of CP-96,345, another highly potent antagonist, CP-99,994, was developed that had reduced affinity for the L-type Ca^{2+} channel.[224] RP-67,580 is less potent than CP-96,345 but is equally selective for the NK1 receptor, and nonspecific actions have not been demonstrated.[225] SR-140,333 is also a potent nonpeptide antagonist at the NK1 receptor with few nonspecific actions.[226] These compounds all have high potency, affinity, selectivity, and enzymatic resistance.

11.2.12   Therapeutic Use of Specific NK1 Receptor Antagonists

The potential use of tachykinin antagonists in human disease conditions has been reviewed by Maggi et al.[7] and Palmer,[2] and only those uses related to nociception are mentioned here. It appeared that the most obvious use of NK1 receptor antagonists was to produce analgesia. As mentioned above, the selective nonpeptide SP antagonists have been shown to have some analgesic actions in behavioral models of nociception in the mouse and rat, and there may be potential for their use in chronic pain states such as arthritis and neuropathy. However, much of this analgesia probably derives from actions of the drugs at peripheral NK1 receptors which mediate the neurogenic component of the inflammatory response.

   The ability of NK1 antagonists to reduce plasma extravasation[227–230] suggests that they may have antimigraine properties.[231–234] They may also block nociceptive transmission mediated by SP released from the central endings of afferent fibers of the trigeminal nerve, which innervate the blood vessels of the dura.

11.2.13   Therapeutic Use of Capsaicin

Capsaicin is a neurotoxin which when administered chronically to adult animals renders them insensitive to painful stimuli due to a depletion of SP from primary afferent C-fiber terminals[49,238,239] which is reversible.[71] Recently, the use of topically applied capsaicin has been shown to provide substantial pain relief in the majority of patients suffering from neuropathic pain states such as trigeminal neuralgia, postherpetic neuralgia, postmastectomy pain syndrome, and diabetic neuropathy (see Ref. 235). Capsaicin has also been shown to be of benefit to patients suffering from osteo- and rheumatoid arthritis.[236] Interestingly, intranasally applied capsaicin is also used in clinical trials for the treatment of migraine and cluster headache.[237] A recently derived isomer of capsaicin, civanide, is more potent than capsaicin at depleting SP, but lacks the potentially degenerative actions at C fibers. This substance should be of even more value to the treatment of neuropathic pain in the future.

11.3   LAMINA I NK1 NEURON ENCODING OF NOXIOUS AND COLD THERMAL STIMULI

There are several ways of monitoring activity induced in spinal cord neurons by acute peripheral stimuli. For example, lamina I NK1 receptors undergo phosphorylation and endocytosis after activation by SP, and this internalization can be monitored immunocytochemically.[104,240] Unfortunately, this type of analysis is specific for NK1 cells in lamina I[104,240,241] and gives no information on the activation of NK1 neurons in laminae III to X or on the distribution of non-NK1 cells that are also activated. An alternative marker of peripheral stimulation is the acute expression of the immediate-early gene c-*fos*.[3–5,243] Within 1 to 2 hours after peripheral stimulation, there is transcription of Fos protein in postsynaptic neurons of the spinal cord. This expression is somatotopic, occurs only following noxious (or prolonged innocuous) stimulation, and is thought to be due to the monosynaptic activation of spinal cord neurons following primary afferent stimulation.

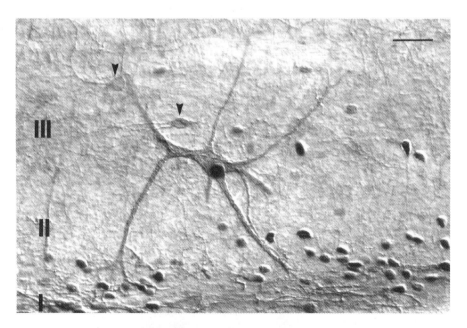

Figure 11.1   Example of a large lamina III neuron that was double labeled for the SP receptor (NK1) and the Fos transcription factor after noxious cutaneous stimulation. Note that NK1-immunoreactivity was present throughout the cell body and dendrites of the neuron, whereas Fos staining, which was more intense, was restricted to the nucleus. This cell has dendrites that project dorsally into laminae I and II and may therefore receive nociceptive input from Aδ and C fibers. Laminae I, II, and III are indicated by Roman numerals. Scale bar: 50 μm.

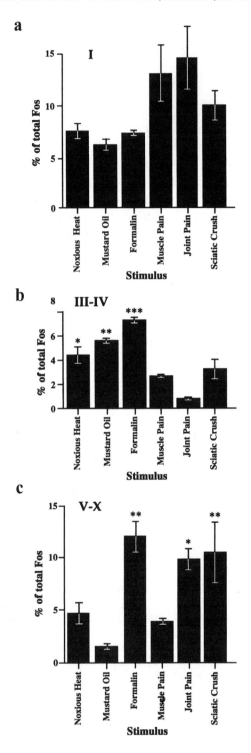

11.3.1   Studies Using a Range of Nociceptive Stimuli

Although SP is implicated in several aspects of nociception, the precise contribution that this peptide makes to nociceptive activity derived from various peripheral tissues or to activity generated by various pain models remains unclear. In these experiments we have used the acute expression of Fos[3,243–250] to monitor the activation of spinal cord neurons during selective stimulation of cutaneous, muscle, or joint nociceptors and during nerve injury and inflammation. When combined with immunostaining for the NK1 receptor, Fos labeling will allow us to assess whether nociceptive signals generated by a noxious stimulus may be selectively modulated by SP.

The density and distribution of NK1 immunostaining, which was robust, intense, and unequivocal, was in accord with that reported in previous studies.[99,101–106,118,242] Briefly, the greatest density of NK1 cell bodies was found in lamina I, lamina III, and the medial third of laminae IV to VI (Fig. 11.1). Similarly, the pattern of Fos expression observed ipsilaterally after each noxious stimulus (Fig. 11.4A,C,E) was in accord with what has been published[3–5,243–250] and was tightly coupled to the termination patterns of nociceptive primary afferents in the spinal cord.[251–254]

Following each noxious stimulus (skin, joint, muscle, inflammation, nerve injury), a subpopulation of NK1 neurons in ipsilateral lamina I and in the deep layers expressed the Fos transcription factor (Fig. 11.1). In lamina I, the proportion of activated (Fos-positive) cells that stained for the NK1 receptor was similar (about 10%) irrespective of the noxious stimulus (Fig. 11.2A). In contrast, in laminae V to X (Fig. 11.2C), stimulation of joint nociceptors and

---

Figure 11.2   Percentage of Fos-positive nuclei in layers I (A), III and IV (B), and V to X of the spinal cord that were present within NK1 receptor–bearing neurons after each acute noxious stimulus. Data are mean ($\pm$ SEM) of three animals. For each stimulus, only a small proportion ($<15\%$) of Fos-positive neurons in the spinal cord stained for the NK1 receptor. In lamina I (A), the frequency of double-labeled cells (ca. 10%) was similar irrespective of the noxious stimulus. In laminae III and IV (B), however, intradermal injection of formalin resulted in the greatest recruitment of NK1 receptor–bearing cells (***$p < 0.001$ compared to noxious muscle and joint stimulation, $p < 0.01$ compared to sciatic crush, and $p < 0.05$ compared to noxious heat), closely followed by noxious chemical (**$p < 0.01$ compared to muscle and joint pain) and thermal (*$p < 0.01$ compared to noxious joint pain) stimulation of the skin. In the deep dorsal horn and ventral horn (C), noxious stimulation of the knee joint produced a greater proportion of Fos/NK1 double-labeled neurons than activation of muscular or cutaneous nociceptors (*$p < 0.05$), suggesting a particular influence of SP on activity derived from this tissue. Formalin-induced inflammation also recruited a disproportionately large number of NK1 cells (**$p < 0.01$ compared to activation of cutaneous and muscular afferents), suggesting that SP may also be an important mediator of inflammatory hyperalgesia. Injury to the sciatic nerve, like intradermal formalin, activates both cutaneous and deep nociceptors and leads to the activation of a similar proportion of lamina V to X NK1–positive neurons (**$p < 0.01$ compared to activation of cutaneous and muscular afferents).

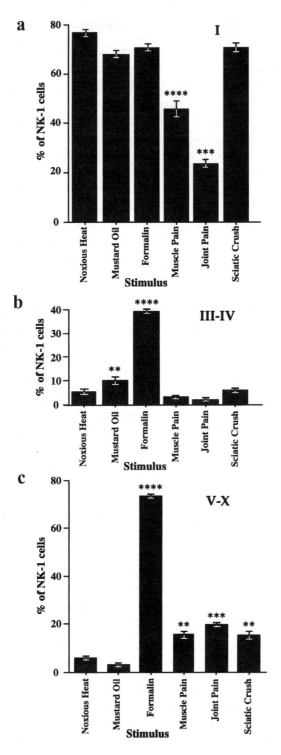

formalin-induced inflammation led to a greater proportion of Fos-reactive NK1 neurons than did noxious stimulation of skin and muscle. Formalin-induced inflammation was again the most effective stimulus at recruiting the NK1 population in laminae III and IV.

When the results were analyzed from the perspective of NK1 cells, it was found that noxious stimulation of the skin, intradermal formalin, and nerve injury activated significantly more lamina I NK1 neurons than did stimulation of muscular and articular nociceptors (Fig. 11.3A). Interestingly, the proportion of lamina I NK1 cells activated by noxious peripheral stimulation never exceeded 70 to 75%, which is consistent with the observation that 5 min after subcutaneous capsaicin injection, or noxious pinching of the skin, 67 to 70% of lamina I NK1 cells showed activity-dependent internalization of the NK1 receptor.[104] In the deep laminae (III and IV and V–X), formalin-induced inflammation produced by far the greatest incidence of double-labeled NK1 neurons with, on average, 40 and 70% of the total NK1 population in each region being activated (Fig. 11.3B,C). In laminae V to X, noxious stimulation of the knee joint also lead to a disproportionately large number of deep NK1 neurons becoming Fos positive (20%).

It has been shown in many studies that the number of Fos-positive neurons present in the superficial (laminae I and II) and deep (III to X) layers of the spinal cord increases with an increase in the severity of the noxious stimulus.[3,244–250] Thus if the number of Fos-positive neurons is taken as a measure of stimulus intensity, in lamina I the total number of Fos/NK1 double-labeled cells is directly proportional to the intensity of the stimulus ($r^2 = 0.98$) (Fig. 11.4B). This correlation held across noxious thermal and chemical stimulation of the skin, deep nociceptive stimulation of the joint and muscle, formalin-induced peripheral inflammation and crush injury of the sciatic nerve and was also observed for laminae III and IV ($r^2 = 0.87$) (Fig. 11.4D). In contrast,

---

Figure 11.3 Percentage of NK1 neurons in lamina I (A), III and IV (B), and V to X (C) that were reactive for Fos. Data are mean ($\pm$ SEM) of three animals. Stimulation of skin nociceptors, intradermal formalin and sciatic crush activated most (70 to 80%) lamina I NK1 cells (A). Lower incidences occurred after stimulation of muscle (****$p < 0.0001$) and joint ($p < 0.0001$ compared to muscle) afferents. (B) In layers III and IV, intradermal injection of formalin produced the greatest recruitment of NK1 receptor–bearing neurons (40%; ****$p < 0.0001$ compared to all other sensory stimuli). Cutaneous application of mustard oil produced a greater proportion of Fos/NK1 double-labeled neurons than activation of muscular and articular nociceptors (**$p < 0.01$). (C) In laminae V to X, formalin-induced inflammation (***$p < 0.0001$ compared to all other sensory stimuli) and stimulation of knee joint afferents (***$p < 0.001$ compared to activation of cutaneous afferents) produced the greatest proportion of Fos/NK1 double-labeled neurons, further suggesting particular influences of SP on inflammatory hyperalgesia and joint pain. Activation of muscular nociceptors and sciatic nerve injury were more effective stimuli at recruiting NK1 positive neurons in this region than activation of cutaneous afferents (**$p < 0.01$).

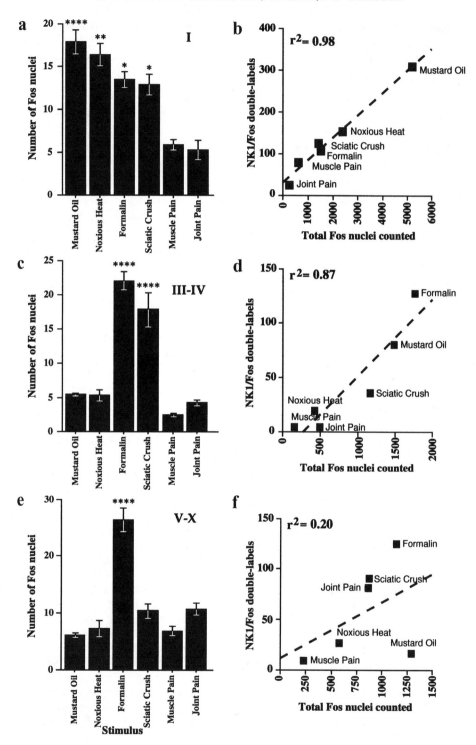

the correlation did not hold for Fos labeling of NK1 neurons in layers V to X, where noxious stimulation of the knee joint and formalin-induced inflammation lead to a far larger proportion of Fos-positive NK1 neurons than would have been predicted from the total Fos count (Fig. 11.4F).

Comparing Fos induction with the morphological subtypes of NK1 cells present in the spinal cord produced some interesting findings. Not unsurprisingly, both large and small lamina I neurons, including NK1-bearing marginal cells of Waldeyer, were frequently Fos reactive. Similarly, the sparse population of NK1 cells in lamina II, which are sometimes considered to be displaced lamina I neurons,[101] were also often Fos positive. Throughout the deeper layers, a proportion of most subtypes of NK1 neuron expressed Fos immunoreactivity, and this was most commonly observed in the large lamina III and IV neurons, which projected dendrites into the superficial dorsal horn (Fig. 11.1); in the NK1 cells in the medial third of laminae III to V; and in the cluster of NK1 cells at the lateral margin of lamina V. The population of lamina III neurons with denrites that extend in the rostrocaudal plane never stained for Fos.

11.3.2   Studies Using a Range of Intensities of Cold Thermal Stimuli

In these experiments we examined whether there is also a graded recruitment of lamina I (or deep) NK1 neurons in response to increasing intensities of cold thermal stimulation (20, 10, and 4°C) of the hind-paw skin. Again, Fos immunohistochemistry was used as the label for spinal cord neurons that responded to skin cooling.[255–264]

In lamina I there was a gradual increase in the number of Fos-positive cells as the intensity of the cold stimulus was increased (Fig. 11.5). Thus, compared

---

Figure 11.4   (A,C,E) Average number of Fos-reactive nuclei in each region of a single 40-μm transverse section following each noxious stimulus. (Data are mean ± SEM of 16 to 48 sections.) In lamina I (A), noxious chemical and thermal stimulation of the skin produced the greatest amount of Fos staining (****$p < 0.0001$, **$p < 0.01$ compared to muscle and joint pain), closely followed by intraplantar injection of formalin and sciatic nerve injury (*$p < 0.05$ compared to muscle and joint pain). (B) Regression analysis showed that in lamina I the number of double-labeled neurons was positively correlated with the intensity of the stimulus ($r^2 = 0.98$) and was not directly related to any particular peripheral target. In laminae III and IV (C), intradermal formalin and sciatic crush produced the greatest Fos induction (****$p < 0.0001$ compared to all other stimuli), and regression analysis (D) showed that the number of double-labeled neurons was, again, positively correlated with the intensity of the stimulus ($r^2 = 0.87$). In contrast, this relationship did not hold for activation of NK1 neurons in laminae V to X (F), where formalin produced the greatest numbers of Fos-positive nuclei (E, ****$p < 0.0001$ compared to all other stimuli), and noxious stimulation of the knee joint and formalin-induced inflammation lead to a far larger proportion of Fos-positive NK1 neurons than would have been predicted from the total Fos count (F).

a

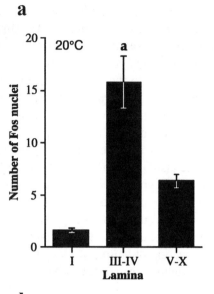

b

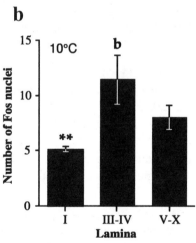

c

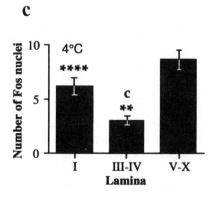

to 20°C, Fos expression in lamina I was significantly greater at 10 and 4°C. Innocuous cooling (20°C) and moderately cold stimulation (10°C) induced unexpectedly large amounts of Fos in laminas III and IV (Fig. 11.5A,B), whereas only weak Fos expression was observed after intense (4°C) cold stimulation (Fig. 11.5C). Thus, as the cold stimulus intensity increased, the amount of Fos present in laminas III and IV fell. In the deep laminas (V to X), the number of Fos nuclei present at each temperature was not significantly different.

Skin cooling induced Fos within NK1 neurons throughout the ipsilateral spinal cord (Fig. 11.6). In lamina I, the proportion of cells that costained for the NK1 receptor increased as the thermal stimulus became more intense and noxious (Fig. 11.6A). In contrast, in laminae III and IV (Fig. 11.6B) and V to X (Fig. 11.6C) there was no correlation between the proportion of Fos-reactive NK1 neurons and stimulus intensity, and the Fos/NK1 double-labeled population never exceeded about 2% of the total Fos count in these layers.

When the results were analyzed from the perspective of the NK1 cells, it was found that as the intensity of cooling increased, there was a progressive rise in the frequency of activated lamina I NK1 neurons (Fig. 11.7A). Thus at 20, 10, and 4°C, 2, 25, and 47%, respectively, of the total lamina I NK1 population was activated. In layers III and IV and V to X, there was no relationship between stimulus intensity and recruitment of NK1 neurons.

11.3.3 Function of Lamina I NK1 Neurons

It is well established that neurons in lamina I transmit nociceptive and thermoreceptive information to the brain (for an excellent review on this subject, see Ref. 48). The population of NK1 cells in this region, which comprises less than 10% of all lamina I neurons,[265] is nociceptive,[104,265] ascends to the thalamus and parabrachial nucleus,[105,106] and has been shown to encode the intensity of noxious thermal stimuli.[148] In the latter study, the authors found that

---

Figure 11.5 The relationship between stimulus temperature and mean number of Fos-IR nuclei present in laminae I, III and IV, and V to X of a single 40-µm transverse section. Data are mean (± SEM) of three animals. In lamina I, the number of Fos-IR nuclei present increased as the cold stimulus became more intense (**$p < 0.01$, ****$p < 0.0001$ compared to stimulation at 20°C). Innocuous cooling (20°C, A) and moderately cold stimulation (10°C, B) produced unexpectedly large amounts of Fos in laminas III and IV, whereas only weak labeling was observed after intense cold (4°C) stimulation (C, **$p < 0.01$ compared to stimulation at 20°C). In the deep laminae (V to X), the mean number of Fos nuclei present at 20°C, 10°C and 4°C were not significantly different. a, Innocuous cooling at 20°C produced significantly more Fos staining in laminae III and IV than lamina I ($p < 0.0001$) or laminae V to X ($p < 0.001$); b, moderate cold stimulation (10°C) also produced heavy Fos expression in layers III and IV ($p < 0.05$ compared to lamina I), although it was less marked than at 20°C; c, intense cold stimulation (4°C) resulted in only minor Fos staining in laminae III and IV ($p < 0.01$ comapred to laminae V to X).

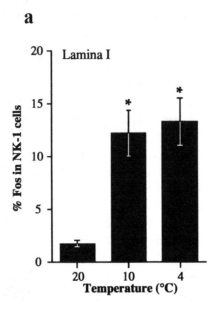

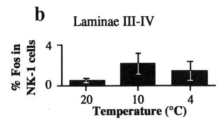

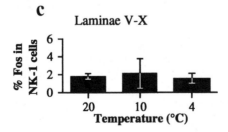

Figure 11.6   Percentage of Fos-positive nuclei in layers I (A), III and IV (B) and V to X (C) of the spinal cord that were present within NK1 receptor–bearing neurons after each thermal stimulus. Data are mean (± SEM) of three animals. (A) In lamina I, the proportion of activated (Fos-positive) cells which stained for the NK1 receptor increased as the thermal stimulus became more intense and noxious (*$p < 0.05$ compared to 20°C). In contrast, in laminae III and IV (B) and V to X (C), there was no correlation between the proportion of Fos-reactive NK1 neurons and stimulus intensity.

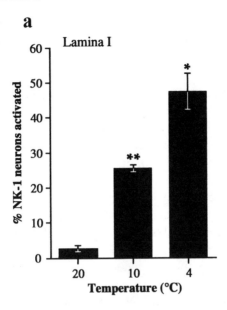

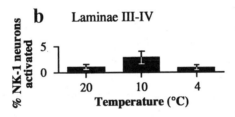

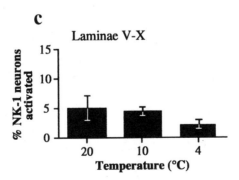

Figure 11.7   Percentage of NK1 neurons in layers I (A), III and IV (B), and V to X (C) that were reactive for Fos. Data are mean (± SEM) of three animals. (A) As the intensity of the cold stimulus was increased, there was a graded increase in the frequency of activated lamina I NK1 neurons (**$p < 0.01$ compared to 20°C, *$p < 0.05$ compared to 10°C). In layers III and IV and V to X, there was no relationship between stimulus intensity and recruitment of NK1 neurons.

gradually raising the intensity of noxious heat (43 to 55°C) or cold (10 to −20°C) increased internalization of the NK1 receptor in lamina I neurons, which was graded with respect to the number of lamina I NK1 neurons recruited and the number of NK1 endosomes within each neuron. Our studies, which use several different types of noxious stimuli or a range of intensities of cold stimulation, also conclude that lamina I NK1 neurons are critical for the accurate discrimination of stimulus intensity. This is in agreement with our recent electrophysiological observations of mice in which the NK1 gene has been disrupted[6] and which will be described in detail in the next section. This correlation also held for Fos labeling of nociceptive NK1 neurons in laminae III and IV, presumably because many of the NK1 cells in this region are activated via their distal dendrites in laminae I and II. In marked contrast, the correlation between stimulus intensity and labeling of NK1-positive neurons did not hold for Fos labeling of NK1 neurons in deeper laminae, where for experiments investigating Fos induction after a range of noxious stimuli, recruitment of the NK1 population was more related to peripheral target. In these layers of the spinal cord (III–IV and V–X), acute inflammation (formalin) and activation of articular nociceptors lead to the greatest recruitment of NK1 neurons. This result suggests that deep NK1 neurons may influence the signaling of joint pain and inflammatory hyperalgesia, and is consistent with data from behavioral studies showing that NK1 antagonism can reduce inflammatory hyperalgesia.[154,182–185,187]

Acute inflammation induced by intradermal injection of formalin[170] or terpentine oil[167] and axotomy[168,169] produces up-regulation of SP in a subpopulation of primary afferent neurons and a large increase in NK1 and SP mRNA[170] in many lamina I and II spinal cord neurons. This has lead to the suggestion that increased expression of SP generates the behavioral changes that accompany inflammation and nerve injury. However, recent data suggest that other mechanisms may also be involved. Our studies with NK1 gene knockout mice (see Ref. 6 and later) have shown that inflammatory hyperalgesia develops normally following an ipsilateral hind-paw injection of complete Freund's adjuvant. Moreover, using a technique that selectively destroys the lamina I NK1-positive projection neurons, Mantyh et al.[265] have shown that capsaicin-induced hyperalgesia is, to a considerable extent, dependent on the presence of these cells. Taken together, these data suggested an alternative model for the role of SP in hyperalgesia, in which *NK1-bearing lamina I projection neurons control the excitability of the dorsal horn of the spinal cord through reciprocal projections with the brainstem.*[6] Hyperalgesia therefore becomes a reflection of the excitatory activity in the ascending pathway and the closely coupled descending inhibitory and excitatory pathways terminating within the dorsal horn of the spinal cord.[266–269] Noxious stimulation results in the co-release of SP and glutamate from primary afferent terminals into the superficial dorsal horn.[123,125] Thus although glutamate release would still result in the activation of dorsal horn neurons, disruption of the NK1 receptor gene[6] would compromise sensitization of the lamina I NK1 neurons, result in a compensatory reduction in descending inhibition on the spinal cord, and maintain a hyperalgesic state. Ablation of lamina I NK1 neurons[265] abolishes the ascending drive from lamina I NK1 neurons to the brain stem. This would severely disrupt descending modulation of spinal excitability, resulting in reduced behavioral hypersensitivity in the presence of peripheral injury. The role of deep NK1 receptor-bearing neurons and of changes in SP and NK1 mRNA in the dorsal horn during peripheral inflammation in the development of behavioral pain states remains enigmatic. Conceivably, long-term changes in the excitability of these neurons, as a result of both primary afferent and descending influences, could provide a complementary molecular substrate for the behavioral manifestations of peripheral inflammation.

11.3.4 Role of Laminae III–IV NK1 Receptor–Negative Neurons in Thermoreception

Innocuous (20°C) and mildly noxious (10°C) skin cooling induced unexpectedly large numbers of Fos-positive nuclei in laminas III and IV. This labeling, which was probably due to activity in cold-sensitive Aαβ mechanoreceptors,[271–274] was not observed in earlier skin cooling experiments,[247,270] although it has been seen after gentle mechanical stimulation of the skin.[5,249] The failure of cold stimulation to induce Fos in laminae III and IV in previous studies may be explained by the shorter stimulation paradigm used by the authors[247] or by a lower sensitivity to cooling of facial mechanoreceptors.[270]

It has been suggested that the thermal responses of cold-sensitive Aαβ mechanoreceptors are too weak to be significant in thermoreception.[273,275–277] However, on the basis that dorsal column lesions result in an increase in temperature (and pain) sensation[278] and that 30 to 40% of the axons in the dorsal columns originate from laminae III and IV projection neurons[279] which receive a strong synaptic input from cold-sensitive Aαβ mechanoreceptors (type I and type II slowly adapting mechanoreceptors),[280,281] it is possible that these cells play an important regulatory role in thermoreception.

11.4 NOCICEPTION, ANALGESIA, AND AGGRESSION IN MICE LACKING THE SUBSTANCE P RECEPTOR

Homologous recombination in embryonic stem cells was used to create a mouse line in which the NK1 receptor gene was disrupted in exon 1[282] (Fig. 11.8a). Interbreeding of mice heterozygous for the disrupted allele resulted in

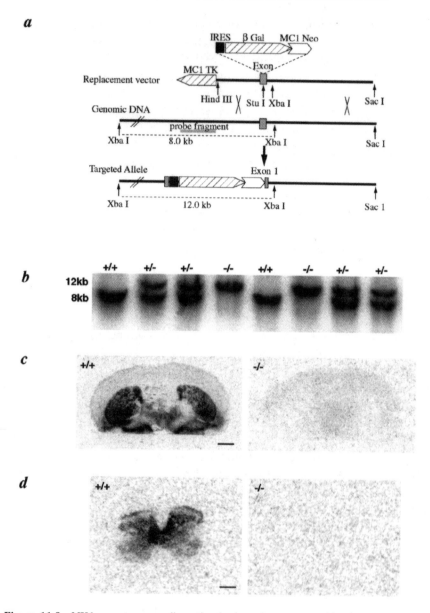

Figure 11.8 NK1 receptor gene disruption by homologous recombination. (a) Schematic drawing of the region of the wild-type NK1 locus containing exon 1, the targeting (replacement) vector and the predicted structure of the targeted NK1 receptor gene. The 5′ external probe used for Southern blot analysis and the sizes of the restriction fragments detected with this probe in the wild-type and targeted alleles are indicated. (b) Southern blot analysis of offspring from an NK1[+/−] intercross by *Xba*I digestion of tail DNA and hybridization with the probe. Homozygous (12 kb), heterozygous (12 kb and 8 kb) and wild-type (8 kb) mice were generated with a ratio of 1:2:1. (c,d) Autoradiographic mapping of SP-binding sites in forebrain (c) and spinal cord (d) sections of NK1[−/−] and NK1[+/+] mice. Scale bars: 1 mm (c) and 0.5 mm (d).

healthy homozygous mutant mice (Fig. 11.8b) which bred normally and did not exhibit impaired maternal behavior. Two studies have disrupted the pre-protachykinin gene itself, resulting in the absence of both SP and NKA. Each of these mice present a different array of deficits, although the NK1 knockout mouse resembles antagonist-treated wild-type mice the most closely.

11.4.1 NK1 Receptor Gene Knockout Mouse

Receptor autoradiography, using [^{125}I] Bolton–Hunter SP, indicated that SP binding sites were absent in brain and spinal cord of NK1$^{-/-}$ mice (Fig. 11.8c,d). This demonstrated that no receptor was available to mediate the actions of SP in the central nervous system (CNS) of NK1$^{-/-}$ mice. This was confirmed by immunohistochemistry using a specific antibody to the C-terminus of the NK1 receptor. Using in situ hybridization, levels of NK3 receptor mRNA in the CNS were found to be similar in both NK1$^{-/-}$ and NK1$^{+/+}$ mice, while NK2 receptor mRNA was undetectable in the brain and spinal cord of both genotypes as reported previously.[78,115] Immunohistochemical analysis of SP, CGRP, and the μ opioid receptor found no detectable differences in the intensity or distribution of peptide staining within the spinal cord and brain of NK1$^{+/+}$ and NK1$^{-/-}$ mice. These results indicate that the general morphology and neurochemistry of the brain and spinal cord had not been perturbed in NK1$^{-/-}$ mice and that there were no compensatory changes in the levels of tachykinins or their receptors.

Electrophysiological evidence implicates the NK1 receptor in spinal cord sensitization following injury or inflammation, and in the amplification of postsynaptic responses following repetitive high-threshold nerve stimulation.[175,177,283] This was investigated by recording electromyographic activity[284] in the anaesthetized mouse while applying electrical or mechanical stimulation to the hind paw. The responses observed to noxious mechanical stimulation at graded intensities were remarkable in that NK1$^{-/-}$ mice showed no evidence of intensity encoding. In NK1$^{+/+}$ mice, increasing the stimulus intensity induced a progressive increase in the responses recorded ($p < 0.05$); for example, a force of 100 mN above threshold produced an average increase of 101%, while a suprathreshold force of 300 mN induced an average increase of 381%. In contrast, in NK1$^{-/-}$ mice, no clear differences were observed using stimuli 100 to 600 mN above threshold.

We also examined *windup*, where repetitive activation of C fibers but not A fibers leads to an augmented response to subsequent C fiber input. This effect is reduced by NK1 and NMDA receptor antagonists.[175,177,186,283,285] In NK1$^{-/-}$ mice, windup was not observed at any of the stimulation intensities used. We therefore conclude that the NK1 receptor is essential for the expression of a normal *windup* response.

Behaviorally, acute nociceptive thresholds were not affected by the gene disruption. Tail pinch tests showed no significant differences in thresholds between the two groups of animals (Fig. 11.9a). In paw withdrawal reflex experiments, the thresholds were again not significantly different between the two groups of animals, either for noxious mechanical or electrical stimulation (Fig. 11.9a). Tail flick and hot plate assays were used to assess heat thresholds. Tail flick is primarily a spinal reflex, whereas hot plate has a substantial supraspinal input to the response which involves lifting and licking the hind paw.[286,287] Latencies were comparable in NK1[-/-] and NK1[+/+] animals (Fig. 11.9b,c). Our interpretation of these data is that SP does not mediate acute pain sensation.

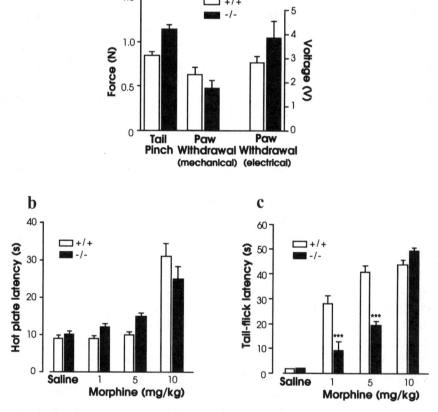

Figure 11.9 Acute nociceptive responses and sensitivity to morphine. (a) Tail pinch and paw withdrawal thresholds to noxious mechanical (force) or electrical (voltage) stimulation measured under anesthesia (NK1[+/+], $n = 6$; NK1[-/-], $n = 7$). (b,c) Effects of intraperitoneal morphine sulfate on hot plate (b) and tail flick (c) latency (NK1[+/+], $n = 10$; NK1[-/-], $n = 10$). *** $p < 0.001$ compared to NK1[+/+]. Data are mean ± SEM and were analyzed using the Mann–Whitney U-test.

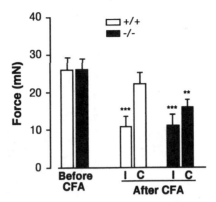

Figure 11.10 Adjuvant-induced inflammation. Hyperalgesia measured with Von Frey hairs 60 h after ipsilateral (I) hind paw injection of CFA. C, contralateral. (NK1[+/+], $n = 12$; NK1[-/-], $n = 12$). **$p < 0.01$ compared to NK1[-/-] before CFA, ***$p < 0.001$ compared to same phenotype before CFA. Data are mean ± SEM and were analyzed by the Wilcoxon signed rank test.

The up-regulation of SP expression in subsets of sensory and spinal cord neurons following inflammatory lesion of the hind paw has implied that the increased release of SP may be responsible for the central sensitization and hyperalgesia associated with inflammation.[167,170,288] We investigated this possibility following injection of complete Freund's adjuvant (CFA) into the left hind paw of mice. Twenty-four or sixty hours after injection of CFA, the inflammatory process was comparable in both groups of mice, with similar degrees of erythema and swelling of the ipsilateral paw (NK1[+/+] = 3.48 ± 0.11 mm, NK1[-/-] = 3.29 ± 0.09 mm; data are mean ± SEM). The development of ipsilateral mechanical hyperalgesia was similar in both groups of mice (Fig. 11.10). However, there was significant contralateral hyperalgesia ($p < 0.01$) in NK1[-/-] mice but not NK1[+/+] mice (Fig. 11.10), although no obvious swelling of the right paw was present (NK1[+/+] = 2.16 ± 0.09 mm, NK1[-/-] = 2.10 ± 0.07 mm; data are mean ± SEM). These data indicate that hyperalgesia can develop in the absence of SP activity.

Nociceptive behaviors following formalin injection were also disrupted in the NK1[-/-] mice. Injection of formalin into the paw results in two phases of nociceptive behavior. The second phase of nociceptive behavior is the result of an inflammation-induced increase in primary afferent activity[289,290] and a central change in neuronal excitability.[184] The second phase of nociceptive behavior was significantly attenuated in mutant mice (>40%, Fig. 11.11a). Spinal cords were also removed from these mice 2 h after the injection of formalin and examined for Fos immunoreactivity. Numbers of Fos-positive neurons were reduced by 30% within the superficial laminae (I and II) in NK1[-/-] compared to NK1[+/+] mice (Fig. 11.11b) as in antagonist-treated animals.[243]

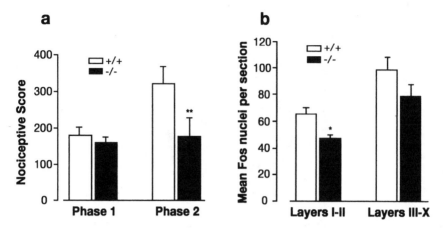

Figure 11.11   Formalin test. (a) Nociceptive score (total duration of biting and licking behavior) during phases 1 and 2 of the formalin response. (NK1$^{+/+}$, $n = 6$; NK1$^{-/-}$, $n = 6$). **$p < 0.01$ compared to NK1$^{+/+}$ phase 2. (b) Mean number of Fos-positive nuclei in the superficial laminae (I and II) and deep layers (III to X) of the spinal cord 2 h after injection of 2% formalin in the hind paw. These data were obtained from the same animals as in (a). *$p < 0.05$ compared to NK1$^{+/+}$ laminae I and II. Data are mean ± SEM and were analyzed by the two-tailed Student's t-test.

These data imply a decrease in central excitability and reduced nociceptor sensitization in the NK1$^{-/-}$ mice.

We next examined the analgesic response of mice exposed to either morphine or to a period of stress induced by a short forced swim. The effects of morphine were assessed on tail flick and hot plate thresholds. Hot plate thresholds increased comparably in both NK1$^{+/+}$ and NK1$^{-/-}$ animals (Fig. 11.9b), whereas the increase in tail flick thresholds with low doses of morphine was significantly reduced in NK1$^{-/-}$ mice (Fig. 11.9c). Previous work has indicated that tail flick and hot plate responses are modulated by different opioid mechanisms within the CNS.[291–293] We conclude that the modulation of tail flick spinal reflex by opiates is mediated, in part, by SP, as suggested previously[294]

Previous work has shown that cold water (4 to 15°C) produces a nonopiate, NMDA-dependent analgesia, whereas warmer water (33°C) results in opiate-dependent analgesia.[291,292] Both types of analgesia are thought to be mediated by descending supraspinal pathways. Following a swim at 4°C (tail flick test) or 10°C (hot plate test), there was a marked reduction in the amount of analgesia that developed in the NK1$^{-/-}$ mice compared to NK1$^{+/+}$ mice: a 45% reduction was seen in hot plate latency (Fig. 11.12a) and a 70% reduction was seen in tail flick latency (Fig. 11.12b). To confirm that this was not the result of a neurochemical compensation brought on by the absence of NK1 recep-

tors during development, we tested NK1$^{+/+}$ animals in the hot plate paradigm
after pretreatment with the NK1-specific antagonist RP67580. A comparable
reduction in the amount of analgesia to that seen in NK1$^{-/-}$ mice was found
in antagonist-treated NK1$^{+/+}$ mice (Fig. 11.12c), demonstrating that activation
of stress-induced analgesia was indeed one function of SP. We also pretreated
NK1$^{+/+}$ and NK1$^{-/-}$ mice with the NMDA receptor antagonist MK-801, which
has been shown to reduce stress-induced analgesia produced by cold water

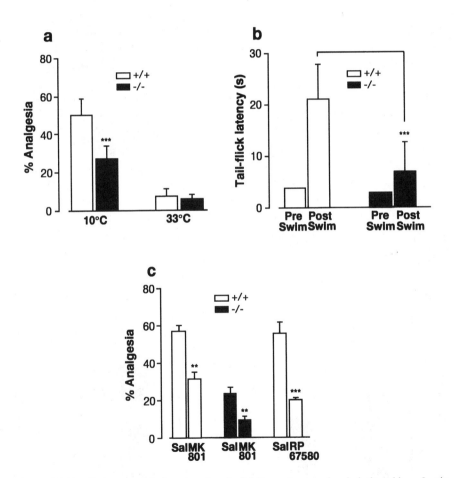

Figure 11.12 Swim stress–induced analgesia. (a) Percentage analgesia induced by a 3-min
swim at 10 or 33°C assessed using the hot plate assay (NK1$^{+/+}$, $n = 16$; NK1$^{-/-}$, $n = 16$). ***$p <$
0.001 compared to 10°C swim NK1$^{+/+}$. (b) Tail flick latency measured following a 90-s swim
in water at 4°C (NK1$^{+/+}$, $n = 10$; NK1$^{-/-}$, $n = 10$). ***$p < 0.001$ compared to postswim NK1$^{+/+}$.
(c) Effect of MK-801 (0.075 mg/kg intraperitoneally) or RP 67580 (0.04 mg/kg intravenously)
on swim stress–induced analgesia at 10°C using the hot plate assay (NK1$^{+/+}$, $n = 6$; NK1$^{-/-}$,
$n = 6$). Sal, saline. **$p < 0.01$, ***$p < 0.001$ compared to saline. Data are mean ± SEM.
Analyzed by the two-tailed Student's t-test.

swim.[293] The two groups of mice were equally sensitive to the antagonist in the hot plate assay (Fig. 11.12c) and a comparable decline in the amount of analgesia was seen in both groups (ca. 40%), implying that the neural mechanisms that generate NMDA analgesia are intact in the NK1[-/-] mouse. Finally, mice were pretreated with naloxone, which abolishes the opiate-sensitive, stress-induced analgesia that follows a swim at 33°C. Both groups of animals showed similar analgesia and, following naloxone treatment, a comparable reduction in analgesia, indicating that opiate-mediated stress-induced analgesia was intact in NK1[-/-] mice. Collectively, these data indicated that there was a pharmacologically distinct route for the generation of stress-induced analgesia by SP. We proposed that SP played a central role in the control of spinal excitability primarily through the activation of central inhibitory pathways from the brainstem.

The NK1 receptor is also found throughout the brain, notably within the limbic system and hypothalamus,[78,89] suggesting a role for SP in emotional behavior. Activity was evaluated in the open field assay.[286] No differences between groups were detected and no preferences for the sides or the center of the field were noticed (Fig. 11.13a), demonstrating that levels of anxiety were similar in NK1[-/-] and NK1[+/+] animals. Aggression was assessed using the resident-intruder test, in which isolated males of either phenotype are exposed to NK1[+/+] mice housed communally.[286] NK1[-/-] mice were considerably less aggressive (Fig. 11.13b). Consistent with these data, defensive

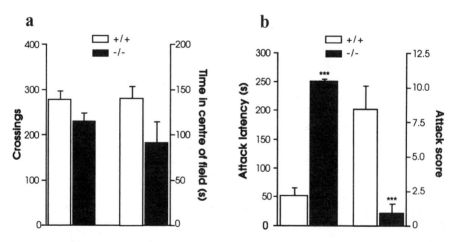

Figure 11.13   Anxiety and aggression. (a) Open field assay. Number of line crossings and time spent in center field were measured (NK1[+/+], $n = 10$; NK1[-/-], $n = 10$). (b) Aggressive behavior of mice in the resident–intruder assay. Attack latencies and total fighting scores of NK1[+/+] ($n = 8$) and NK1[-/-] ($n = 8$) mice. ***$p < 0.001$ compared to NK1[+/+]. Data are mean ± SEM and were analyzed by the Mann–Whitney U-test.

rage provoked by medial hypothalamic stimulation can also be blocked by NK1 antagonists.[295]

11.4.2 Preprotachykinin Gene Knockout Mice

Two groups[296,297] have produced animals that do not express SP and NKA, but the behavioral results are remarkably different between the two studies. The response to formalin injection was completely absent in one study[297] but was only slightly reduced in the other.[296] Similarly, visceral pain responses to intraperitoneal acetic acid injection were unaffected in one study,[297] but were profoundly affected in the other.[296] In the hot plate nociceptive assay, knockout mice showed an increased response latency to mildly painful heat (52°C) in one study[297] but in the other, the responses of wild-type and mutant mice were similar, and it was only when the plate temperature became moderately painful (55.5°C) that the mutant mice showed a decreased response latency.[296] In the study, which concluded that only moderate to severe pain is signaled by SP,[296] it was found that CFA-induced hyperalgesia and allodynia was similar in both wild and knockout animals, as was the case with the NK1 knockout animal.

Taken together these data are extremely confusing. We are of the opinion that the NK1 antagonist studies tend to support the NK1 receptor gene disruption analysis rather than the inconsistent results produced by preprotachykinin gene disruption. Whether these differences reflect genetic background or experimental approaches remains to be determined.

11.5 CONCLUSIONS

The results from the NK1 gene disruption analysis indicated that SP, while not primarily concerned with signaling pain, is critical to the survival response of the mouse in dangerous situations: due to either actual bodily harm or potential harm following the appearance of an aggressor in the environment. The animals reception of danger triggers numerous responses that have survival value. In the wild, a short period of analgesia following injury facilitates execution of a "fight or flight" response, while the aggressive response secures the territorial rights and social status of the animal. This increased vigilance that follows the appearance of danger in the environment is a form of anxiety that directs the animal's attention toward potential dangers in the environment. It is of some interest that previous studies with NK1 antagonists had identified a possible role for SP in the generation of anxiety and stress,[298–302] and indicate a role for NK1 antagonists, not as analgesics, but in the control of anxiety and, perhaps, depression.

REFERENCES

1. Otsuka, M., and Yoshioka, K. (1993). Neurotransmitter functions of mammalian tachykinins. Physiol. Rev. 73:229–308.

2. Palmer, J. (1996). The expression and regulation of the neurokinin-1 receptor in the rat central nervous system. Ph.D. thesis, Cambridge University.

3. Doyle, C. A., and Hunt, S. P. (1997). Fos co-localizes with the substance P receptor (NK-1) in a sub-population of rat spinal cord neurons following noxious peripheral stimulation. J. Physiol. 501:16.

4. Doyle, C. A., Palmer, J. A., Munglani, R., et al. (1997). Molecular consequences of noxious stimulation. In: Molecular aspects of the neurobiology of pain, ed. Borsook, D., Progress in pain research and management, Vol 9, IASP Press, Seattle, Wash., pp. 145–169.

5. Hunt, S. P., Pini, A., and Evan, G. (1987). Induction of c-*fos*-like protein in spinal cord neurons following sensory stimulation. Nature 328:632–634.

6. De Felipe, C., Herrero, J. F., O'Brien, J. A., et al. (1998). Nociception, analgesia and aggression are disrupted in mice lacking the substance P receptor. Nature 392:394–397.

7. Maggi, C. A., Patacchini, R., Rovero, P., et al. (1993). Tachykinin receptors and tachykinin antagonists. J. Auton. Pharmacol. 13:23–93.

8. Lee, C.-M., Iversen, L. L., Hanley, M. R., et al. (1982). The possible existence of multiple receptors for substance P. Naunyn Schmiedebergs Arch. Pharmacol. 318:281–287.

9. Pernow, B. (1983). Substance P. Pharmacol. Rev. 35:85–141.

10. Bonner, T., Affolter, H.-U., Young, A. C., et al. (1987). A cDNA encoding the precursor of the rat neuropeptide, neurokinin B. Mol. Brain Res. 2:243–249.

11. Kawaguchi, Y., Hoshimaru, M., Nawa, H., et al. (1986). Sequence analysis of cloned cDNA for rat substance P precursor: existence of a third substance P precursor. Biochem. Biophys. Res. Commun. 139:1040–1046.

12. Nawa, H., Hirose, T., Takashima, H., et al. (1983). Nucleotide sequences of cloned cDNAs for two types of bovine brain substance P precursor. Nature 306:32–36.

13. Nawa, H., Kotani, H., and Nakanishi, S. (1984). Tissue-specific generation of two preprotachykinin mRNAs from one gene by alternative RNA splicing. Nature 312:729–734.

14. Kotani, H., Hoshimaru, M., Nawa, H., et al. (1986). Structure and gene organization of bovine neuromedin K precursor. Proc. Natl. Acad. Sci. USA 83:7074–7078.

15. Nakanishi, S. (1986). Structure and regulation of the preprotachykinin gene. TINS 9:41–44.

16. Nakanishi, S. (1987). Substance P precursor and kininogen: their structures, gene organizations, and regulation. Physiol. Rev. 67:1117–1142.

17. Krause, J. E., Chirgwin, J. M., Carter, M. S., et al. (1987). Three rat prepro-tachykinin mRNAs encode the neuropeptides substance P and neurokinin A. Proc. Natl. Acad. Sci. USA 84:881–885.

18. Nilsson, G., Hökfelt, T., and Pernow, B. (1974). Distribution of substance P–like immunoreactivity in the rat central nervous system as revealed by immunohis-tochemistry. Med. Biol. 52:424–427.

19. Hökfelt, T., Kellerth, J. O., Nilsson, P. G., et al. (1975). Substance P: localiza-tion in central nervous system and in some primary sensory neurons. Science 190:889–890.

20. Hökfelt, T., Elde, R., Johansson, O., et al. (1976). Immunohistochemical evi-dence for separate populations of somatostatin-containing and substance P–containing primary afferent neurons in the rat. Neuroscience 1:131–136.

21. Hökfelt, T., Meyerson, B., Nilsson, G., et al. (1976). Immunochemical evidence for SP-containing nerve endings in the human cortex. Brain Res. 104:181–186.

22. Hökfelt, T., Johansson, O., Kellerth, J. O., et al. (1977). Immunohistochemical distribution of substance P. In: Substance P, ed. von Euler, U. S., and Pernow, B., Raven Press, New York, pp. 117–145.

23. Hökfelt, T., Ljungdahl, Å., Terenius, L., et al. (1977). Immunohistochemical analysis of peptide pathways possibly related to pain and analgesia: enkephalin and substance P. Proc. Natl. Acad. Sci. USA 74:3081–3085.

24. Hökfelt, T., Ljungdahl, Å., Steinbusch, H., et al. (1978). Immunohistochemical evidence of substance P–like immunoreactivity in some 5-hydroxytrypta-mine–containing neurons in the rat central nervous system. Neuroscience 3:17–38.

25. Hökfelt, T., Pernow, B., Nilsson, G., et al. (1978). Dense plexus of substance P immunoreactive nerve terminals in eminentia medialis of the primate hypothal-amus. Proc. Natl. Acad. Sci. USA 75:1013–1015.

26. Hökfelt, T., Schultzberg, M., Elde, R., et al. (1978). Peptide neurons in periph-eral tissues including the urinary tract: immunohistochemical studies. Acta Pharmacol. Toxicol. 43:79–89.

27. Hökfelt, T., Zhang, X., and Wiesenfeld-Hallin, Z. (1994). Messenger plasticity in primary sensory neurons following axotomy and its functional implications. TINS 17:22–30.

28. Brownstein, M. J., Mroz, E. A., Kizer, J. S., et al. (1976). Regional distribution of substance P in the brain of the rat. Brain Res. 116:299–305.

29. Chan-Palay, V., and Palay, S. L. (1977). Ultrastructural identification of sub-stance P cells and their processes in rat sensory ganglia and their terminals in the spinal cord by immunocytochemistry. Proc. Natl. Acad. Sci. USA 74:4050–4054.

30. Chan-Palay, V., Jonsson, G., and Palay, S. L. (1978). Serotonin and substance P coexist in neurons of the rat's central nervous system. Proc. Natl. Acad. Sci. USA 75:1582–1586.

31. Cuello, A. C., and Kanazawa, I. (1978). The distribution of substance P immunoreactive fibers in the rat central nervous system. J. Comp. Neurol. 178:129–156.

32. Schultzberg, M., Dreyfus, C. F., Gershon, M. D., et al. (1978). VIP-, enkephalin-, substance P-, and somatostatin-like immunoreactivity in neurons intrinsic to the intestine: immunohistochemical evidence from organotypic cultures. Brain Res. 155:239–248.

33. Ljungdahl, Å., Hökfelt, T., and Nilsson, G. (1978). Distribution of substance P–like immunoreactivity in the central nervous system of the rat. I. Cell bodies and nerve terminals. Neuroscience 3:861–943.

34. Ljungdahl, Å., Hökfelt, T., Nilsson, G., et al. (1978). Distribution of substance P–like immunoreactivity in the central nervous system of the rat. II. Light microscopic localization in relation to catecholamine-containing neurons. Neuroscience 3:945–976.

35. Hunt, S. P., Kelly, J. S., Emson, P. C., et al. (1981). An immunohistochemical study of neuronal populations containing neuropeptides or γ-aminobutyrate within the superficial layers of the rat dorsal horn. Neuroscience 6:1883–1898.

36. Barber, R. P., Vaughn, J. E., Slemmon, J. R., et al. (1979). The origin, distribution, and synaptic relationships of substance P axons in the rat spinal cord. J. Comp. Neurol. 184:331–351.

37. DiFiglia, M., Aronin, N., and Leeman, S. E. (1982). Light microscopic and ultrastructural localization of immunoreactive substance P in the dorsal horn of monkey spinal cord. Neuroscience 7:1127–1139.

38. DeLanerolle, N. C., and LaMotte, C. C. (1982). The human spinal cord: substance P and methionine-enkephalin immunoreactivity. J. Neurosci. 2:1369–1386.

39. Warden, M. K., and Young, W. S. (1988). Distribution of cells containing mRNA's encoding substance P and neurokinin B in the rat central nervous system. J. Comp. Neurol. 272:90–113.

40. Lima, D., Avelino, A., and Coimbra, A. (1993). Morphological characterization of marginal (lamina I) neurons immunoreactive for substance P, enkephalin, dynorphin and gamma-aminobutyric acid in the rat spinal cord. J. Chem. Neuroanat. 6:43–52.

41. Senba, E., Yanaihara, C., Yanaihara, N., et al. (1988). Co-localization of substance P and met-enkephalin-arg-gly-leu in the intraspinal neurons of the rat, with special reference to the neurons of the substantia gelatinosa. Brain Res. 453:110–116.

42. Menetrey, D., and Basbaum, A. I. (1987). The distribution of substance P-, enkephalin- and dynorphin-immunoreactive neurons in the medulla of the rat and their contribution to bulbospinal pathways. Neuroscience 23:173–187.

43. Ogawa, T., Kanazawa, I., and Kimura, S. (1985). Regional distribution of substance P, neurokinin-1 and neurokinin-2 in rat spinal cord, nerve roots and dorsal root ganglia, and the effects of dorsal root section or spinal transection. Brain Res. 359:152–157.

44. Jessell, T., Tsunoo, A., Kanazawa, I., et al. (1979). Substance P: depletion in the dorsal horn of the rat spinal cord after section of the peripheral processes of primary sensory neurons. Brain Res. 168:247–259.

45. Lawson, S. N., and McCarthy, P. W. (1989). Cell type and conduction velocity of rat primary sensory neurons with substance P–like immunoreactivity. Neuroscience 28:745–753.

46. Light, A. R., and Perl, E. R. (1979). Spinal termination of functionally identified primary afferent neurons with slowly conducting myelinated fibres. J. Comp. Neurol. 186:133–150.

47. Sugiura, Y., Lee, C. L., and Perl, E. R. (1986). Central projections of identified unmyelinated (C) afferent fibres innervating mammalian skin. Science 234:358–361.

48. Craig, A. D. (1994). Spinal and supraspinal processing of specific pain and temperature. In: Touch, temperature and pain in health and disease: mechanisms and assessments, ed. Boivie, J., Hansson, P., and Lindblom, U., Progress in pain research and management, Vol. 3, IASP Press, Seattle, Wash. pp. 421–437.

49. Janscó, G., Kiraly, E., and Jancsó-Gábor, A. (1977). Pharmacologically induced selective degeneration of chemosensitive primary sensory neurones. Nature 270:741–743.

50. Nagy, J. I., and Hunt, S. P. (1983). The termination of primary afferents within the rat dorsal horn: evidence for rearrangement following capsaicin treatment. J. Comp. Neurol. 218:145–158.

51. Nagy, J. I., Hunt, S. P., Iversen, L. L., et al. (1981). Biochemical and anatomical observations on the degeneration of peptide-containing primary afferent neurons after neonatal capsaicin. Neuroscience 6:1923–1934.

52. Nagy, J. I., Iversen, L. L., Goedert, M., et al. (1983). Dose-dependent effects of capsaicin on primary sensory neurons in the neonatal rat. J. Neurosci. 3:399–406.

53. Kanagawa, K., Minamino, N., Fukada, A., et al. (1983). Neuromedin K: a novel mammalian tachykinin identified in porcine spinal cord. Biochem. Biophys. Res. Commun. 114:533–540.

54. Kimura, S., Okada, M., Sugita, Y., et al. (1983). Novel neuropeptides, neurokinins a and b, isolated from porcine spinal cord. Proc. Jpn. Acad. Ser. B 59:101–104.

55. Kimura, S., Goto, K., Ogawa, T., et al. (1984). Pharmacological characterization of novel mammalian tachykinin a and neurokinin b. Neurosci. Res. 2:97–104.

56. Maggio, J. E., Sandberg, B. E. B., Bradley, C. V., et al. (1983). Substance K: a novel tachykinin in mammalian spinal cord. In: Substance P, ed. Skrabanek, P., and Powell, D., Boole Press, Dublin, pp. 20–21.

57. Minamino, N., Kanagawa, K., Fukada, A., et al. (1984). Neuromedin L: a novel mammalian tachykinin identified in porcine spinal cord. Neuropeptides 4:157–166.

58. Hua, X.-Y., Theodorsson-Norheim, E., Brodin, E., et al. (1985). Multiple tachykinins (neurokinin A, neuropeptide K and substance P) in capsaicin-sensitive sensory neurons in the guinea-pig. Regul. Pept. 13:1–19.

59. Lee, J., McLean, S., Maggio, J. E., et al. (1986). The localization and characterization of substance P and substance K in striatonigral neurons. Brain Res. 370:152–154.

60. Helke, C. J., and Niederer, A. J. (1990). Studies on the coexistence of substance P with other putative transmitters in the nodose and petrosal ganglia. Synapse 5:144–151.

61. Duggan, A. W., Hope, P. J., Jarrot, B., et al. (1990). Release, spread and persistence of immunoreactive neurokinin A in the dorsal horn of the cat following noxious cutaneous stimulation: studies with antibody microprobes. Neuroscience 35:195–202.

62. Duggan, A. W., Schaible, H.-G., Hope, P. J., et al. (1992). Effect of peptidase inhibition on the pattern of intraspinally released immunoreactive substance P detected with antibody microprobes. Brain Res. 579:261–269.

63. Duggan, A. W., Morton, C. R., Zhao, Z. Q., et al. (1987). Noxious heating of the skin releases immunoreactive substance P in the substantia gelatinosa of the cat: a study with antibody microprobes. Brain Res. 403:345–349.

64. Duggan, A. W., Hendry, I. A., Morton, C. R., et al. (1988). Cutaneous stimuli releasing immunoreactive substance P in the dorsal horn of the cat. Brain Res. 451:261–273.

65. Duggan, A. W., and Hendry, I. (1986). Laminar localization of the sites of release of immunoreactive substance P in the dorsal horn with antibody coated microelectrodes. Neurosci. Lett. 68:134–140.

66. Kanazawa, I., Ogawa, T., Kimura, S., et al. (1984). Regional distribution of substance P, neurokinin A and neurokinin B in rat central nervous system. Neurosci. Res. 2:111–120.

67. Arai, H., and Emson, P. C. (1986). Regional distribution of neuropeptide K and other tachykinins (neurokinin A, neurokinin B and substance P) in rat central nervous system. Brain Res. 399:240–249.

68. Helke, C. J., Krause, J. E., Mantyh, P. W., et al. (1990). Diversity in mammalian tachykinin peptidergic neurons: multiple peptides, receptors, and regulatory mechanisms. FASEB J. 4:1606–1615.

69. Otsuka, M., and Konishi, S. (1976). Release of substance P–like immunoreactivity from isolated spinal cord of newborn rat. Nature 264:83–84.

70. Akagi, H., Otsuka, M., and Yanagisawa, M. (1980). Identification by high-performance liquid chromatography of immunoreactive substance P released from isolated rat spinal cord. Neurosci. Lett. 20:259–263.

71. Gamse, R., Molnar, A., and Lembeck, F. (1979). Substance P release from spinal cord slices by capsaicin. Life Sci. 25:629–636.

72. Theriault, E., Otsuka, M., and Jessell, T. (1979). Capsaicin-evoked release of substance P from primary sensory neurons. Brain Res. 170:209–213.

73. Takano, M., Takano, Y., and Yaksh, T. L. (1993). Release of calcitonin gene–related peptide (CGRP), substance P, and vasoactive intestinal polypeptide (VIP) from rat spinal cord: modulation by a-2 agonists. Peptides 14:371–378.

74. Yaksh, T. L., Jessell, T. M, Gamse, R., et al. (1980). Intrathecal morphine inhibits substance P release from mammalian spinal cord in vivo. Nature 286:155–157.

75. Mudge, A. W., Leeman, S. E., and Fischbach, G. D. (1979). Enkephalin inhibits release of substance P from sensory neurons in culture and decreases action potential duration. Proc. Natl. Acad. Sci. USA 76:526–530.

76. Kuraishi, Y., Hirota, N., Sato, M., et al. (1985). Noradrenergic inhibition of the release of substance P from the primary afferents in the rabbit spinal dorsal horn. Brain Res. 359:177–182.

77. Hershey, A. D., and Krause, J. E. (1990). Molecular characterization of a functional cDNA encoding the rat substance P receptor. Science 247:958–961.

78. Mantyh, P. W., Gates, T., Mantyh, C. R., et al. (1989). Autoradiographic localization and characterization of tachykinin receptor binding sites in the rat brain and peripheral tissues. J. Neurosci. 9:258–279.

79. Mantyh, P. W., and Hunt, S. P. (1985). The autoradiographic localization of substance P receptors in the rat and bovine spinal cord and the rat and cat trigeminal nucleus pars caudalis and the effects of neonatal capsaicin. Brain Res. 332:315–324.

80. Ninkovic, M., Beaujouan, J. C., Torrens, Y., et al. (1985). Differential localization of tachykinin receptors in rat spinal cord. Eur. J. Pharmacol. 106:463–464.

81. Maurin, Y., Buck, S. H., Wamsley, J. K., et al. (1984). Light microscopic autoradiographic localization of [^{3}H]substance P binding sites in rat thoracic spinal cord. Life Sci. 34:1713–1716.

82. Mantyh, P. W., Hunt, S. P., and Maggio, J. E. (1984). Substance P receptors: localization by light microscope autoradiography in rat brain using [^{3}H]SP as the radioligand. Brain Res. 307:147–165.

83. Schults, C. W., Quirion, R., Jense, R. T., et al. (1982). Autoradiographic localization of substance P receptors using [^{125}I]substance P. Peptides 3:1073–1075.

84. Schults, C. W., Quirion, R., Chronwell, B., et al. (1984). A comparison of the anatomical distribution of substance P and substance P receptors in the rat central nervous system. Peptides 5:1097–1128.

85. Charlton, C. G., and Helke, C. J. (1985). Autoradiographic localization and characterization of spinal cord substance P binding sites: high densities in sensory, autonomic, phrenic, and Onuf's motor nuclei. J. Neurosci. 5:1653–1661.

86. Dam, T.-V., and Quirion, R. (1986). Pharmacological characterization and autoradiographic localization of substance P receptors in guinea pig brain. Peptides 7:855–864.

87. Quirion, R., Schults, C. W., Moody, T. W., et al. (1983). Autoradiographic distribution of substance P receptors in rat central nervous system. Nature 303:714–716.

88. McLean, S., Ganong, A. H., Seeger, T. F., et al. (1991). Activity and distribution of binding sites in brain of a nonpeptide substance P (NK-1) antagonist. Science 251:437–439.

89. Buck, S. H., Helke, C. J., Burche, E., et al. (1986). Pharmacologic characterization and autoradiographic distribution of binding sites for iodinated tachykinins in rat central nervous system. Peptides 7:1109–1120.

90. Mussap, C. J., Geraghty, D. P., and Burche E. (1993). Tachykinin receptors: a radioligand binding perspective. J. Neurochem. 60:1987–2009.

91. Dam, T.-V., and Quirion, R. (1994). Comparative distribution of receptor types in the mammalian brain. In: The tachykinin receptors, ed. Buck, S. H., Humana Press, Totowa, N.J., pp. 101–123.

92. Yokota, Y., Akazaw, C., Ohkub, H., et al. (1992). Delineation of structural domains involved in the subtype specificity of tachykinin receptors through chimeric formation of substance P/substance K receptors. EMBO J. 11:3585–3591.

93. Moussaoui, S. M., Hermans, E., Mathieu, A. M., et al. (1992). Polyclonal antibodies against the rat NK-1 receptor: characterization and localization in the spinal cord. Neuroreport 3:1073–1076.

94. Shigemoto, R., Nakaya, Y., Nomura, S., et al. (1993). Immunocytochemical localization of rat substance P receptor in the striatum. Neurosci. Lett. 153:157–160.

95. Bret-Dibat, J. L., Zouaoui, D., Déry, O., et al. (1994). Antipeptide polyclonal antibodies that recognize a substance P–binding site in mammalian tissues: a biochemical and immunocytochemical study. J. Neurochem. 63:333–343.

96. Vigna, S. R., Bowden, J. J., McDonald, D. J., et al. (1994). Characterization of antibodies to the rat substance P (NK-1) receptor and to a chimeric substance P receptor expressed in mammalian cells. J. Neurosci. 14:834–845.

97. Kaneko, T., Shigemoto, R., Nakanishi, S., et al. (1993). Substance P receptor-immunoreactive neurons in the rat neostriatum are segregated into somatostatinergic and cholinergic aspiny neurons. Brain Res. 631:297–303.

98. Kaneko, T., Shigemoto, R., Nakanishi, S., et al. (1994). Morphological and chemical characteristics of substance P receptor-immunoreactive neurons in the rat neocortex. Neuroscience 60:199–211.

99. Nakaya, Y., Kaneko, T., Shigemoto, M., et al. (1994). Immunohistochemical localization of substance P receptor in the central nervous system of the adult rat. J. Comp. Neurol. 347:249–274.

100. Brown, J. L., Liu, H., Maggio, J. E., et al. (1995). Morphological characterization of substance P receptor-immunoreactive neurons in rat spinal cord and trigeminal nucleus caudalis. J. Comp. Neurol. 356:327–344.

101. Bleazard, L., Hill, R. G., and Morris, R. (1994). The correlation between the distribution of the NK-1 receptor and the actions of tachykinin agonists in the dorsal horn of the rat indicates that substance P does not have a functional role on substantia gelatinosa (lamina II) neurons. J. Neurosci. 14:7655–7664.

102. Littlewood, N. K., Todd, A. J., Spike, R. C., et al. (1995). The types of neuron in spinal dorsal horn which possess neurokinin-1 receptors. Neuroscience 66:597–608.

103. Liu, H., Brown, J. L., Jasmin, L., et al. (1994). Synaptic relationships between substance P and electron microscopic characterization of the mismatch between neuropeptides and their receptors. Proc. Natl. Acad. Sci. USA 91:1009–1013.

104. Mantyh, P. W., DeMaster, E., Malhotra, A., et al. (1995). Receptor endocytosis and dendrite reshaping in spinal neurons after somatosensory stimulation. Science 268:1629–1632.

105. Marshall, G. E., Shehab, S. A. S., Spike, R. C., et al. (1996). Neurokinin-1 receptors on lumbar spinothalamic neurons in the rat. Neuroscience 72:255–263.

106. Ding, Y.-Q., Takada, M., Shigemoto, R., et al. (1995). Spinoparabrachial tract neurons showing substance P receptor–like immunoreactivity in the lumbar spinal cord of the rat. Brain Res. 674:336–340.

107. Yokota, Y., Sasai, Y., Tanaka, K., et al. (1989). Molecular characterization of a functional cDNA for rat substance P receptor. J. Biol. Chem. 264:17649–17652.

108. Gerfen, C. R. (1991). Substance P (neurokinin-1) receptor mRNA is selectively expressed in cholinergic neurons in the striatum and basal forebrain. Brain Res. 556:165–170.

109. Matute, C., Wahle, P., Gutiérrez-Igarza, K., et al. (1993). Distribution of neurons expressing substance P receptor messenger RNA in immature and adult cat visual cortex. Exp. Brain Res. 97:295–300.

110. Aubry, J.-M., Schulz, M.-F., Pagliusi, S., et al. (1993). Coexpression of dopamine D_2 and substance P (neurokinin-1) receptor messenger RNAs by a subpopulation of cholinergic neurons in the rat striatum. Neuroscience 53:417–424.

111. Aubry, J.-M., Lundström, K., Kawashima, E., et al. (1994). NK-1 receptor expression by cholinergic interneurons in human striatum. Neuroreport 5:1597–1600.

112. Whitty, C. J., Walker, P. D., Goebel, D. J., et al. (1995). Quantitation, cellular localization and regulation of neurokinin receptor gene expression within the rat substantia nigra. Neuroscience 64:419–425.

113. Maeno, H., Kiyama, H., and Tohyama, M. (1993). Distribution of the substance P receptor (NK-1 receptor) in the central nervous system. Mol. Brain Res. 18:43–58.

114. Schäfer, M. K.-H., Nohr, D., Krause, J. E., et al. (1993). Inflammation-induced upregulation of NK-1 receptor mRNA in dorsal horn neurones. Neuroreport 4:1007–1010.

115. Tsuchida, K., Shigemoto, R., Yokota, Y., et al. (1990). Tissue distribution and quantification of the mRNAs for three rat tachykinin receptors. Eur. J. Biochem. 193:751–757.

116. Mantyh, P. W., Maggio, J. E., and Hunt, S. P. (1984). The autoradiographic distribution of kassinin and substance K binding sites is different from the distribution of substance P binding sites in rat brain. Eur. J. Pharmacol. 102:361–364.

117. Herkenham, M. (1987). Mismatches between neurotransmitter and receptor localizations in brain: observations and implications. Neuroscience 23:1–38.

118. Naim, M., Spike, R. C., Watt, C., et al. (1997). Cells in laminae III and IV of the rat spinal cord that possess the neurokinin-1 receptor and have dorsally directed dendrites receive a major synaptic input from tachykinin-containing primary afferents. J. Neurosci. 17:5536–5548.

119. Lee, Y., Kawai, Y., Shiosaka, S., et al. (1985). Coexistence of calcitonin gene–related peptide and substance P–like peptide in single cells of the trigeminal ganglion of the rat: immunohistochemical analysis. Brain Res. 330:194–196.

120. Lee, Y., Takami, K., Kawai, Y., et al. (1985). Distribution of calcitonin gene–related peptide in the rat peripheral nervous system with reference to its coexistence with substance P. Neuroscience 15:1227–1237.

121. Skofitsch, G., and Jacobwitz, D. M. (1985). Calcitonin gene–related peptide coexists with substance P in capsaicin sensitive neurons and sensory ganglia of the rat. Peptides 6:747–754.

122. Wiesenfeld-Hallin, Z., Hökfelt, T., Jundberg, L. M., et al. (1984). Immunoreactive calcitonin gene–related peptide and substance P coexist in sensory neurons to the spinal cord and interact in spinal behavioral responses of the rat. Neurosci. Lett. 52:199–204.

123. Battaglia, G., and Rustioni, A. (1988). Co-existence pf glutamate and substance P in dorsal root ganglion neurons of the rat and monkey. J. Comp. Neurol. 277:302–312.

124. Maxwell, D. J., Christie, W. M., Short, A. D., et al. (1990). Central boutons of glomeruli in the spinal cord of the cat are enriched with L-glutamate-like immunoreactivity. Neuroscience 36:83–104.

125. De Biasi, S., and Rustioni, A. (1988). Glutamate and substance P coexist in primary afferent terminals in the superficial laminae of spinal cord. Proc. Natl. Acad. Sci. USA 85:7820–7824.

126. Merighi, A., Polak, J. M., and Theodosis, D. T. (1991). Ultrastructural visualization of glutamate and aspartate immunoreactivities in the rat dorsal horn, with special reference to the co-localization of glutamate, substance P and calcitonin gene–related peptide. Neuroscience 40:67–80.

127. Yoshimura, M., and Jessell, T. M. (1989). Primary afferent-evoked synaptic responses and slow potential generation in rat substantia gelatinosa neurons in vitro. J. Neurophysiol. 62:96–108.

128. Rusin, K. I., Bleakman, D., Chard, P. S., et al. (1993). Tachykinins potentiate N-methyl-D-aspartate responses in acutely isolated neurons from the dorsal horn. J. Neurochem. 60:952–960.

129. Johansson, O., Hökfelt, T., Pernow, B., et al. (1981). Immunohistochemical support for three putative transmitters in one neuron: coexistence of 5-hydroxytryptamine, substance P–and thyrotropin releasing hormone–like immunoreactivity in medullary neurons projecting to the spinal cord. Neuroscience 6: 1857–1881.

130. Martin, R. F., Jordan, L. M., and Willis, W. D. (1978). Differential projections of cat medullary raphe neurons demonstrated by retrograde labelling following spinal cord lesions. J. Comp. Neurol. 182:77–88.

131. Fields, H. L., and Basbaum, A. I. (1979). Brain-stem control of spinal pain transmission neurons. Annu. Rev. Physiol. 40:193–221.

132. Tashiro, T., and Ruda, M. A. (1988). Immunocytochemical identification of axons containing coexistent serotonin and substance P in the cat lumbar spinal cord. Peptides 9:383–391.

133. Sasek, C. A., Wessendorf, M. W., and Helke, C. J. (1990). Evidence for coexistence of thyrotropin-releasing hormone, substance P and serotonin in ventral medullary neurons that project to the intermediolateral cell column in the rat. Neuroscience 35:105–119.

134. Björkland, A., Emson, P. C., Gilbert, R. F. T., et al. (1979). Further evidence for the possible co-existence of 5-hydroxytryptamine and substance P in medullary raphe neurons of rat brain. Br. J. Pharmacol. 66:112.

135. Gilbert, R. F. T., Emson, P. C., Hunt, S. P., et al. (1982). The effects of monoamine neurotoxins on peptides in the rat spinal cord. Neuroscience 7:69–87.

136. Besson, J.-M., and Chaouch, A. (1987). Peripheral and spinal mechanisms of nociception. Physiol. Rev. 67:67–187.

137. Kosaka, K., Hama, K., Nagatsu, I., et al. (1988). Possible coexistence of amino acid (γ-aminobutyric acid), amine (dopamine) and peptide (substance P): neurons containing immunoreactivities for glutamic acid decarboxylase, tyrosine hydroxylase and substance P in the hamster main olfactory bulb. Exp. Brain Res. 71:633–642.

138. Murakami, S., Kubota, Y., Kito, S., et al. (1989). The coexistence of substance P– and glutamic acid decarboxylase–like immunoreactivity in entopeduncular neurons of the rat. Brain Res. 485:403–406.

139. Penny, G. R., Afsharpour, S., and Kitai, S. T. (1986). The glutamate decarboxylase–, leucine enkephalin–, methione enkephalin– and substance P–immunoreactive neurons in the neostriatum of the rat and cat: evidence for partial population overlap. Neuroscience 17:1011–1045.

140. Penny, G. R., Afsharpour, S., and Kitai, S. T. (1986). Substance P–immunoreactive neurons in the neocortex of the rat: a subset of the glutamic acid decarboxylase-immunoreactive neurons. Neurosci. Lett. 65:53–59.

141. Vincent, S. R., Satoh, K., Armstrong, D. M., et al. (1983). Substance P in the ascending cholinergic reticular system. Nature 306:688–691.

142. Murakami, S., Inagaki, S., Shimada, S., et al. (1989). The colocalization of substance P– and somatostatin–like peptides in neurons of the entopeduncular nucleus of rats. Peptides 10:973–977.

143. Cameron, A. A., Leah, J. D., and Snow, P. J. (1988). The coexistence of neuropeptides in feline sensory neurons. Neuroscience 27:969–979.

144. Anderson, K. D., and Reiner, A. (1990). Extensive co-occurrence of substance P and dynorphin in striatal projection neurons: an evolutionarily conserved feature of basal ganglia organization. J. Comp. Neurol. 295:339–369.

145. Skirboll, L., Hökfelt, T., Rehfeld, J., et al. (1982). Coexistence of substance P– and cholecystokinin–like immunoreactivity in neurons of the mesencephalic periaqueductal central gray. Neurosci. Lett. 28:35–39.

146. Skirboll, L., Hökfelt, T., Dockray, G., et al. (1983). Evidence for periaqueductal cholecystokinin–substance P neurons projecting to the spinal cord. J. Neurosci. 3:1151–1157.

147. Ma, W., Ribeiro-da-Silva, A., De Koninck, Y., et al. (1997). Substance P and enkephalin immunoreactivities in axonal boutons presynaptic to physiologically identified dorsal horn neurons: an ultrastructural multiple-labelling study in the cat. Neuroscience 77:793–811.

148. Allen, B. J., Rogers, S. D., Ghilardi, J. R., et al. (1997). Noxious cutaneous thermal stimuli induce a graded release of endogenous substance P in the spinal cord: imaging peptide action in vivo. J. Neurosci. 17:5921–5927.

149. Schaible, H.-G., Jarrott, B., Hope, P. J., et al. (1990). Release of immunoreactive substance P in the spinal cord during development of acute arthritis in the knee joint of the cat: a study with antibody microprobes. Brain Res. 529:214–223.

150. Liu, X.-G., and Sandkühler, J. (1995). The effects of extrasynaptic substance P on nociceptive neurons in laminae I and II in rat lumbar spinal dorsal horn. Neuroscience 68:1207–1218.

151. Salter, M. W., and Henry, J. L. (1991). Responses of functionally identified neurones in the dorsal horn of the cat spinal cord to substance P, neurokinin A and physalaemin. Neuroscience 43:601–610.

152. Willcockson, W. S., Chung, J. M., Hori, Y., et al. (1984). Effect of ionophoretically released peptides on primate spinothalamic tract cells. J. Neurosci. 4:741–750.

153. Urban, L., Thompson, S. W. N., and Dray, A. (1994). Modulation of spinal excitability: cooperation between neurokinin and excitatory amino acid neurotransmitters. TINS 17:432–438.

154. Chapman, V., and Dickenson, A. H. (1993). The effect of intrathecal administration of RP 67580, a potent neurokinin 1 antagonist on nociceptive transmission in the rat spinal cord. Neurosci. Lett. 157:149–152.

155. Kantner, R. M., Kirby, M. L., and Goldstein, B. D. (1985). Increase in substance P release in the dorsal horn during a chemogenic nociceptive stimulus. Brain Res. 338:196–199.

156. Nagy, I., Miller, B. A., and Woolf, C. J. (1994). NK-1 and NK-2 receptors contribute to C-fibre evoked slow potentials in the spinal cord. Neuroreport 5:2105–2108.

157. Dougherty, P. M., and Willis, W. D. (1991). Enhancement of spinothalamic neuron responses to chemical and mechanical stimuli following combined micro-

ionophoretic application of *N*-methyl-D-aspartate and substance P. Pain 47:85–93.

158. Dougherty, P. M., Palacek, J., Palaceková, V., et al. (1995). Infusion of substance P or neurokinin A by microdialysis alters responses of primate spinothalamic tract neurons to cutaneous stimuli and to iontophoretically released amino acids. Pain 61:411–425.

159. Heppenstall, P. A., and Fleetwood-Walker, S. M. (1996). Mediators of tachykinin-NMDA interactions in nociception. J. Physiol. 495:15.

160. Headley, P. M., Chitz, B. A., and Cumberbatch, M. J. (1996). Interactions between neuropeptides and excitatory amino acids in vivo. J. Physiol. 495:13.

161. Schaible, H,-G. (1996). Changes in spinal processing of nociception during peripheral inflammation. J. Physiol. 495:16–17.

162. Woolf, C. J. (1983). Evidence for a central component of post-injury pain hypersensitivity. Nature 306:686–688.

163. Womack, M. D., MacDermott, A. B., and Jessell, T. M. (1988). Sensory transmitters regulate intracellular calcium in dorsal horn neurons. Nature 334:351–353.

164. Chen, L., and Huang, L. Y. (1992). Protein kinase C reduces Mg^{2+} block of NMDA receptor channels as a mechanism of modulation. Nature 356:521–523.

165. Randic, M., Jiang, M. C., Rusin, K. I., et al. (1993). Interactions between excitatory amino acids and tachykinins and long-term changes of synaptic responses in the rat spinal dorsal horn. Regul. Pept. 46:418–420.

166. Woolf, C. J., and King, A. E. (1990). Dynamic alterations in the cutaneous mechanoreceptive fields of dorsal horn neurons in the rat spinal cord. J. Neurosci. 10:2717–2726.

167. Neumann, S., Doubell, T. P., Leslie, T., et al. (1996). Inflammatory pain hypersensitivity mediated by phenotypic switch in myelinated primary sensory neurons. Nature 384:360–364.

168. Noguchi, K., Dubner, R., DeLeon, M., et al. (1994). Axotomy induces preprotachykinin gene expression in a subpopulation of dorsal root ganglion neurons. J. Neurosci. Res. 37:596–603.

169. Noguchi, K., Kawai, Y., Fukuoka, T., et al. (1995). Substance P induced by peripheral nerve injury in primary afferent sensory neurons and its effect on dorsal column nucleus neurons. J. Neurosci. 15:7633–7643.

170. McCarson, K. E., and Krause, J. E. (1994). NK-1 and NK-3 type tachykinin receptor mRNA expression in the rat spinal dorsal horn is increased during adjuvant or formalin-induced nociception. J. Neurosci. 14:712–720.

171. Smith, G. D., Harmar, A. J., McQueen, D. S., et al. (1992). Increase in substance P and CGRP, but not somatostatin content of innervating dorsal root ganglia in adjuvant monoarthritis in the rat. Neurosci. Lett. 137:257–260.

172. Abbadie, C., Brown, J. L., Mantyh, P. W., et al. (1996). Spinal cord substance P receptor immunoreactivity increases in both inflammatory and nerve injury models of persistent pain. Neuroscience 70:201–209.

173. Marlier, L., Poulat, P., Rajaofetra, N., et al. (1991). Modifications of serotonin–, substance P– and calcitonin gene–related peptide-like immunoreactivities in the dorsal horn of the spinal cord of arthritic rats: a quantitative immunocytochemical analysis. Exp. Brain Res. 85:482–490.

174. Noguchi, K., and Ruda, M. A. (1992). Gene regulation in an ascending nociceptive pathway: inflammation-induced increase in preprotachykinin mRNA in rat lamina I spinal projection neurons. J. Neurosci. 12:2563–2580.

175. Ma, Q.-P., and Woolf, C. J. (1995). Involvement of neurokinin receptors in the induction but not the maintainance of mechanical allodynia in rat flexor motoneurons. J. Physiol. 486:769–777.

176. Woolf, C. J., and Wiesenfeld-Hallin, Z. (1986). Substance P and calcitonin gene–related peptide synergistically modulate the gain of the nociceptive flexor withdrawal reflex in the rat. Neurosci. Lett. 66:226–230.

177. Laird, J. M. A., Hargreaves, R. J., and Hill, R. G. (1993). Effect of RP 67580, a non-peptide neurokinin$_1$ receptor antagonist, on facilitation of a nociceptive spinal flexion reflex in the rat. Br. J. Pharmacol. 109:713–718.

178. Björkman, R., Hallman, K., Hedner, J., et al. (1994). Acetaminophen blocks spinal hyperalgesia induced by NMDA and substance P. Pain 57:259–264.

179. Wilcox, G. L. (1988). Pharmacological studies of grooming and scratching behaviour elicited by spinal substance P and excitatory amino acids. Ann. N.Y. Acad. Sci. 525:228–236.

180. Malmberg, A. B., and Yaksh, T. L. (1992). Hyperalgesia mediated by spinal glutamate or substance P receptor blocked by spinal cyclooxygenase inhibition. Science 257:1276–1279.

181. Jung, M., Calassi, R., Maruani J., et al. (1994). Neuropharmacological characterization of SR 140333, a non peptide antagonist of NK-1 receptors. Neuropharmacology 33:167–179.

182. Garret, C., Caruette, A., Fardin, V., et al. (1991). Pharmacological properties of a potent and selective nonpeptide substance P antagonist. Proc. Natl. Acad. Sci. USA 88:10208–10212.

183. Seguin, L., Le Marouille-Girardon, S., and Millan, M. J. (1995). Antinociceptive profiles of non-peptidergic neurokinin$_1$ and neurokinin$_2$ antagonists: a comparison to other classes of antinociceptive agent. Pain 61:325–343.

184. Rupniak, N. M. J., Carlson, E., Boyce, S., et al. (1996). Enantioselective inhibition of the formalin paw late phase by the NK-1 receptor antagonist L-733,060 in gerbils. Pain 67:189–195.

185. Traub, R. J. (1996). The spinal contribution of substance P to the generation and maintainance of inflammatory hyperalgesia in the rat. Pain 67:151–161.

186. Thompson, S. W. N., King, A. E., and Woolf, C. J. (1990). Activity-dependant changes in rat ventral horn neurones in vitro: summation of prolonged afferent evoked postsynaptic depolarizations produce a D-AP5 sensitive windup. Eur. J. Neurosci. 2:638–649.

187. Ren, K., Iadarola, M. J., and Dubner, R. (1996). An isobolographic analysis of the effects of N-methyl-D-aspartate and NK-1 tachkinin receptor antagonists on inflammatory hyperalgesia in the rat. Br. J. Pharmacol. 117:196–202.

188. Amman, R., Schuligoi, R., Holzer, P., et al. (1995). The nonpeptide NK-1 receptor antagonist SR 140333 produces long-lasting inhibition of neurogenic inflammation, but does not influence acute chemonociception or thermonociception in rats. Naunyn Schmiedebergs Arch. Pharmacol. 352:201–205.

189. Le Greves, P., Nyberg, F., Terenius, L., et al. (1985). Calcitonin gene-related peptide is a potent inhibitor of substance P degradation. Eur. J. Pharmacol. 115:309–311.

190. Oku, R., Satoh, M., Fujii, N., et al. (1987). Calcitonin gene–related peptide promotes mechanical nociception by potentiating release of substance P from the spinal dorsal horn in rats. Brain Res. 403:350–354.

191. Kangrga, I., and Randic, M. (1990). Tachykinins and calcitonin gene–related peptide enhance release of endogenous glutamate and aspartate from the rat spinal dorsal horn slice. J. Neurosci. 10:2026–2038.

192. Gamse, R., and Saria, A. (1985). Potentiation of tachykinin-induced plasma protein extravasation by calcitonin gene–related peptide. Eur. J. Pharmacol. 114:61–66.

193. Henry, J. L. (1976). Effects of substance P on functionally identified units in cat spinal cord. Brain Res. 114:439–451.

194. Nowak, L. M., and MacDonald, R. L. (1982). Substance P: ionic basis for depolarizing responses of mouse spinal cord neurons in cell culture. J. Neurosci. 2:1119–1128.

195. Lynn, B., and Hunt, S. P. (1984). Afferent C-fibres: physiological and biochemical correlations. TINS 7:186–188.

196. Iversen, L. L., Jessell, T., and Kanazawa, I. (1976). Release and metabolism of substance P in rat hypothalamus. Nature 264:81–83.

197. Segawa, T., Nakata, Y., Yajima, H., et al. (1977). Further observation of the lack of active uptake system for substance P in the central nervous system. Jpn. J. Pharmacol. 27:573–580.

198. Nakata, Y., Kusaka, Y., Yajima, H., et al. (1981). Active uptake of substance P carboxy-terminal heptapeptide (5-11) into rat brain and rabbit spinal cord slices. J. Neurochem. 37:1529–1534.

199. Matsas, R., Kenny, A. J., and Turner, A. J. (1984). The metabolism of neuropeptides: the hydrolysis of peptides, including enkephalins, tachykinins and their analogues, by endopeptidase-24.11. Biochem. J. 223:433–440.

200. Hall, M. E., Miley, F., and Stewart, J. M. (1989). The role of enzymatic processing in the biological actions of substance P. Peptides 10:895–901.

201. Pollard, H., Bouthenet, M. L., Moreau, J., et al. (1989). Detailed immunoautoradiographic mapping of enkephalinase (EC 3.4.24.11) in rat central nervous

system: comparison with enkephalins and substance P. Neuroscience 30:339–376.

202. Chubb, I. W., Hodgson, A. J., and White, G. H. (1980). Acetylcholinesterase hydrolyzes substance P. Neuroscience 5:2065–2072.

203. Benuck, M., Grynbaum, A., and Marks, N. (1977). Breakdown of somatostatin and substance P by cathepsin D purified from calf brain by affinity chromatography. Brain Res. 143:181–185.

204. Lee, C.-M., Sandberg, B. E. B., Hanley, M. R., et al. (1981). Purification and characterisation of a membrane-bound substance-P-degrading enzyme from human brain. Eur. J. Biochem. 114:315–327.

205. Laufer, R., Ewenson, A., Gilon, C., et al. (1985). Inhibition of substance P degradation in rat brain preparations by peptide hydroxamic acids. Eur. J. Biochem. 150:135–140.

206. Probert, L., and Hanley, M. R. (1987). The immunocytochemical localisation of "substance-P–degrading enzyme" within the rat spinal cord. Neurosci. Lett. 78:132–137.

207. Taylor, C. W., Merritt, J. E., Putney, J. W., et al. (1986). A guanine nucleotide–dependent regulatory protein couples substance P receptors to phospholipase C in rat parotid gland. Biochem. Biophys. Res. Commun. 136:362–368.

208. Suh, P. G., Ryu, S. H., Moon, K. H., et al. (1988). Inositol phospholipid–specific phospholipase-C–complete cDNA and protein sequences and sequence homology to tyrosine kinase–related oncogene products. Proc. Natl. Acad. Sci. USA 85:5419–5423.

209. Reeh, S. G., Suh, P. G., Ryu, S. H., et al. (1989). Studies of inositol phospholipid specific phospholipase-C. Science 244:546–550.

210. Berridge, M. J., and Irvine, R. F. (1989). Inositol phosphates and cell signalling. Nature 341:197–205.

211. Berridge, M. J. (1993). Inositol trisphosphate and calcium signalling. Nature 361:315–325.

212. Mantyh, P. W., Pinnock, R. D., Downes, C. P., et al. (1984). Correlation between inositol phospholipid hydrolysis and substance P receptors in rat CNS. Nature 309:795–797.

213. Torrens, Y., Daguet de Montety, M. C., El Etr, M., et al. (1989). Tachykinin receptors of the NK-1 type (substance P) coupled positively to phospholipase C on cortical astrocytes from newborn mouse in primary culture. J. Neurochem. 52:1913–1918.

214. Supattapone, S., Worley, P. F., Baraban, J. M., et al. (1988). Solubilization, purification, and characterization of an inositol trisphosphate receptor. J. Biol. Chem. 263:1530–1534.

215. Womack, M. D., MacDermott, A. B., and Jessell, T. M. (1988). Sensory transmitters regulate intracellular calcium in dorsal horn neurons. Nature 334:351–353.

216. Bury, R. W., and Mashford, M. L. (1976). Biological activity of C-terminal partial sequences of substance P. J. Med. Chem. 19:854–856.

217. Piercey, M. F., Dobry-Schreur, P. J. K., Masiques, N., et al. (1985). Stereospecificity of SP_1 and SP_2 substance P receptors. Life Sci. 36:777–780.

218. Drapeau, G., D'Orléans-Juste, P., Dion, S., et al. (1987). Selective agonists for substance P and neurokinin receptors. Neuropeptides 10:43–54.

219. Engberg, G., Svensson, T. H., Rosell, S., et al. (1981). A synthetic peptide as an antagonist of substance P. Nature 293:222–223.

220. Hökfelt, T., Vincent, S., Hellsten, L., et al. (1981). Immunohistochemical evidence for a "neurotoxic" action of $(D\text{-}Pro^2,D\text{-}Trp^{7,9})$–substance P, an analogue with substance P antagonistic activity. Acta Physiol. Scand. 113:571–573.

221. Snider, R. M., Constantine, J. W., Lowe, J. A., et al. (1991). A potent nonpeptide antagonist of the substance P (NK-1) receptor. Science 251:435–437.

222. Schmidt, A. W., McLean, S., and Heym, J. (1992). The substance P receptor antagonist CP-96,345 interacts with Ca^{2+} channels. Eur. J. Pharmacol. 219: 491–492.

223. Guard, S., and Watling, K. J. (1992). Interaction of the non-peptide NK-1 tachykinin receptor antagonist (±)CP 96,345 with L-type calcium channels in rat cerebral cortex. Br. J. Pharmacol. 106:37.

224. McLean, S., Ganong, A., Seymour, P. A., et al. (1993). Pharmacology of CP-99,994: a nonpeptide antagonist of the tachykinin neurokinin-1 receptor. J. Pharmacol. Exp. Ther. 267:472–479.

225. Garret, C., Carruette, A., Fardin, V., et al. (1991). Pharmacological properties of a potent and selective nonpeptide substance P antagonist. Proc. Natl. Acad. Sci. USA 88:10208–10212.

226. Emonds-Alt, X., Doutremepuich, J. D., Heaulme, M., et al. (1993). In vitro and in vivo biological activities of SR 140333, a novel potent non-peptide tachykinin NK-1 receptor antagonist. Eur. J. Pharmacol. 250:403–413.

227. Birch, P. J., Harrison, S. M., Hayes, A. G., et al. (1992). The nonpeptide NK-1 receptor antagonist (±)CP 96,345, produces antinociceptive and antioedema effects in the rat. Br. J. Pharmacol. 105:508–510.

228. Lembeck, F., Donnerer, J., Tsuchuiya, M., et al. (1992). The nonpeptide tachykinin antagonist, CP-96,345 is a potent inhibitor of neurogenic inflammation. Br. J. Pharmacol. 105:527–530.

229. Nagahisa, A., Kanai, Y., Suga, O., et al. (1992). Antiinflammatory and analgesic activity of a nonpeptide substance P receptor antagonist. Eur. J. Pharmacol. 217:191–195.

230. Xu, X. J., Dalsgaard, C. J., Maggi, C. A., et al. (1992). NK-1, but not NK-2, tachykinin receptors mediate plasma extravasation induced by antidromic C-fiber stimulation in rat hindpaw: demonstrated with NK-1 antagonist CP 96,345 and NK-2 antagonist MEN 10207. Neurosci. Lett. 139:249–252.

231. Beattie, D. T., Stubbs, C. M., Conner, H. E., et al. (1993). Neurokinin-induced changes in pial artery diameter in the anaesthetized guinea-pig. Br. J. Pharmacol. 108:146–149.

232. Moussaoui, S. M., Philippe, L., LePrado, N., et al. (1993). Inhibition of neurogenic inflammation in the meninges by a non-peptide NK-1 receptor antagonist, RP 67580. Eur. J. Pharmacol. 238:421–424.

233. O'Shaughnessy, C. T., and Connor, H. E. (1993). Neurokinin NK-1 receptors mediate plasma protein extravasation in guinea-pig dura. Eur. J. Pharmacol. 236:319–321.

234. Shepheard, S. L., Williamson, D. J., Williams, J., et al. (1995). Comparison of the effects of sumatriptan and the NK-1 antagonist CP-99,994 on plasma extravasation in dura mater and c-fos mRNA expression in trigeminal nucleus caudalis of rats. Neuropharmacology 34:255–261.

235. Bernstein, J. E. (1994). Substance P and substance P antagonists. Curr. Opin. Anaesthesiol. 7:462–464.

236. Deal, C. L., Schnitzer, T. J., Lipstein, E., et al. (1991). Treatment of arthritis with topical capsaicin: a double-blind study. Clin. Ther. 13:383–395.

237. Fusco, B., Fiore, G., Gallo, F., et al. (1994). Capsaicin-sensitive sensory neurons in cluster headache: pathophysiological aspects and therapeutic indication. Headache 34:132–137.

238. Jessell, T. M., Iversen, L. L., and Cuello, A. C. (1978). Capsaicin-induced depletion of substance P from primary sensory neurones. Brain Res. 152:183–188.

239. Bevan, S., and Szolcsányi, J. (1990). Sensory neuron–specific actions of capsaicin: mechanisms and applications. TIPS 11:330–333.

240. Allen, B. J., Rogers, S. D., Ghilardi, J. R., et al. (1997). Noxious cutaneous thermal stimuli induce a graded release of endogenous substance P in the spinal cord: imaging peptide action in vivo. J. Neurosci. 17:5921–5927.

241. Abbadie, C., Trafton, J., Liu, H., et al. (1997). Inflammation increases the distribution of dorsal horn neurons that internalize the neurokinin-1 receptor in response to noxious and non-noxious stimulation. J. Neurosci. 17:8049–8060.

242. Liu, H., Brown, J. L., Jasmin, L., et al. (1994). Synaptic relationships between substance P and electron microscopic characterization of the mismatch between neuropeptides and their receptors. Proc. Natl. Acad. Sci. USA 91:1009–1013.

243. Chapman, V., Buritova, J., Honoré, P., et al. (1996). Physiological contributions of neurokinin 1 receptor activation, and interactions with NMDA receptors, to inflammatory-evoked spinal c-Fos expression. J. Neurophysiol. 76:1817–1827.

244. Williams, T. S.C. (1991). C-Fos induction in spinal neurons by sensory stimulation. Ph.D. thesis, Cambridge University.

245. Williams, S., Pini, A., Evan, G., et al. (1989). Molecular events in the spinal cord following sensory stimulation. In: Processing of sensory information in the superficial dorsal horn of the spinal cord, ed. Cervero, F., Bennett, G. J., and Headley, P. M., NATO ASI series, Plenum Press, New York, pp. 273–284.

246. Abbadie, C., Honore, P., Fourniezaluski, M. C., et al. (1994). Effects of opioids and nonopioids on c-fos–like immunoreactivity induced in rat lumbar spinal cord neurons by noxious heat stimulation. Eur. J. Pharmacol. 258:215–227.

247. Abbadie, C., Honore, P., and Besson, J.-M. (1994). Intense cold noxious stimulation of the rat hindpaw induces c-fos expression in lumbar spinal cord neurons. Neuroscience 59:457–468.

248. Bester, H., Matsumoto, N., Besson, J.-M., et al. (1997). Further evidence for the involvement of the spinoparabrachial pathway in nociceptive processes: a c-fos study in the rat. J. Comp. Neurol. 383:439–458.

249. Bullitt, E., Lee, C. L., Light, A. R., et al. (1992). The effect of stimulus duration on noxious-stimulus induced c-fos expression in the rodent spinal cord. Brain Res. 580:172–179.

250. Willcockson, H. H., Taylorblake, B., and Light, A. R. (1995). Induction of Fos-like immunoreactivity by electrocutaneous stimulation of the rat hindpaw. Somatosens. Motor Res. 12:151–161.

251. Craig, A. D., Heppelmann, B., and Schaible, H.-G. (1988). The projection of the medial and posterior articular nerves of the cat's knee to the spinal cord. J. Comp. Neurol. 276:279–288.

252. Craig, A. D., and Mense, S. (1983). The distribution of afferent fibres from the gastrocnemius-soleus muscle in the dorsal horn of the cat, as revealed by the transport of horseradish peroxidase. Neurosci. Lett. 41:233–238.

253. Light, A. R., and Perl, E. R. (1979). Spinal termination of functionally identified primary afferent neurons with slowly conducting myelinated fibRes. J. Comp. Neurol. 186:133–150.

254. Sugiura, Y., Lee, C. L., and Perl, E. R. (1986). Central projections of identified unmyelinated (C) afferent fibres innervating mammalian skin. Science 234:358–361.

255. Cervero, F., Iggo, A., and Ogawa, H. (1976). Nociceptor-driven dorsal horn neurons in the lumbar spinal cord of the cat. Pain 2:5–14.

256. Christensen, B. N., and Perl, E. R. (1970). Spinal neurons specifically excited by noxious or thermal stimuli: marginal zone of the dorsal horn. J. Neurophysiol. 33:293–307.

257. Craig, A. D, and Hunsley, S. J. (1991). Morphine enhances the activity of thermoreceptive cold-specific lamina I spinothalamic neurons in the cat. Brain Res. 58:93–97.

258. Craig, A. D, and Kniffki, K.-D. (1985). Spinothalamic lumbosacral lamina I cells responsive to skin and muscle stimulation in the cat. J. Physiol. 365:197–221.

259. Kumazawa, T., and Perl, E. R. (1978). Excitation of marginal and substantia gelatinosa neurons in the primate spinal cord: indications of their place in dorsal horn functional organization. J. Comp. Neurol. 177:417–434.

260. Light, A. R., Trevino, D. L., and Perl, E. R. (1979). Morphological features of functionally defined neurons in the marginal zone and substantia gelatinosa of the spinal dorsal horn. J. Comp. Neurol. 186:151–172.

261. Menétrey, D., Giesler, G. J., and Besson, J.-M. (1977). An analysis of response properties of spinal cord dorsal horn neurons to non-noxious and noxious stimuli in the spinal rat. Exp. Brain Res. 27:15–33.

262. Price, D. D., Dubner, R., and Hu, J. W. (1976). Trigeminothalamic neurons in nucleus caudalis responsive to tactile, thermal and nociceptive stimulation of monkey's face. J. Neurophysiol. 39:936–953.

263. Rèthelyi, M., Light, A. R., and Perl, E. R. (1989). Synaptic ultrastructure of functionally and morphologically characterized neurons of the superficial spinal dorsal horn of cat. J. Neurosci. 9:1846–1863.

264. Woolf, C. J., and Fitzgerald, M. (1983). The properties of neurones recorded in the superficial dorsal horn of the rat spinal cord. J. Comp. Neurol. 221:313–328.

265. Mantyh, P. W., Rogers, S. D., Honore, P., et al. (1997). Ablation of lamina I spinal neurons expressing the substance P receptor profoundly inhibits hyperalgesia. Science 278:275–279.

266. McMahon, S. B., and Wall, P. D. (1988). Descending excitation and inhibition of spinal cord lamina I projection neurons. J. Neurophysiol. 59:1204–1219.

267. Rees, H., Terenzi, M. G., and Roberts, M. H. T. (1995). Anterior pretectal nucleus facilitation of superficial dorsal horn neurones and modulation of deafferentation pain in the rat. J. Physiol. 489:159–169.

268. Ren, K., and Dubner, R. (1996). Enhanced descending modulation of nociception in rats with persistent hindpaw inflammation. J. Neurophysiol. 76: 3025–3037.

269. Schaible, H.-G., Neugebauer, V., Cervero, F., and Schmidt, R. F. (1991). Changes in tonic descending inhibition of spinal neurons with articular input during the development of acute arthritis in the cat. J. Neurophysiol. 66: 1021–1032.

270. Strassman, A. M., Vos, B. P., Mineta, Y., et al. (1993). Fos-like immunoreactivity in the superficial medullary dorsal horn induced by noxious and innocuous thermal stimulation of facial skin in the rat. J. Neurophysiol. 70:1811–1821.

271. Hensel, H., and Zotterman, Y. (1951). The response of mechanoreceptors to thermal stimulation. J. Physiol. 115:16–24.

272. Burton, H., Terashima, S. I., and Clark, J. (1972). Response properties of slowly adapting mechanoreceptors to temperature stimulation in cats. Brain Res. 45:401–416.

273. Duclaux, R., and Kenshalo, D. R. (1972). The temperature sensitivity of the type I slowly adapting mechanoreceptors in cats and monkeys. J. Physiol. 224:647–664.

274. Iggo, A. (1969). Cutaneous thermoreceptors in primates and sub-primates. J. Physiol. 200:403–430.

275. Johnson, K. O., Darian-Smith, I., and LaMotte, C. (1973). Peripheral neural determinants of temperature discrimination in man: a correlative study of responses to cooling of the skin. J. Neurophysiol. 36:347–370.

276. Konietzny, F. (1984). Peripheral neural correlates of temperature sensations in man. Human Neurobiol. 3:21–32.

277. Werner, G., and Mountcastle, V. B. (1965). Neural activity in mechanoreceptive cutaneous afferents: stimulus–response relations, Weber functions and information transmission. J. Neurophysiol. 28:359–397.

278. Nathan, P. W., Smith, M. C., and Cook, A. W. (1986). Sensory effects in man of lesions of the posterior columns and of some other afferent pathways. Brain 109:1003–1041.

279. Giesler, G. J., Nahin, R. L., and Madsen, A. M. (1984). Postsynaptic dorsal column pathway of the rat. I. Anatomical studies. J. Neurophysiol. 51:260–275.

280. Angaut-Petit, D. (1975). The dorsal column system. I. Existence of long ascending postsynaptic fibres in the cat's fasciculus gracilis. Exp. Brain Res. 2: 457–470.

281. Angaut-Petit, D. (1975). The dorsal column system. II. Functional properties and bulbar relay of the postsynaptic fibres of the cat's fasciculus gracilis. Exp. Brain Res. 22:471–493.

282. Nehls, M., et al. (1996). Two genetically separable steps in the differentiation of thymic epithelium. Science 272:886–889.

283. Xu, X.-J., Dalsgaard, C.-J., and Wiesenfeld-Hallin, Z. (1992). Intrathecal CP-96,345 blocks reflex facilitation induced in rats by substance P and C-fiber–conditioning stimulation. Eur. J. Pharmacol. 216:337–344.

284. Herrero, J. F., and Headley, P. M. (1993). Functional evidence for multiple receptor activation by k-ligands in the inhibition of spinal nociceptive reflexes in the rat. Br. J. Pharmacol. 110:303–309.

285. Woolf, C. J., and Thompson, S. W. N. (1991). The induction and maintenance of central sensitization is dependent on N-methyl-D-aspartic acid receptor activation: implications for the treatment of post-injury pain hypersensitivity states. Pain 44:293–299.

286. König, M., Zimmer, A. M., Steiner, H., et al. (1996). Pain responses, anxiety and aggression in mice deficient in preproenkephalin. Nature 383:535–538.

287. Yaksh, T. L., and Malmberg, A. B. (1994). In: The textbook of pain. ed. Wall, P. D., and Melzack, R., Churchill-Livingstone, London, pp. 165–200.

288. Noguchi, K., and Ruda, M. A. (1992). Gene regulation in an ascending nociceptive pathway: inflammation-induced increase in preprotachykinin mRNA in rat lamina I spinal projection neurons. J. Neurosci. 12:2563–2572.

289. Abbadie, C., Taylor, B. K., Peterson, M. A., et al. (1997). Differential contribution of the two phases of the formalin test to the pattern of c-*fos* expression in the rat spinal cord: studies with remifentanil and lidocaine. Pain 69:101–110.

290. Bozic, C. R., Lu, B., Höpken, U. E., et al. (1996). Neurogenic amplification of immune complex inflammation. Science 273:1722–1725.

291. Rubinstein, M., et al. (1996). Absence of opioid stress-induced analgesia in mice lacking β-endorphin by site-directed mutagenesis. Proc. Natl. Acad. Sci. USA 93:3995–4000.

292. Marek, P., Mogil, J. S., Sternberg, W. F., et al. (1992). N-Methyl-D-aspartic acid (NMDA) receptor antagonist MK-801 blocks non-opioid stress-induced analgesia. II. Comparison across three swim-stress paradigms in selectively bred mice. Brain Res. 578:197–202.

293. Vanderah, T. W., et al. (1992). Mediation of swim-stress antinociception by the opioid *delta*$_2$ receptor in the mouse. J. Pharmacol. Exp. Ther. 262:190–197.

294. Jessell, T. M., and Iversen, L. L. (1977). Opiate analgesics inhibit substance P release from rat trigeminal nucleus. Nature 268:549–551.

295. Siegel, A., Schubert, K., and Shaiku, M. B. (1995). Neurochemical mechanisms underlying amygdaloid modulation of aggressive-behaviour in the cat. Aggressive Behav. 21:49–62.

296. Cao, Y. Q., et al. (1998). Primary afferent tachykinins are required to experience moderate to intense pain. Nature 392:390–394.

297. Zimmer, A., et al. (1998). Hypoalgesia in mice with a targeted deletion of the tachykinin 1 gene. Proc. Natl. Acad. Sci. USA 95:2630–2635.

298. File, S. E. (1997). Anxiolytic action of a neurokinin 1 receptor antagonist in the social interaction test. Pharmacol. Biochem. Behav. 58:747–752.

299. Culman, J., and Unger, T. (1995). Central tachykinins: mediators of defence reaction and stress reactions. Can. J. Physiol. Pharmacol. 73: 885–891.

300. Ikeda, K., Miyata, K., Orita, A., Kubota, H., Yamada, T., and Tomioka, K. (1995). RP67580, a neurokinin 1 receptor antagonist, decreased restraint stress-induced defaecation in rat. Neurosci. Lett. 198:103–106.

301. Culman, J., et al. (1997). Effect of tachykinin receptor inhibition in the brain on cardiovascular and behavioural responses to stress. J. Pharmacol. Exp. Ther. 280:238–246.

302. Teixera, R. M., et al. (1996). Effects of central administration of tachykinin receptor agonists and antagonists on plus-maze behaviour in mice. Eur. J. Pharmacol. 311:7–14.

CHAPTER 12

Molecular Basis of Peripheral Hyperalgesia

STEVEN ENGLAND

Pfizer Central Research
Sandwich, Kent, England

12.1   INTRODUCTION

Tissue damage or infection results in a number of physiological responses. Changes in local blood flow result from the concerted action of a number of locally acting mediators. Increased vascular permeability leads to the site of tissue injury being invaded by a host of immune cells, which in turn stimulate the release of other active substances. Associated with this series of events is hyperalgesia due to the stimulation of the nociceptors, the sensory neurones that convey "painful" afferent information to the spinal cord. This orchestrated series of events underlies the symptoms of pain and inflammation well recognized by humans.

Probably the best characterized of all the inflammatory mediators are the prostaglandins. The analgesic effect of aspirin has been known for centuries, and we now know that this property can be explained by the inhibition of the cyclooxygenase enzyme and a reduction in the production of some inflammatory products of the arachidonic acid cascade. There is some controversy surrounding whether the prostaglandins are overtly excitatory, and historically, the prostaglandins have not generally been regarded as nociceptive when applied alone. However, the sensitizing effect of this type of substance is well recognized, and the algogenic actions of agents such as 5-hydroxytryptamine (5-HT) and bradykinin are markedly enhanced when applied together with a prostaglandin. Surprisingly, the precise mechanism of action of the prostaglandins in enhancing sensory neuron excitability is unclear.

Molecular Basis of Pain Induction, Edited by John N. Wood
ISBN 0-471-34607-1   Copyright © 2000 by Wiley-Liss, Inc. All rights reserved.

However, recent studies have shown that alterations in the function of a number of ion channels expressed by sensory neurons, especially voltage-gated sodium channel activity, may underlie the cellular mode of action of some prostanoids. This review aims to summarize the current state of knowledge regarding the cellular basis for the nociceptive properties of the prostaglandins. The focus is largely on the effects of prostaglandin E_2 (PGE_2), since this is the most widely studied of this group of mediators.

12.2 PGE_2 ACTION ON SENSORY NEURONS

Historically, the prostaglandins have not been regarded as overtly excitatory when applied in the absence of other pronociceptive agents, and there are many examples in the literature. The intradermal injection of PGE_1 or PGE_2 into human skin does not evoke a sensation of pain, despite producing a pronounced wheal and flare response.[1] In the neonatal rat, isolated spinal cord-tail preparation (where ventral root potentials are measured as an indirect indicator of sensory neuron activation) PGE_2 application also failed to evoke a response.[2] PGE_2 has been shown to excite polymodal nociceptors in canine testicular afferents only at very high concentrations.[3,4] Such studies have led to the belief that prostaglandins are not able to activate sensory neurons directly. However, a number of studies both in vivo and in vitro have shown that under certain experimental conditions, PGE_2 and PGI_2 can excite nociceptors. In monkeys, PGE_2 applied subcutaneously to the tail produced a thermal allodynia,[5] while in the rat paw, PGE_2 alone evoked a mechanical hyperalgesia.[6,7] These in vivo studies do not provide compelling evidence for the direct effects of the prostaglandins since the local application of these agents almost certainly provokes the release of other inflammatory mediators. More convincing evidence has emerged from simpler experimental systems.

Sections of vagus nerve isolated from the rat and mounted in a "grease gap" recording apparatus give robust depolarizations in response to exogenously applied E-type prostaglandins (Fig. 12.1A). The sciatic and saphenous nerves are also depolarized by PGE_2 (S. England, unpublished observations). It is not clear from this type of preparation which fibers are depolarized since the nerve trunks contains axons other than those originating from the dorsal root ganglia. However, in identified single Aδ fibers teased from rat saphenous nerve, administration of PGE_2 increased the frequency of spontaneous firing.[8]

Extending these observations to the single-cell level, 1-μM PGE_2 will produce depolarization of rat isolated dorsal root ganglion neurons (DRG) under conditions of current clamp, but only in a small subpopulation (ca. 15%) of cells[9] (Fig. 12.1B). Data from studies where populations of single DRG neurons have been used also support a direct excitatory effect of some

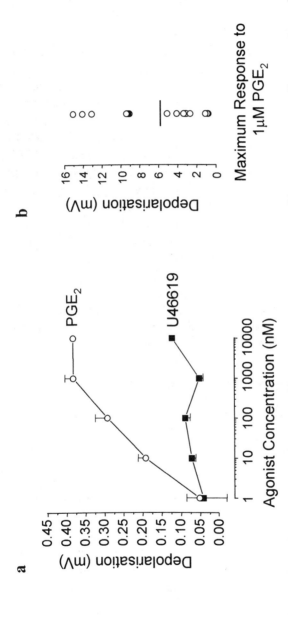

Figure 12.1 (A) PGE_2-dependent depolarization of rat vagus nerve. Vagus nerves were mounted in a grease-gap recording apparatus, and PGE_2 or U46619 (A thromboxane A_2-mimetic) added at 15-min intervals. PGE_2, but not U46619 produced a concentration-dependent depolarization of the nerves. Data shown are mean ± standard error of the mean, from eight different nerves (S. England, unpublished observations). (B) Depolarization of rat dorsal root ganglion neurons evoked by 1 μM PGE_2. Recordings were made in current-clamp mode, and the plot shows the maximum depolarization recorded from 17 responsive cells. The bar indicates the mean response.

263

prostaglandins. Using a substance P release assay from avian sensory neurons in culture, 1- and 5-μM PGE_2 has been shown to increase neuropeptide release by two- and fourfold respectively.[10] PGI_2 also evoked neuropeptide release in the same preparation.[11] In each of these studies the precise mechanism of action of the prostaglandins in evoking overt excitation of sensory neurons has not been investigated further. However, a clearer picture emerges when one considers the sensitizing actions of prostaglandins.

There are many examples in the literature both in vivo and in vitro, demonstrating that the responsiveness of sensory neurons to some nociceptive agents is increased dramatically when these agents are administered in the presence of a prostaglandin. For example, in the rat ankle joint, bradykinin-evoked hyperalgesia was markedly enhanced when applied in the presence of PGE_2.[12] In the neonatal rat isolated spinal cord tail preparation, bradykinin-evoked excitation of the primary afferents was enhanced by both PGE_2 and PGI_2,[2] while a similar effect was observed in canine testicular afferents.[3,4] In these examples, sensitization is apparent in experimental preparations that clearly include cell types other than sensory neurons. However, potentiation of the excitatory action of bradykinin on sensory neurons by PGE_2 has also been observed at the single-cell level.[13] In rat DRG neurons, the bradykinin-evoked increase in action potential frequency was increased when applied with PGE_2.[14,15] As well as cross-sensitization between these two inflammatory mediators, there is evidence to suggest that the algogenic and inflammatory actions of bradykinin are due, in greater part, to the local release of prostaglandins.[5,16]

12.2.1 Sensitization and Cyclic AMP

There is a large family of prostanoid receptors coupled to an array of intracellular transduction mechanisms (see Ref. 17 for review). The EP- and IP-type receptors (which have, respectively, E-series prostaglandins and prostacyclin as their preferred ligands) are positively linked to adenylate cyclase, presumably via the G-protein G_s, and occupation of these receptors raises intracellular cyclic adenosine monophosphate (cAMP) levels. It seems that the increase in intracellular cAMP is crucial to the sensitizing process in sensory neurons, since the greatest effect is observed with those prostaglandins positively coupled to adenylate cyclase. Receptors for these proinflammatory prostaglandins have been identified on the primary afferent neurons. Binding sites for iloprost (a stable analog of PGI_2) have been described on the unmyelinated or small myelinated fibers in the dorsal horn, with PGE_2 binding sites found in the same region.[18] In situ hybridization studies have also shown that IP, EP1, EP3, and EP4 receptor mRNA is localized in mouse dorsal root ganglia,[19] but this may not necessarily reflect what is happening at the protein level. Using a transgenic approach, Murata and colleagues demonstrated that mice lacking the receptor for PGI$_2$ showed a marked reduction in pain scores in response to acetic acid–induced writhing compared to wild-type mice,[20] demonstrating the involvement of the IP receptor in this model of inflammatory pain. With regard to other functional studies, PGE$_2$ and PGI$_2$ have been shown on numerous occasions to be the most potent of the prostanoids at enhancing primary afferent excitability both in vivo and in vitro.

In the neonatal rat spinal cord-tail preparation, PGE$_2$ and PGI$_2$ increased the responsiveness of the sensory neurons to capsaicin, bradykinin, and submaximal thermal stimulation, whereas PGF$_{2\alpha}$ was less effective.[2] Receptors for PGD$_2$ are also coupled positively to adenylate cyclase, but interestingly, this prostaglandin was without effect in this preparation. Substance P release from rat DRG neurons in culture is enhanced on exposure of the cells to an analog of cAMP, and more dramatically with forskolin,[21] a direct activator of adenylate cyclase. In an adult rat model, the inflammatory hyperalgesia evoked by PGE$_2$ was prolonged by the coapplication of an inhibitor of phosphodiesterase,[7,22] further implicating the adenylate cyclase–cAMP pathway in the sensitizing process. There appears to be no involvement of cyclic guanosine monophosphate (GMP) in sensitization since application of analogs of cGMP to rat skin failed to evoke sensitization, whereas analogs of cAMP produced marked effects.[23] However, it has been suggested that cGMP may have a role in termination of the PGE$_2$-dependent sensitization. Treatment of rat sensory neurons with PGE$_2$ produced a two- to threefold increase in the magnitude of capsaicin-evoked inward currents.[24] This effect was transient but was reversed by treatment of the cells with an analog of cGMP, suggesting that cGMP-dependent protein kinase may act to oppose the sensitization produced by protein kinase A.

Thus it would appear that although under some experimental conditions prostaglandins other than those of the E and I types can excite sensory neurons, those whose receptors are positively linked to the cellular generation of cAMP are most effective. In this context it is noteworthy that the antinociceptive action of μ and δ opioid receptor agonists are thought to be due to a reduction in levels of cAMP in the spinal cord. Thus the analgesia evoked by morphine (a μ receptor agonist) can be overcome by the administration of an analog of cAMP into the spinal cord,[25] further emphasizing the central role played by the adenylate cyclase cascade in mechanisms of nociception.

12.2.2 Sensory Neurons Synthesize and Release Prostaglandins

The concept that the excitability of sensory neurons is modulated by the chemical environment or "inflammatory soup"[26] that is in contact with the neurons is beyond question. However, it is clear that the sensory neurons can themselves be the source of prostaglandins, and that release of these substances may play an important role in nociceptive signaling, possibly at the level of the spinal cord. The constitutively active form of cyclooxygenase, cyclooxygenase–1 (COX-1), like immunoreactivity is present in the small- to medium-diameter neurons in the dorsal root ganglia of rat.[27] More important, capsaicin has been shown to stimulate PGE_2 release from a rat spinal cord slice preparation.[28] In addition, formalin injected into the paw of adult rats elicits an increase in the spinal release of PGE_2-like immunoreactivity.[29] This release of PGE_2 appears to be confined to the putative nociceptors since application of capsaicin to neonatal rats (around 24 h after birth) selectively destroys the capsaicin-sensitive sensory neurons and dramatically reduces spinal PGE_2 release in response to an inflammatory insult of the hind paw at 10 weeks of age.[30] In a single-cell study, the bradykinin-evoked increase in excitability in nodose neurons was shown to be dependent on the generation of PGI_2 in the neuronal membrane, since inhibitors of PGI_2 synthesis abolished the effect of bradykinin.[31] This raises the intriguing possibility that the sensory neurons themselves may be the source of some inflammatory prostaglandins, which could positively regulate the excitability of those same neurons. The excitability of sensory neurons may therefore also be under the influence of both exogenously and endogenously produced inflammatory prostanoids.

12.3   PROSTAGLANDIN ACTION ON SENSORY NEURON ION CHANNELS

12.3.1   Potassium Currents

A subpopulation of sensory neurons, especially those whose cell bodies are to be found in the visceral ganglia, exhibits a hyperpolarizing current after periods of repetitive firing.[32–34] More specifically, the after-hyperpolarization (AHP) is composed of two distinct conductances, a fast AHP that lasts for less than 500 ms and a slow AHP whose duration can be measured in seconds.[35,36] These currents can be found only in subtypes of C cells.[35] The slow AHP occurs as a result of the activation of a calcium-dependent potassium conductance[35] and is blocked by apamin.[36] The fast AHP shows dependence on extracellular calcium in only about 50% of cells.[35]

Collectively, the AHP contributes to the refractory period in neurons, controlling the frequency of neuronal firing and is thus involved in the process of spike frequency adaptation.[37] Inhibition of the AHP abolishes the refractory period between bursts of firing, and hence the neurons are converted to a state that promotes repetitive firing.[38] PGD_2,[38] PGE_1,[35] PGE_2,[36,38] and bradykinin[31] have been shown to attenuate the slow AHP in sensory neurons. $PGF_{2\alpha}$ was without effect, while forskolin produced suppression of the slow AHP and an increase in excitability indistinguishable from those evoked by E-type prostaglandins.[38]

It is worth noting that abolition of the AHP by bradykinin may not be a direct effect of the peptide, since as mentioned above, it appears to depend on the generation of PGI_2 within the neurons.[31] This hypothesis that inhibition of AHP leads to promotion of repeated firing can explain the excitatory action of prostaglandins in some sensory neurons, especially the visceral afferents, which show marked expression of this channel (see below) but cannot explain the sensitizing phenomena in the broader group of neurons. The reason for this is a mismatch between the relatively small number of primary afferents that exhibit an AHP and the much larger number of neurons that are sensitized to PGE_2.[36,39] In a separate study using DRG neurons isolated from the guinea pig, PGE_2 was shown to inhibit I_h, an inward current evoked following hyperpolarization of the membrane.[40] However, the effect was seen in cells isolated from the nodose and trigeminal ganglia, but not in the small cells of the dorsal root ganglia since these cells do not express I_h (see also Ref. 41). Strictly speaking, I_h results from activation of a nonspecific cation conductance rather than a "pure" potassium current, but is dealt with here for simplicity. Even so, because of the limited distribution of this channel, inhibition of I_h cannot explain the sensitization phenomenon seen in small-cell DRG neurons, the putative nociceptors.

Another proposed mechanism of action of PGE_2 and other agents that enhance cellular levels of cAMP is inhibition of outward potassium conductances, which since potassium currents are largely responsible for the repolarizing phase of the action potential,[37] may underpin the excitatory and sensitizing actions of this class of compounds. Sensory neurons of the rat express a large number of voltage-gated potassium currents.[42] PGE_2 does produce inhibition of voltage-gated potassium currents in isolated DRG neurons, but the effect is marked only at relatively positive membrane potentials[43] (Fig. 12.2). It would appear that the potassium current most affected by PGE_2 in sensory neurons is the noninactivating "delayed rectifier"-like current. The more rapidly inactivating "A-like" current was largely unaffected by the prostaglandin.[44] In this study a stable prostacyclin analog produced effects similar to those of PGE_2. Analogs of cAMP also produce a small degree of inhibition of potassium currents in DRG.[45] Forskolin, which activates adenylate cyclase directly, produces more marked effects: It increases the action potential duration in chick DRG[46] and produces a greater inhibition of potassium current in rat DRG, but this effect appears to be due only in part to direct activation of adenylate cyclase.[45] Figure 12.3 shows that forskolin can produce depolarization of DRG neurons and an increase in action potential firing, but the rapidity of the response would suggest that this effect is independent of activation of adenylate cyclase and probably results from partial block of a potassium conductance.

Taken collectively, these data suggest that abolition of an AHP or inhibition of some other potassium conductances is insufficient to fully explain the

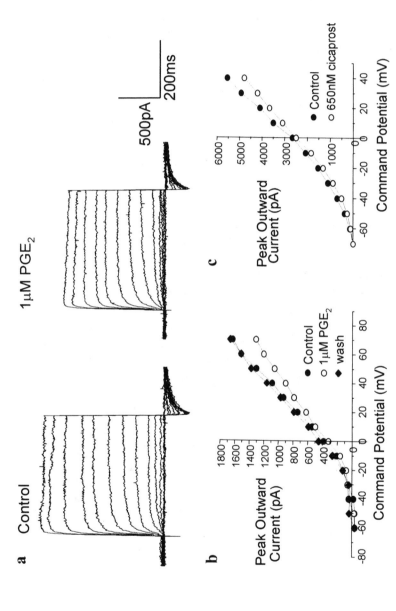

Figure 12.2 (A) Family of potassium currents recorded from rat dorsal root ganglion neuron under control conditions (left panel) and in the presence of 1 μM PGE₂ (right panel). The currents were evoked by stepping the command potential from a holding potential of −90 mV (in 10-mV increments), to potentials between −60 and +70 mV. (B) Current–voltage relationship for the cell shown in (A), together with the current recorded after recovery from the effect of PGE₂. The PGI₂ analog cicaprost also inhibited voltage-gated potassium currents. (C) Current–voltage relationship recorded from a different cell, before and during application of 650 nM cicaprost (see also Ref. 43).

sensitizing properties of the prostaglandins. However, these phenomena must contribute to the excitatory effects of the prostaglandins, if only in subpopulations of sensory neurons.

12.3.2 Calcium Currents

Not many data exist concerning the effects of prostaglandins on voltage-activated calcium currents. Calcium current in chick DRG neurons was enhanced following treatment with PGE_2 and was accompanied by an increase in the release of substance P.[10] These workers suggested that it was the L-type channel that was sensitive to PGE_2. Vasko and colleagues[47] have also shown that the release of neuropeptide from DRG neurons in culture is enhanced if the cultures are treated with the phosphatase inhibitor okadaic acid, and these workers proposed that this phenomenon may be due to phosphorylation-dependent facilitation of calcium channels. However, this effect is probably mediated at least in part by protein kinase C, since stimulation of constitutively active PKC enhances high-threshold calcium currents in rat DRG neurons.[48]

In mouse isolated DRG neurons, PGE_1, forskolin, and dibutyryl cAMP enhanced action potential duration, which these workers concluded was due

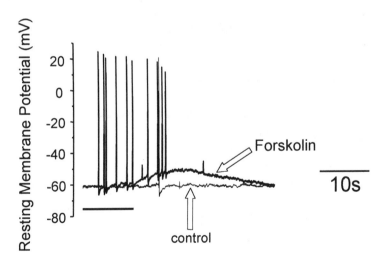

Figure 12.3 Current-clamp recording made from a rat dorsal root ganglion neuron. The membrane potential was recorded under control conditions, and during a short exposure (ca. 10 s) to 10 μM forskolin, shown at the bar. Note that the resting membrane potential (lower, thin trace) was steady at around –60 mV but that the neuron fired an occasional action potential. Forskolin caused a rapid 10-mV depolarization in the membrane potential and provoked the firing of a number of action potentials. Note also that the excitability of the neuron was enhanced prior to as well as during the depolarization phase. Small deflections are due to action potentials in the neurites. (From S. England, unpublished.)

primarily to inhibition of a potassium current but which may have involved enhancement of an unidentified calcium conductance.[49] However, these agents appeared to have a time-dependent effect such that action potential duration was initially enhanced and then shortened with prolonged drug application. This later shortening of action potential duration was found to be due to a decrease in the N-type calcium conductance,[50,51] although the effect of these agents was not particularly large. Inhibition of cAMP-dependent protein kinase (PKA) inhibits opioid-dependent prolongation of action potential duration in mouse DRG neurons, which was interpreted as being due to an increase in the calcium component of the waveform.[52] However, these authors did not rule out a possible effect of the PKA inhibitor on the tetrodotoxin-resistant sodium current. How this collection of observations concerning the modulation of calcium conductances relates to changes in the overall level of excitability in sensory neurons is as yet unclear.

12.3.3   Tetrodotoxin-Insensitive Sodium Currents

Studies undertaken 20 years ago suggested that there was some evidence for competition between prostaglandins and local anaesthetics at a common site on nerve cell membranes,[53,54] implicating sodium channels as a possible cellular target for this group of mediators. Models of neuronal activity based on the Hodgkin–Huxley equation for electrogenesis in the squid giant axon have shown that even small changes in sodium conductance can produce dramatic effects on the firing rate of the simulated neurons.[55] More important, the electrophysiological characteristics of the tetrodotoxin (TTX)-resistant sodium current mean that an increase in this conductance would lead to more dramatic effects on neuronal discharge than would a similar degree of change to the TTX-S current.[56] Recent studies have indeed shown that modulation of a sensory neuron–specific voltage-gated sodium current by certain prostaglandins and other proinflammatory mediators is probably the major mechanism for increasing sensory neuron excitability.

12.4   SNS

SNS is a sensory neuron–specific voltage-gated sodium channel expressed in a subpopulation of sensory neurons, and the molecular properties of this channel have recently been described[57] (see Chapter 6). The channel is also known as PN3.[58] For a number of years, electrophysiologists have recorded a sodium current from sensory neurons that shows resistance to block by tetrodotoxin. The characteristics of this tetrodotoxin-resistant sodium current (TTX-R I_{Na}) have been reported in detail previously,[59,60] and it seems likely that SNS comprises either all or the greater part of the TTX-R I_{Na} in sensory neurons. The link between the expression of a TTX-R I_{Na} and capsaicin sensitivity in small-diameter sensory neurons has become well established. It is the Aδ and C fibers that are thought to have a major role in the input of noxious stimuli to the spinal cord, and these fibers derive from small-diameter cell bodies found in the sensory ganglia. These fibers are relatively slowly conducting and are selectively activated by capsaicin.[61] Single-cell electrophysiological studies have shown that the capsaicin-sensitive population of DRG expresses the TTX-R I_{Na} preferentially in comparison to the TTX-sensitive current(s),[62,63] although there is considerable overlap between the subpopulations of cells. More important, the capsaicin-sensitive population of sensory neurons is that which exhibits greatest sensitivity to the actions of prostaglandins.[16,39] These data therefore place the receptors for the proinflammatory prostaglandins and TTX-R I_{Na} (or SNS) on those capsaicin-sensitive small-diameter sensory neurons responsible for transmission of nociceptive information. In addition to a possible role in inflammatory pain states, a recent study has suggested that SNS channels accumulate at the site of peripheral nerve injury and that these channels may contribute to the hyperexcitability associated with neuropathic pain.[64] Evidence implicating SNS in nociceptive signal processing is therefore mounting.

Recently, evidence for a further TTX-R sodium channel in small-diameter sensory neurons has been obtained.[65,66] This channel may underlie some of the TTX-R currents observed in DRG neurons in culture.[67] However, given the claimed electrophysiological properties of this channel named NaN or SNS2,[66] it seems unlikely that it contributes greatly to excitability in DRG neurons, since at around the resting membrane potential of the cell the channel is largely inactivated.

12.4.1   Electrophysiological Evidence for Modulation of SNS

Application of 1-μM PGE_2 to neonatal rat DRG under conditions of current clamp produces two major effects. First, there is a reduction in the threshold for firing of action potentials, and second, there can be conversion from a rapidly adapting mode (i.e., single action potentials or short bursts of spikes) to prolonged and sustained trains of action potentials[43] (Fig. 12.4). Because of the expression of high levels of the tetrodotoxin-resistant sodium channel in some sensory neurons, this behavior (i.e., the increased excitability in response to PGE_2) is apparent even in the presence of tetrodotoxin. This demonstrates two important points: First, that sensory neurons can utilize TTX-R I_{Na} for repetitive firing, at least under experimental conditions, and second, that the excitatory action of PGE_2 does not depend on an interaction with the TTX-sensitive sodium channel(s). In addition, the increased excitability evoked by the prostaglandin is not accompanied by any dramatic change in

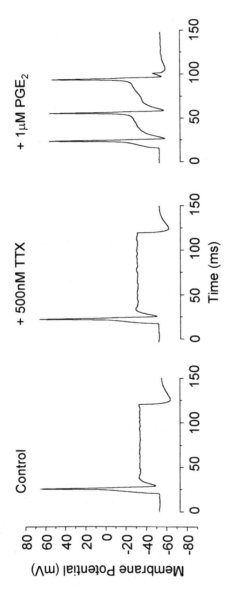

Figure 12.4 Current-clamp recording from a rat dorsal root ganglion neuron. The left-hand panel shows a recording where a single action potential was evoked in response to the injection of 100 pA of current. The center panel shows a record from the same cell using the same clamp protocol, but in this instance 500 nM tetrodotoxin was included in the extracellular medium. Note that the cell remains able to fire an action potential in response to the same degree of current injection, because of the expression of the tetrodotoxin-resistant sodium channel by the neuron. The right panel shows the increase in excitability in response to 1 μM PGE$_2$, in the presence of extracellular tetrodotoxin. The increase in firing frequency was not accompanied by depolarization in the membrane potential nor by a significant broadening in the spike width. (See also Ref. 43.)

the width of the individual spikes, as may be expected if there was significant inhibition of the potassium conductances responsible for the repolarizing or falling phase of the action potential. Investigation of the effect of PGE_2 on TTX-R I_{Na} under voltage-clamp conditions showed that the prostaglandin produced a number of important effects. Most noticeable is a modest increase (of about 15%) in the maximal amplitude of TTX-R I_{Na}, but on plotting the current–voltage (I–V) relationship for the current, a hyperpolarizing shift in the relationship for the current is also apparent (Fig. 12.5). This leftward shift presumably reflects an increase in the voltage sensitivity of the channel. It is easy to understand why the sensory neurons become so excitable in response to PGE_2 when one considers that at potentials just positive to the threshold for activation of TTX-R I_{Na}, the size of the currents may be

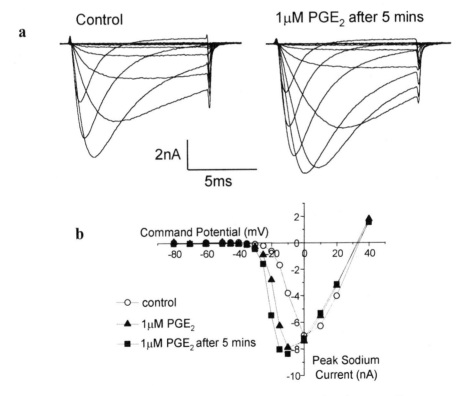

Figure 12.5 Whole-cell voltage-clamp recordings from a rat dorsal root ganglion neuron. (A) Families of tetrodotoxin-resistant sodium currents recorded under control conditions and in the presence of 1 μM PGE_2. Currents were evoked in the continued presence of tetrodotoxin by stepwise increments in the command potential from a holding potential of –90 mV, to potentials between –80 and +40 mV. (B) Current–voltage relationship for the cell in (A). PGE_2 caused a modest increase in the peak amplitude of the current and a hyperpolarizing shift in the peak current of approximately 15 mV.

increased four- to sixfold. The effect of PGE_2 can be mimicked by an analog of cAMP and by forskolin, implicating cAMP in the effect on TTX-R I_{Na}. In addition, prior treatment of the DRG by an analog of cAMP abolishes the effect of subsequent exposure to PGE_2, suggesting a common intracellular mechanism of action. As may be expected, protein kinase A (PKA) was also involved in this pathway, since intracellular perfusion of neurons with a peptide inhibitor of PKA blocked the effect of PGE_2 on TTX-R I_{Na}.

In a similar study using adult rat DRG, PGE_2 caused similar effects to those detailed above.[68] Moreover, these workers also showed that the effect of the prostaglandin was mimicked by 5-HT and adenosine, but not by thromboxane B_2, an agent that does not promote hyperalgesia. The mechanism of action of PGE_2, 5-HT, and adenosine was not investigated further in this study, but a more recent study has suggested that 5-HT$_4$ receptors seem to be involved in increasing the amplitude of TTX-R I_{Na} in DRG.[69] Thus it seems likely that modulation of TTX-R I_{Na} may be a common mechanism utilized by a number of inflammatory mediators.

The findings from these single-cell studies therefore mirror very closely those from in vivo experiments. As touched on previously, an analog of cAMP has been shown to produce hyperalgesia in an adult rat model of primary afferent hyperalgesia,[70] and mechanical hyperalgesia in the rat in response to PGE_2 can be prolonged by the administration of a phosphodiesterase inhibitor.[7,22] Moreover, in the rat, PGE_2-mediated hyperalgesia is attenuated by WIPTIDE, an inhibitor of PKA.[71,72] Further supporting evidence is provided by the observation that application of 8-bromo cAMP into the spinal cord of freely moving rats evoked hyperalgesia and allodynia which was attenuated by an inhibitor of PKA.[73]

It should be noted that with these in vivo experiments it is not possible to say categorically that these agents are actually acting at the primary afferent nerve endings because of the complexity of the preparations. However, taken in conjunction with findings from the single-cell studies, it seems the most likely explanation. Support for this hypothesis comes from a recently published study. In mice carrying a null mutation for RIβ, which is a neuronally specific isoform of the type I regulatory subunit of PKA, the mice exhibited a reduction in experimentally induced inflammatory hyperalgesia, thermal sensitivity, and plasma extravasation.[74] Pain behaviors associated with nerve damage were identical in the mutant and wild-type mice.

There is therefore evidence from both in vitro and in vivo studies to suggest that the adenylate cyclase, cAMP, and PKA system has a key role in the sensitizing process involving a number of mediators. Central to the common effects of these mediators may be the facilitation of TTX-R I_{Na}. Under some circumstances this may be sufficient to produce overt excitation of the primary afferents alone, but if not, will certainly lower their threshold for firing in response to other chemical activators, such as bradykinin, capsaicin (and hence noxious heat[75]), ATP, and protons.[26]

12.4.2 Phosphorylation-Dependent Control of TTX-R I_{Na}/SNS

There is evidence in the literature concerning the phosphorylation-dependent control of neuropeptide release from sensory neurons. Using a substance P and calcitonin gene–related peptide in vitro release assay, Hingten and Vasko[47] showed that pretreatment of DRG cultures with the phosphatase inhibitor okadaic acid enhanced peptide release in response to bradykinin, capsaicin, or high-extracellular potassium solution. The increase in peptide release was accompanied by increased incorporation of ^{32}P into the neurons, but clearly, with this preparation it is impossible to ascertain which cellular proteins are under phosphorylation-dependent control, or whether ion channels in the membrane are phosphorylated, and to what extent. Experiments of this type, but including specific ion channel blockers with and without okadaic acid, would hopefully identify those ion channels associated with peptide release. From these experiments it seems likely that phosphorylation of the channel by PKA or an as yet unidentified intermediate is the primary mechanism for modulating its function.

There are marked differences between the effects of phosphorylation of the TTX-R sodium channel in DRG and other sodium channels found in the CNS. Phosphorylation of sodium channels found in the CNS (see, e.g., Refs. 76 and 77), and also those of the heart,[78] result in inhibition of the whole-cell currents, whereas activation of PKA results in an increase and a modulation of the voltage-dependent characteristics of the sodium current in sensory neurons. Phosphorylation of other sodium channels, notably the rat brain type IIA channel, which has been most widely studied, appears to occur in the intracellular loop between domains I and II of the α subunit[79–82] and produces a reduction in current amplitude.

Possibly the best to model to explain what is happening with SNS may be provided by studies using the human cardiac sodium channel α-subunit. The cAMP and protein kinase A–dependent phosphorylation of this channel results in marked enhancement in the magnitude of the sodium current, when the channel is expressed in *Xenopus* oocytes.[83] Formation of chimeric channels again pinned down the important structural determinant for phosphorylation to the cytosolic loop connecting domains I and II.[80] It may not be surprising that phosphorylation of voltage-gated sodium channels can produce completely opposite effects, depending on the channel type, given that one of the least conserved regions of such channels is the intracellular loop between domains I and II.[84]

In common with other voltage-gated sodium channels, SNS includes five serine residues on the major intracellular loop of the channel, and these are located within PKA phosphorylation motifs.[57] Recent studies[85] have demonstrated that phosphorylation of SNS by PKA in a heterologous expression system enhances sodium fluxes, providing a mechanistic basis for the in vivo effects of PKA described above. However, we still do not know whether PKA directly phosphorylates the TTX-resistant sodium channel or whether it initiates a phosphorylation cascade that ultimately modifies the channel. It will be useful to determine whether or not the kinase itself is able to modify the single-channel behavior in a manner analogous to those of the whole-cell recordings. Evidence for the involvement of an intermediate in PKA-dependent phosphorylation of an ion channel can be found in another system. A recent study has suggested that β-adrenoceptor-mediated inhibition of L-type calcium current requires the presence of a PKA-anchoring protein AKAP79, which binds PKA and facilitates phosphorylation of the channel.[86] It seems possible that a similar system may control the phosphorylation of voltage-gated sodium channels, although at present such a mechanism has not been described in sensory neurons. It is also important to note that PKC also has a function in the modulation of sensory neuron function by PGE_2.[87]

12.4.3   Chronic Modulation of TTX-R I_{Na}

Although evidence has been provided for increased excitability in sensory neurons in response to the acute application of PGE_2, it is likely that in vivo there is probably a more complex series of events. In chronic inflammatory conditions, such as rheumatoid arthritis, sensory neurons could well be exposed to inflammatory mediators for very long periods, maybe even decades. This could potentially lead to phenotypic changes in the neurons. Long-term exposure (7 to 9 days) of DRG neurons to an analog of cAMP (dbcAMP) dramatically enhanced the size of the sodium currents. The peak amplitude of the TTX-R I_{Na} was increased around twofold compared with time-matched control cultures (Fig. 12.6).[88] Interestingly, the TTX-sensitive current was also increased by a similar amount. This was not a result of increased cell size, since when the cell capacitances of the groups were compared, they were not significantly different. At present it is unclear whether this phenomenon occurs as a result of increased channel expression, or whether the channel density is similar in the two experimental groups but that in dbcAMP-treated cells there is some modulation to single-channel behavior. If there were increased channel expression, it would be interesting to see whether this is reflected at the level of the mRNA (for SNS) (i.e., increased transcription) or if the change occurred as a result of enhanced insertion of channels in the membrane.

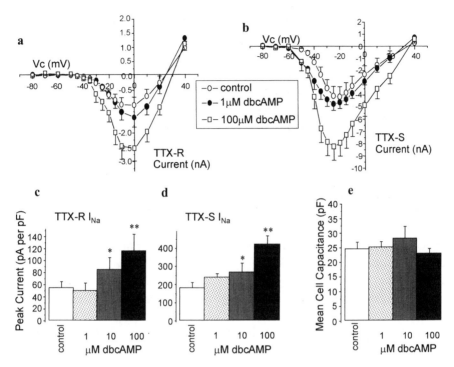

Figure 12.6   Chronic treatment with dibutyryl cAMP (dbcAMP) enhances sodium current amplitude in rat dorsal root ganglion neurons. Cells were treated with dbcAMP at concentrations of 1, 10, or 100 μM for 7 to 9 days, and the magnitude of the sodium currents compared with time-matched untreated controls. Cells were washed for at least 30 min in extracellular solution, prior to making recordings. (A,B) Mean current–voltage relationships for the tetrodotoxin-resistant and sensitive current, respectively. In both cases the currents were increased by about 110% in response to 100 μM dbcAMP. The increase in size of the whole-cell currents was not due to an overall increase in cell size in response to the treatment. (C,D) Whole cell currents represented as current densities. It can be seen that there is a concentration-dependent increase in the current density despite the fact that there was no significant difference in the sizes (as measured by cell capacitance) of the cells from which recordings were made (E). $*p < 0.01$, $**p < 0.001$, $n > 35$.

12.5   PROSTAGLANDINS AND NERVE GROWTH FACTOR PATHWAYS

At present little is known about the possible transduction mechanisms that may be mediating the cellular effects detailed above. However, signal transduction pathways also regulated by nerve growth factor (NGF) may be involved. NGF is a well-recognized hyperalgesic agent and is increased in inflammatory states. Acting via the tyrosine kinase (Trk) receptor, NGF is known to increase the expression of a number of genes in primary afferent neurons (see Ref. 89 for review).

In PC12 cells, NGF-dependent expression of the type II/IIA sodium channel was found to be dependent on the activation of PKA.[90] This activity of PKA may not necessarily involve an increase in sodium channel mRNA levels but may be important at a posttranslational step allowing the expression of fully functional sodium channels.[91] NGF also seems to be important for the expression of SNS in sensory neurons. Axotomy of peripheral nerves leads to a reduction in the levels of mRNA that codes for the α subunit of SNS, in the corresponding DRG,[92] and results in down-regulation of TTX-R currents.[93] The most likely mechanism for this is a reduction in the retrograde transport of growth factors necessary for the maintenance of normal levels of channel expression. Findings from in vitro studies tend to support this hypothesis, since DRG neurones deprived of NGF show reduced levels of mRNA coding for the α subunit of SNS.[94] It would not be surprising to find in sensory neurons a situation akin to that in PC12 cells, where there is a PKA-dependent step in NGF-dependent regulation of channel expression. While considering NGF-dependent effects on PC12 cells, it is also worth noting that NGF also enhances the expression of cyclooxygenase (type 1) in this cell line.[95] As mentioned earlier in the chapter, the sensory neurons themselves synthesize and release prostaglandins, suggesting that enhanced activity of cyclooxygenase by NGF may contribute to its pronociceptive properties. NGF is unlikely to be the only growth factor regulating the level of expression of SNS. GDNF as well as NGF has been shown to enhance SNS expression through transcriptional regulation.[96,97]

12.6   CONCLUSIONS AND FUTURE DIRECTIONS

Cyclic AMP appears to have a central role in inflammatory hyperalgesia. The increase in excitability produced by the prostaglandins results from positive regulation of some ion channels, and an inhibition of others (Fig. 12.7). The precise relationship between cAMP, the activation of protein kinase A, and effects (both inhibitory and excitatory) on the respective ion channels needs to be determined. The roles of the other kinases in sensory neuron excitability are unclear. There are some observations which suggest that PKG may oppose the effects of PKA, while the function of PKC, which has been shown to play a role in sensory neuron sensitization, needs further investigation. In addition, the cellular mechanisms involved in the potentiating interactions of the inflammatory mediators remain something of a mystery.

It is clear that primary afferent neurons express cyclooxygenase, and it seems that prostanoids released in the spinal cord may have a signaling function. Whether the peripheral terminals of the neurons also synthesize and re-

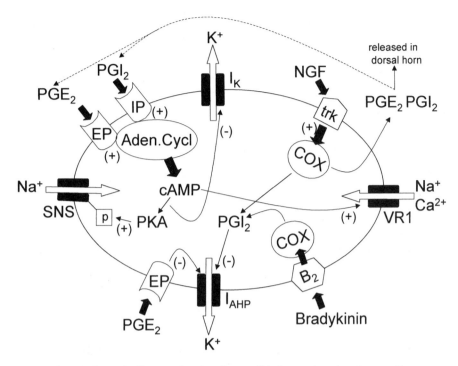

Figure 12.7 Schematic diagram showing the possible interactions in primary afferent neurons that may result in increased cell excitability. Inhibitory effects are shown (–); excitatory events are represented by (+). Some EP and IP receptors for the prostaglandins are linked positively to adenylate cyclase. Occupation of these receptors raises cellular cAMP that in turn activates protein kinase A. This pathway has a positive modulating effect on SNS and the capsaicin receptor (vanilloid receptor VR1) but inhibits potassium channels carrying outward current, further promoting excitability. Bradykinin acting via the B_2 receptor stimulates cyclooxygenase (COX), releasing PGI_2, which suppresses the after-hyperpolarization. Nerve growth factor (NGF) can upregulate COX, leading to the release of PGE_2 and I_2, which may have a signaling role in the dorsal horn. It has yet to be established whether a similar phenomenon occurs at the peripheral end of the neurons. NGF also probably enhances the expression of a number of ion channels in sensory neurons.

lease prostaglandins is not known. If prostanoids are released at the peripheral ends of the sensory neurons, do they feed back onto the terminals and enhance their own excitability? Evidence is emerging that there are phenotypic changes in the neurons in response to chronic exposure to some of the inflammatory mediators. The evidence for NGF-dependent regulation of gene expression is strong, while it is not clear whether other mediators will have a similar effect. Sensory neurons show a high degree of plasticity in respect to the expression pattern of a number of ion channels and receptors. Studies that investigate this phenomenon tend to focus on the DRG. Is there localized plasticity at the level of the peripheral terminals, and do local inflammatory and hyperalgesic agents influence the level of expression of membrane proteins in the nerves? There are clearly more questions than answers, and the control of sensory neurone excitability continues to be a fruitful area of research.

REFERENCES

1. Crunkhorn, P., and Willis, A. L. (1971). Cutaneous reactions to intradermal prostaglandins. Br. J. Pharmacol. 41:49–56.

2. Rueff, A., and Dray, A. (1993). Sensitization of peripheral afferent fibres in the in vitro neonatal rat spinal cord-tail by bradykinin and prostaglandins. Neuroscience 54:527–535.

3. Mizumura, K., Sato, J., and Kumazawa, T. (1987). Effects of prostaglandins and other putative chemical intermediaries on the activity of canine testicular polymodal receptors studied in vitro. Pflugers Arch. 408:565–572.

4. Mizumura, K., Sato, J., and Kumazawa, T. (1991). Comparison of the effects of prostaglandins E_2 and I_2 on testicular nociceptor activities studied in vitro. Naunyn Schmiedebergs Arch. Pharmacol. 344:368–376.

5. Negus, S. S., Butelman, E. R., Gatch, M. B., and Woods, J. H. (1995). Effects of morphine and ketorolac on thermal allodynia induced by prostaglandin E_2 and bradykinin in *Rhesus* monkeys. J. Pharmacol. Exp. Ther. 274:805–814.

6. Ferreira, S. H., and Nakamura, M. (1979). Prostaglandin hyperalgesia: the peripheral analgesic activity of morphine, enkephalin and opioid-antagonists. Prostaglandins 18:191–200.

7. Taiwo, Y. O., and Levine, J. D. (1991). Further confirmation of the role of adenyl cyclase and of cAMP-dependent protein kinase in primary afferent hyperalgesia. Neuroscience 44:131–135.

8. Martin, H. A., Basbaum, M., Kwiat, G. C., Goetzl, E. J., and Levine, J. D. (1987). Leukotriene and prostaglandin sensitization of cutaneous high threshold C- and A-delta mechanoreceptors in the hairy skin of rat hind limbs. Neuroscience 22:651–659.

9. Yanagisawa, M., Otsuka, M., and Garcia-Arraras, J. E. (1986). E-type prostaglandins depolarise primary afferent neurons of the neonatal rat. Neurosci. Lett. 68:351–355.

10. Nicol, G. D., Klingberg, D. K., and Vasko, M. R. (1992). Prostaglandin E_2 increases calcium conductance and stimulates release of substance P in avian sensory neurons. J. Neurosci. 12:1917–1927.

11. Hingtgen, C. M., and Vasko, M. R. (1994). Prostacyclin enhances the evoked-release of substance P and calcitonin gene–related peptide from rat sensory neurons. Brain Res. 655:51–60.

12. Birrel, G. J., McQueen, D. S., Iggo, A., and Grubb, B. D. (1993). Prostanoid-induced potentiation of the excitatory and sensitizing effects of bradykinin on articular mechanonociceptors in the rat ankle joint. Neuroscience 54:537–544.

13. Pitchford, S., and Levine, J. D. (1991). Prostaglandins sensitize nociceptors in cell culture. Neurosci. Lett. 132:105–108.

14. Cui, M., and Nicol, G. D. (1995). Cyclic AMP mediates the prostaglandin E_2–induced potentiation of bradykinin excitation in rat sensory neurones. Neuroscience 66:459–466.

15. Nicol, G. D., and Cui, M. (1994). Enhancement by prostaglandin E_2 of bradykinin activation of embryonic rat sensory neurones. J. Physiol. 480:485–492.

16. Schuligoi, R., Donnerer, J., and Amann, R. (1994). Bradykinin-induced sensitization of afferent neurons in the rat paw. Neuroscience 59:211–215.

17. Coleman, R. A., Smith, W. L., and Narumiya, S. (1994). International Union of Pharmacology classification of prostanoid receptors: properties, distribution, and structure of the receptors and their subtypes. Pharmacol. Rev. 46:205–229.

18. Matsumura, K., Watanabe, Y., Onoe, H., and Watanabe, Y. (1995). Prostacyclin receptor in the brain and central terminals of the primary sensory neurons: an autoradiographic study using a stable prostacyclin analogue [^{3}H]Iloprost. Neuroscience 65:493–503.

19. Oida, H., Namba, T., Sugimoto, Y., Ushikubi, F., Ohishi, H., Ichikawa, A., and Narumiya, S. (1995). In situ hybridization studies of prostacyclin receptor mRNA expression in various mouse organs. Br. J. Pharmacol. 116:2828–2837.

20. Murata, T., Ushikubi, F., Matsuoka, T., Hirata, M., Yamasaki, A., Sugimoto, Y., Ichikawa, A., Aze, Y., Tanaka, T., Yoshida, N., Ueno, A., Oh-Ishi, S., and Narumiya, S. (1997). Altered pain perception and inflammatory response in mice lacking prostacyclin receptor. Nature 388:678–682.

21. Hingtgen, C. M., Waite, K. J., and Vasko, M. R. (1995). Prostaglandins facilitate peptide release from rat sensory neurons by activating the adenosine 3′,5′–cyclic monophosphate transduction cascade. J. Neurosci. 15:5411–5419.

22. Ouseph, A. K., Khasar, S. G., and Levine, J. D. (1995). Multiple second messenger systems act sequentially to mediate rolipram-induced prolongation of prostaglandin E_2–induced mechanical hyperalgesia in the rat. Neuroscience 64:769–776.

23. Kress, M., Rodl, J., and Reeh, P. W. (1996). Stable analogues of cyclic AMP but not cyclic GMP sensitize unmyelinated primary afferents in rat skin to heat stimulation but not to inflammatory mediators in vitro. Neuroscience 74:609–617.

24. Lopshire, J. C., and Nicol, G. D. (1997). Activation and recovery of the PGE_2–mediated sensitization of the capsaicin response in rat sensory neurons. J. Neurophysiol. 78:3154–3164.

25. Wang, J. F., Ren, M. F., Xue, J. C., and Han, J. S. (1993). Cyclic AMP mediates mu and delta, but not kappa opioid analgesia in the spinal cord of the rat. Life Sci. 52:1955–1960.

26. Dray, A. (1994). Tasting the inflammatory soup: the role of peripheral neurones. Pain Rev. 1:153–171.

27. Willingale, H. L., Gardiner, N. J., McLymont, N., Giblett, S., and Grubb, B. D. (1997). Prostanoids synthesized by cyclo-oxygenase isoforms in rat spinal cord

and their contribution to the development of neuronal hyperexcitability. Br. J. Pharmacol. 122:1593–1604.

28. Malmberg, A. B., and Yaksh, T. L. (1994). Capsaicin-evoked prostaglandin E_2 release in spinal cord slices: relative effect of cyclooxygenase inhibitors. Eur. J. Pharmacol. 271:293–299.

29. Malmberg, A. B., and Yaksh, T.L. (1995). Cyclooxygenase inhibition and the spinal release of prostaglandin E_2 and amino acids evoked by paw formalin injection: a microdialysis study in unanesthetized rats. J. Neurosci. 15:2768–2776.

30. Hua, X.-Y., Calcutt, N. A., and Malmberg, A. B. (1997). Neonatal capsaicin treatment abolishes formalin-induced spinal PGE_2 release. Neuroreport 8:2325–2329.

31. Weinreich, D., Koschorke, G. M., Undem, B. J., and Taylor, G. E. (1995). Prevention of the excitatory actions of bradykinin by inhibition of PGI_2 formation in nodose neurones of the guinea-pig. J. Physiol. 483:735–746 .

32. Higashi, H., Morita, K., and North, R. A. (1984). Calcium-dependent afterpotentials in visceral afferent neurones of the rabbit. J. Physiol. 355:479–492.

33. Fowler, J. C., Wonderlin, W. F., and Weinreich, D. (1985). Prostaglandins block a Ca^{2+}-dependent slow spike afterhyperpolarization independent of effects on Ca^{2+} influx in visceral afferent neurons. Brain Res. 345:345–349.

34. Morita, K., and Katayama, Y. (1989). Calcium-dependent slow outward current in visceral primary afferent neurones of the rabbit. Pflugers Arch. 414:171–177.

35. Fowler, J. C., Greene, R., and Weinreich, D. (1985). Two calcium-sensitive spike after-hyperpolarizations in visceral sensory neurones of the rabbit. J. Physiol. 365:59–75.

36. Gold, M. S., Shuster, M. J., and Levine, J. D. (1996). Role of a Ca^{2+}-dependent slow afterhyperpolarization in prostaglandin E_2-induced sensitization of cultured rat sensory neurons. Neurosci. Lett. 205:161–164.

37. Hille, B. (1992). Ionic channels of excitable membranes, 2nd ed., Sinauer Associates, Sunderland, Mass.

38. Weinreich, D., and Wonderlin, W. F. (1987). Inhibition of calcium-dependent spike after-hyperpolarization increases excitability of rabbit visceral sensory neurones. J. Physiol. 394:415–427.

39. Gold, M. S., Dastmalchi, S., and Levine, J. D. (1996). Co-expression of nociceptor properties in dorsal root ganglion neurons from the adult rat in vitro. Neuroscience 71:265–275.

40. Ingram, S. L., and Williams, J. T. (1996). Modulation of the hyperpolarization-activated current (I_h) by cyclic nucleotides in guinea-pig primary afferent neurons. J. Physiol. 492.1:97–106.

41. Tokimasa, T., Shiraishi, M., and Akasu, T. (1990). Morphological and electrophysiological properties of C-cells in bullfrog dorsal root ganglia. Neurosci. Lett. 116:304–308.

42. Gold, M. S., Schuster, M. J., and Levine, J. D. (1996). Characterization of six voltage-gated K^+ currents in adult rat sensory neurons. J. Neurophysiol. 75:2629–2646.

43. England, S., Bevan, S., and Docherty, R. J. (1996). PGE_2 modulates the tetrodotoxin-resistant sodium current in neonatal rat dorsal root ganglion neurones via the cyclic AMP–protein kinase A cascade. J. Physiol. 495.2:429–440.

44. Nicol, G. D., Vasko, M. R., and Evans, A. R. (1997). Prostaglandins suppress an outward potassium current in embryonic rat sensory neurons. J. Neurophysiol. 77:167–176.

45. Akins, P. T., and McClesky, E. W. (1993). Characterisation of potassium currents in adult rat sensory neurons and modulation by opioids and cAMP. Neuroscience 56:759–769.

46. Dunlap, K. (1985). Forskolin prolongs action potential duration and blocks potassium current in embryonic chick sensory neurons. Pflugers Arch. 403: 170–174.

47. Hingtgen, C. M., and Vasko, M. R. (1994). The phosphatase inhibitor, okadaic acid, increases peptide release from rat sensory neurons in culture. Neurosci. Lett. 178:135–138.

48. Hall, K. E., Browning, M. D., Dudek, E. M., and MacDonald, R. L. (1995). Enhancement of high threshold calcium currents in rat primary afferent neurons by constitutively active protein kinase C. J. Neurosci. 15:6069–6076.

49. Grega, D. S., and MacDonald, R. L. (1987). Activators of adenylate cyclase and cyclic AMP prolong calcium-dependent action potentials of mouse sensory neurons in culture by reducing a voltage-dependent potassium conductance. J. Neurosci. 7:700–707.

50. Gross, R. A., and MacDonald, R. L. (1989). Cyclic AMP selectively reduces the N-type calcium current component of mouse sensory neurons in culture by enhancing inactivation. J. Neurophysiol. 61:97–105.

51. Gross, R. A., and MacDonald, R. L. (1988). Reduction of the same calcium current component by A and C kinases: differential pertussis toxin sensitivity. Neurosci. Lett. 88:50–56.

52. Chen, G.-G., Chalazonitis, A., Shen, K.-F., and Crain, S. M. (1988). Inhibitor of cyclic AMP dependent protein kinase blocks opioid-induced prolongation of the action potential of mouse sensory neurons in dissociated cell culture. Brain Res. 462:372–377.

53. Horrobin, D. F., Durand, L. G., and Manku, M. S. (1977). Prostaglandin E_1 modifies nerve conduction and interferes with local anaesthetic action. Prostaglandins 14:103–108.

54. Manku, M. S., and Horrobin,, D. F. (1976). Chloroquine, quinine, procaine, quinidine and clomipramine are prostaglandin agonists and antagonists. Prostaglandins 12:789–801.

55. Matzner, O., and Devor, M. (1992). Na^+ conductance and the threshold for repetitive neuronal firing. Brain Res. 597:92–98.

56. Schild, J. H., and Kunze, D. L. (1997). Experimental and modeling study of Na^+ current heterogeneity in rat nodose neurons and its impact on neuronal discharge. J. Neurophysiol. 78:3198–3209.

57. Akopian, A. N., Sivilotti, L., and Wood, J. N. (1996). A tetrodotoxin-resistant voltage-gated sodium channel expressed by sensory neurons. Nature 379: 257–262.

58. Sangameswaran, L., Fish, L. M., Koch, B. D., Rabert, D. K., Delgado, S. G., Ilnicka, M., Jakeman, L. B., Novakovic, S., Wong, K., Sze, P., Tzoumaka, E., Stewart, G. R., Herman, R. C., Chan, H., Eglen, R. M., and Hunter, J. C. (1997). A novel tetrodotoxin-sensitive, voltage-gated sodium channel expressed in rat and human dorsal root ganglia. J. Biol. Chem. 272:14805–14809.

59. Ogata, N., and Tatebayashi, H. (1992). Comparison of two types of Na^+ currents with low-voltage-activated T-type Ca^{2+} current in newborn rat dorsal root ganglia. Pflugers Arch. 420:590–594.

60. Elliott, A. A., and Elliott, J. R. (1993). Characterisation of TTX-sensitive and TTX-resistant sodium currents in small cells from adult rat dorsal root ganglia. J. Physiol. 463:39–56.

61. Lynn, B. (1994). The fibre composition of cutaneous nerves and the classification and response properties of cutaneous afferents, with particular reference to nociception. Pain Rev. 1:172–183.

62. Pearce, R. J., and Duchen, M. R. (1994). Differential expression membrane currents in dissociated mouse primary afferent neurons. Neuroscience 63:1041–1056.

63. Arbuckle, J. B., and Docherty, R. J. (1995). Expression of tetrodotoxin-resistant sodium channels in capsaicin-sensitive dorsal root ganglion neurons of adult rats. Neurosci. Lett. 185:70–73.

64. Novakovic, S. D., Tzoumaka, E., McGivern, J. G., Haraguchi, M., Sangameswaran, L., Gogas, K. R., Eglen, R. M., and Hunter, J. C. (1998). Distribution of the tetrodotoxin-resistant sodium channel PN3 in rat sensory neurons in normal and neuropathic conditions. J. Neurosci. 18:2174–2187.

65. Dib-Hajj, S. D., Tyrrell, L., Black, J. A., and Waxman, S. G. (1998). NaN, a novel voltage-gated Na channel, is expressed preferentially in peripheral sensory neurons and down-regulated after axotomy. Proc. Natl. Acad. Sci. USA 95(15): 8963–8968

66. Tate, S., Benn, S., Kick, C., Trezise, D., John, V., Mannion, R. J., Costigan, M., Plumpton, C., Grose, D., Gladwell, Z., Kendall, G., Dale, K., Bountra, C., and Woolf, C. J. (1998). Two sodium channels contribute to the TTX-R sodium current in primary sensory neurons. Nature Neurosci. 1:653–655.

67. Rush, A. M., Brau, M. E., Elliott, A. A., and Elliott, J. R. (1998). Electrophysiological properties of sodium current subtypes in small cells from adult dorsal root ganglia. J. Physiol. (Lond.) 511(Pt. 3):771–789.

68. Gold, M. S., Reichling, D. B., Schuster, M. J., and Levine, J. D. (1996). Hyperalgesic agents increase a tetrodotoxin-resistant Na^+ current in nociceptors. Proc. Natl. Acad. Sci. USA 93:1108–1112.

69. Cardenas, C. G., Del Mar, L. P., Cooper, B. Y., and Scroggs, R. S. (1997). 5HT4 receptors couple positively to tetrodotoxin-insensitive sodium channels in a sub-

population of capsaicin-sensitive rat sensory neurons. J. Neurosci. 17: 7181–7189.

70. Taiwo, Y. O., Bjerknes, L. K., Goetzl, E. J., and Levine, J. D. (1989). Mediation of primary afferent peripheral hyperalgesia by the cAMP second messenger system. Neuroscience 44:131–135.

71. Khasar, S. G., Ouseph, A. K., Chou, B., Ho, T., Green, P. G., and Levine, J. D. (1995). Is there more than one prostaglandin E receptor subtype mediating hyperalgesia in the rat hindpaw? Neuroscience 64:1161–1165.

72. Wang, J.-F., Khasar, S. G., Ahlgren, S. C., and Levine, J. D. (1996). Sensitization of C-fibres by prostaglandin E_2 in the rat is inhibited by guanosine 5'-O-(2-thiodiphosphate),2',5'-dideoxyadenosine and Walsh inhibitor peptide. Neuroscience 71:259–262.

73. Sluka, K. A. (1997). Activation of the cAMP transduction cascade contributes to the mechanical hyperalgesia and allodynia induced by intradermal injection of capsaicin. Br. J. Pharmacol. 122:1165–1173.

74. Malmberg, A. B., Brandon, E. P., Idzerda, R. L., Liu, H., McKnight, G. S., and Basbaum, A. J. (1997). Diminished inflammation and nociceptive pain with preservation of neuropathic pain in mice with a targeted mutation of the type I regulatory subunit of cAMP-dependent protein kinase. J. Neurosci. 17:7462–7470.

75. Caterina, M. J., Schumacher, M. A., Tominaga, M., Rosen, T. A., Levine, J. D., and Julius, D. (1997). The capsaicin receptor: a heat-activated ion channel in the pain pathway. Nature 389:816–824.

76. Li, M., West, J. W., Lai, Y., Scheuer, T., and Catterall, W. A. (1992). Functional modulation of brain sodium channels by cAMP-dependent phosphorylation. Neuron 8:1151–1159.

77. Schiffman, S. N., Lledo, P.-M., and Vincent, J.-D. (1995). Dopamine D1 receptor modulates the voltage-gated sodium current in rat striatal neurones through a protein kinase A. J. Physiol. 483.1:95–107.

78. Muramatsu, H., Kiyosue, T., Arita, M., Ishikawa, T., and Hidaka, H. (1994). Modification of cardiac sodium current by intracellular application of cAMP. Pflugers Arch. 426:146–154.

79. Murphy, B. J., Rossie, S., De Jongh, K. S., and Catterall, W. A. (1993). Identification of the sites of selective phosphorylation and dephosphorylation of the rat brain Na^+ channel α subunit by cAMP-dependent protein kinase and phosphoprotein phosphatases. J. Biol. Chem. 268:27355–27362.

80. Smith, R. D., and Goldin, A. L. (1996). Phosphorylation of brain sodium channels in the I–II linker modulates channel function in *Xenopus* oocytes. J. Neurosci. 16:1965–1974.

81. Smith, R. D., and Goldin, A. L. (1997). Phosphorylation at a single site in the rat brain sodium channel is necessary and sufficient for current reduction by protein kinase A. J. Neurosci. 17:6086–6093.

82. Cantrell, A. R., Smith, R. D., Goldin, A. L., Scheuer, T., and Catterall, W. A. (1997). Dopaminergic modulation of sodium current in hippocampal neurons via

cAMP-dependent phosphorylation of specific sites in the sodium channel α-subunit. J. Neurosci. 17:7330–7338.

83. Frohnweiser, B., Chen, L.-Q., Schreibmayer, W., and Kallen, R. G. (1997). Modulation of the human cardiac sodium channel α-subunit by cAMP-dependent protein kinase and the responsible sequence domain. J. Physiol. 498.2:309–318.

84. Cohen, S. A., and Barchi, R. L. (1993). Voltage-dependent sodium channels. Int. Rev. Cytol. 137C:55–103.

85. Fitzgerald, E., Okuse, K., Dolphin, A., Wood, J. N., and Moss, S. J. (____). Cyclic AMP-dependent phosphorylation of the tetrodotoxin-resistant voltage-dependent sodium channel, SNS. J. Physiol 516:433–446.

86. Gao, T., Yatani, A., Dell'Acqua, M. L., Sako, H., Green, S. A., Dascal, N., Scott, J. D., and Hosey, M. M. (1997). cAMP-dependent regulation of cardiac L-type Ca^{2+} channels requires membrane targeting of PKA and phosphorylation of channel subunits. Neuron 19:185–196.

87. Gold, M. S., Levine, J. D., and Corea, A. M. (1998). Modulation of TTX-R INa by PKC and PKA and their role in PGE_2 induced sensitization of rat sensory neurons in vitro. J. Neurosci. 18:10345–10355.

88. England, S., and Bevan, S. (1997). Chronic dbcAMP treatment enhances sodium current in rat DRG neurones. Soc. Neurosci. Abst. 23(363.4):911.

89. McMahon, S. B., Bennett, D. L. H., and Koltzenberg, M. (1997). The biological effects of nerve growth factor on primary sensory neurons. In: Molecular neurobiology of pain, ed. Borsook, D., Progress in pain research and management, Vol. 9, IASP Press, Seattle, Wash., pp. 59–78.

90. D'Arcangelo, G., Paradiso, K., Shepherd, D., Brehm, P., and Halegoua, S. (1993). Neuronal growth factor regulation of two different sodium channel types through distinct signal transduction pathways. J. Cell. Biol. 122:915–921.

91. Ginty, D. D., Fanger, G. R., Wagner, J. A., and Maue, R. A. (1992). The activity of cAMP-dependent protein kinase is required at a posttranslational level for induction of voltage-dependent sodium channels by peptide growth factors in PC12 cell. J. Cell. Biol. 116:1465–1473.

92. Dib-Hajj, S., Black, J. A., Felts, P., and Waxman, S. G. (1996). Down-regulation of transcripts for Na channel α-SNS in spinal sensory neurons following axotomy. Proc. Natl. Acad. Sci. USA 93:14950–14954.

93. Cummins, T. R., and Waxman, S. G. (1997). Downregulation of tetrodotoxin-resistant sodium currents and upregulation of a rapidly repriming tetrodotoxin-sensitive sodium current in small spinal sensory neurons after nerve injury. J. Neurosci. 17:3503–3514.

94. Black, J. A., Langworthy, K., Hinson, A. W., Dib-Hajj, S. D., and Waxman, S. G. (1997). NGF has opposing effects on Na^+ channel III and SNS gene expression in spinal sensory neurons. Neuroreport 8:2331–2335.

95. Kaplan, M. D., Olschowka, J. A., and O'Banion, M. K. (1997). Cyclooxygenase-1 behaves as a delayed response gene in PC12 cells differentiated by nerve growth factor. J. Biol. Chem. 272:18534–18537.

96. Fjell, J., Cummins, T. R., Dib-Hajj, S. D., Fried, K., Black, J. A., and Waxman, S. G. (1999). Differential role of GDNF and NGF in the maintenance of two TTX resistant sodium channels in DRG neurons. Mol. Brain Res. 67:267–282.

97. Okuse, K., Chaplan, S. R., McMahon, S., Luo, Z. D., Calcutt, N. A., Scott, B. P., Akopian, A. N., and Wood, J. N. (1997). Regulation of expression of the sensory neuron specific sodium channel SNS in inflammatory and neuropathic pain. Mol. Cell. Neurosci. 10:1967–2007.

CHAPTER 13

Sensory Neuronal Cell Lines as Tools for Lineage and Functional Studies

DINAH W. Y. SAH

Biogen
Cambridge, Massachusetts

13.1 INTRODUCTION

The molecular and cellular properties of sensory neurons have been studied extensively in primary dorsal root ganglion (DRG) cultures. Such cultures contain neurons that exhibit many of the specialized features of sensory neurons, including nociceptive characteristics. However, the limited number of cells in these cultures represents a substantial drawback for most biochemical and molecular studies, which require more material than such cultures can readily provide. This limitation can be overcome with immortalized cell lines that can be differentiated into neurons exhibiting sensory characteristics, including expected neurotransmitters, functional ion channels and neurotransmitter receptors, growth factor receptors, intracellular proteins, and regulated genes. Moreover, such cell lines can be infected or transfected while proliferating, thereby enabling the efficient introduction of exogenous genes for elucidation of function. This chapter provides an overview of the sensory neuronal-like cell lines that have been described to date in the literature, with the focus on applications of these cell lines to lineage and functional studies.

13.2 CHARACTERISTICS OF AVAILABLE SENSORY NEURONAL CELL LINES

The sensory neuronal-like cell lines that have been described in the literature were established by fusion of postmitotic embryonic (F-11 cell line)[1] or neona-

Molecular Basis of Pain Induction, Edited by John N. Wood
ISBN 0-471-34607-1   Copyright © 2000 by Wiley-Liss, Inc. All rights reserved.

tal (ND cell lines)[2] rat DRG neurons with mouse N18Tg2 neuroblastoma cells. These hybrid cell lines exhibit some DRG-selective properties, including transcription factors, cytoskeletal proteins, neurotransmitters, and neurotransmitter receptors. In addition, voltage-gated currents, synaptic proteins, glycosylphosphatidylinositol-linked molecules, and apoptotic responses in these cells have been reported. These characteristics are discussed below.

13.2.1   Transcription Factors

The POU family transcription factors, Brn-3a, Brn-3b, Oct-1, and Oct-2, as well as Pax-3, have been studied in the ND7 subclone. These studies suggest roles for Brn-3a and Brn-3b in the differentiation of this cell line and illustrate the utility of cell lines for elucidating gene function. Brn-3b was originally identified using ND7 cells.[3] Subsequently, Brn-3a and Brn-3b were found to be regulated in opposite directions by differentiation of ND7 cells with low-serum or serum-free conditions; Brn-3a mRNA increases with neuronal differentiation, whereas Brn-3b mRNA decreases.[4] A role of Brn-3a in specification of mature neuronal phenotype was implicated by induction of neuronal maturation[5] and SNAP-25[5] and neurofilament[6] gene transcription upon overexpression of Brn-3a in undifferentiated ND7 cells, and by inhibition of Brn-3a expression with an antisense approach, which abolished neurite outgrowth in response to serum removal.[7] In contrast, Brn-3b blocks differentiation when overexpressed in ND7 cells.[8] Similarly, studies on the roles of Oct-1 and Oct-2 in regulating viral and cellular gene expression were facilitated with the ND7 cell line,[9–11] as were experiments on the possible role of Pax-3 in neuronal development.[12] Thus the ND7 cell line has been instrumental for assessing the functional roles of transcription factors in directing neuronal differentiation as well as in modulating herpes simplex virus immediate-early gene expression.

13.2.2   Cytoskeletal, Synaptic, and Surface Proteins

Hybrid sensory neuronal-like lines express proteins found in all neurons, as well as markers that are relatively selective for sensory neurons. The expression of neurofilament (200 kD), synaptophysin, and SNAP-25 has been examined by immunocytochemical staining or Western blot analysis. The RT97 antibody, which labels neurofilaments in large cells of the DRG, was reported to stain a subset of F-11 cells.[13] Monoclonal antibodies that recognize specific cell-surface carbohydrates,[13,14] such as stage-specific embryonic antigens SSEA-3 and SSEA-4, also labeled a subset of F-11 cells[13] and ND subclones.[2] Thus cytoskeletal and surface markers characteristic of sensory neurons are expressed in some hybrid cells. In addition, synaptophysin immunoreactivity[15] and SNAP-25 protein[7] have been detected following differentiation of ND7 cells, indicating that these cells express synaptic markers after induction of neuronal phenotype. Other surface markers, such as the glycosylphosphatidylinositol-anchored molecules neural cell adhesion molecule (N-CAM), Thy-1, and F3, were found on ND26 cells and regulated by differentiation.[16] These studies confirm the neuronal phenotype of these cell lines after differentiation.

13.2.3   Neurotransmitters

In vivo, DRG neurons express the neuropeptides substance P, calcitonin gene-related peptide, somatostatin, galanin, and neuropeptide Y under normal and experimental conditions. The expression of these neuropeptides, as well as tyrosine hydroxylase, has been examined in the hybrid cell lines. In general, neuropeptide expression in hybrid cell lines mirrored that in DRG neurons to a limited extent. F-11 cells have been reported to synthesize and release substance P,[17] whereas ND7, ND9, and ND21 cells do not express substance P immunoreactivity.[18] Calcitonin gene-related peptide, galanin, and somatostatin immunoreactivities have not been detected in ND7, ND9, or ND21 cell lines.[18] In contrast, tyrosine hydroxylase and neuropeptide Y immunoreactivities were expressed by ND subclones,[18] suggesting that certain properties exhibited by these clones were derived from the neuroblastoma parent. Neuropeptide Y is found in neurons of the autonomic nervous system,[19] as well as in DRG neurons, particularly in response to pathological conditions such as axotomy (for review, see Ref. 20). The presence of this peptide in the ND subclones may represent a property derived from the neuroblastoma parent, or a sensory neuronal characteristic induced by the specific culture conditions used. It is possible that the neurotransmitter expression profiles reported to date for the hybrid cell lines reflect a subset of the repertoire that they are capable of expressing and that alternative culture conditions would induce different patterns of neurotransmitter expression. Nevertheless, the evidence reported to date indicates that these hybrid cell lines do not express some of the neuropeptides normally present within sensory neuronal populations.

13.2.4   Voltage- and Ligand-Gated Currents

Action potentials can be evoked from differentiated F-11 cells.[21] Sodium, calcium, and potassium currents, as well as responses to capsaicin, bradykinin, and opioids, have been characterized electrophysiologically in F-11 and ND7-23 cells. Moderate tetrodotoxin-sensitive sodium currents were present in F-11 cells after differentiation; the biophysical properties of these currents were similar to those present in the neuroblastoma parent cells.[21] Calcium currents in differentiated F-11 cells contained both low- and high-threshold components, or consisted of low-threshold current only.[21,22] Similarly, ND7-23 cells exhibited calcium currents that were comprised of both low- and high-threshold components or consisted of low-threshold current only.[23] Thus low-threshold calcium current appears to be a more predominant component of calcium current in differentiated hybrid cells than in DRG neurons. Most (81%) of the high-threshold calcium current in F-11 cells was sensitive to ω-conotoxin GVIA, suggesting that this component of calcium current was mediated by N-type calcium channels.[22] Potassium channels in F-11 cells are coupled differently to calcium levels than those in DRG cells, with potassium channels in F-11 cells responding to lower concentrations of calcium than those in DRG cells.[24] Recently, the pharmacological and biophysical properties of the inward rectifier potassium current in F-11 cells[25] were reported to be identical to those of the current encoded by the human ether-a-go-go-related gene (HERG); thus this cell line is likely to be useful for further studies of this particular potassium channel.

Responses to capsaicin, bradykinin, and opioid agonists have also been studied in F-11 cells. Capsaicin- and bradykinin-activated currents were expressed by a subset (30%) of F-11 cells[21] at early passages; however, F-11 cells were reported to lose the ability to express these properties after multiple passages.[21] Bradykinin responses included inductions of IP3 and diacylglycerol production and elevations in intracellular calcium and cyclic GMP.[26–28] Opioid responses have been characterized with respect to radioligand binding, G protein coupling, and coupling to potassium current. These studies indicated that early passage F-11 cells exhibit conventional δ (and also μ) opioid receptors, whereas late passage F-11 cells no longer express these conventional opioid receptors, but instead, express a peptide-insensitive opiate binding site that may correpond to the μ3 receptor subtype.[29] δ and μ opioid agonists at high (μM) concentrations were reported to increase voltage-dependent potassium currents in F-11 cells, whereas low concentrations (nM) decreased these currents.[30] Opioid receptors coupled to both stimulatory and inhibitory G proteins, which were sensitive to cholera toxin and pertussis toxin, respectively.[31]

Nociceptive-specific tetrodotoxin-resistant sodium currents[32,33] do not appear to be expressed by F-11 cells, since voltage-dependent sodium currents in these cells were blocked completely by 1-μM tetrodotoxin.[21] To date, the presence of nociceptive-specific P2X3 receptors[34,35] and low-affinity kainate receptors, found in some sensory neurons,[36] has not been examined in the hybrid cell lines. Thus hybrid cell lines appear to functionally express only a subset of the ion channels and neurotransmitter receptors normally found in sensory neurons.

13.2.5 Apoptotic Responses

The F-11 and ND7 cell lines have also been characterized for apoptosis following serum withdrawal or ceramide treatment. After serum withdrawal, F-11 cells exhibited DNA laddering, followed by a decline in viability.[37] Ceramide also induced apoptosis in these cells, accompanied by DNA laddering, nuclear condensation, and a decrease in viability.[38] In ND7 cells, apoptosis also occured upon serum withdrawal.[39] Thus these hybrid sensory neuronal-like cell lines may have utility for elucidating mechanisms of neuronal apoptosis.

13.3 CONCLUSIONS

The hybrid sensory neuronal-like cell lines that have been described to date in the literature exhibit some sensory neuron–selective properties, as well as properties that are common to all neurons. The phenotypic characteristics that have been reported include transcription factors, cytoskeletal proteins, glycosylphosphatidylinositol-linked molecules, synaptic proteins, voltage-gated currents, neurotransmitters, ligand-gated receptors, and apoptotic responses. Some of these features are not stable with passaging; nevertheless, these cell lines have provided a sensory neuronal-like system that has facilitated lineage and functional studies. It will be useful to develop PNS lines that exhibit stable properties, specific to subsets of sensory neurons. Such cell lines would be even more valuable than the hybrid sensory neuronal-like cell lines for studying the molecular and cellular properties of sensory neurons.

The hybrid sensory neuronal-like cell lines that have been described to date in the literature exhibit some sensory neuron–selective properties, as well as properties that are common to all neurons. The phenotypic characteristics that have been reported include transcription factors, cytoskeletal proteins, glycosylphosphatidylinositol-linked molecules, synaptic proteins, voltage-gated currents, neurotransmitters, ligand-gated receptors, and apoptotic responses. Some of these features are not stable with passaging; nevertheless, these cell lines have provided a sensory neuronal-like system that has facilitated lineage and functional studies.

It will be useful to develop peripheral nervous system (PNS) lines that exhibit stable properties specific to subsets of sensory neurons. Human[40] and rodent[41] central nervous system (CNS) lines have been successfully immortalized with the tetracycline-repressible v-myc oncogene. These CNS lines are stable, behaving in a reproducible manner over multiple passages and can be rapidly differentiated into postmitotic functional neurons for basic research and drug discovery. The immortalization strategy used for establishing the CNS lines has now been applied to the development of human PNS lines.[42]

Such PNS lines have been shown to exhibit nociceptor properties and may prove to be even more valuable than the hybrid sensory neuronal-like cell lines for studying the molecular and cellular properties of sensory neurons.

ACKNOWLEDGMENTS

I thank David W. Anderson and Alan Lewis for their support.

REFERENCES

1. Platika, D., Boulos, M. H., Baizer, L., and Fishman, M. C. (1985). Neuronal traits of clonal cell lines derived by fusion of dorsal root ganglia neurons with neuroblastoma cells. Proc. Natl. Acad. Sci. USA 82:3499–3503.

2. Wood, J. N., Bevan, S. J., Coote, P. R., Dunn, P. M., Harmar, A., Hogan, P., Latchman, D. S., Morrison, C., Rougon, G., Theveniau, M., and Wheatley, S. (1990). Novel cell lines display properties of nociceptive sensory neurons. Proc. R. Soc. Lond. B 241:187–194.

3. Lillycrop, K. A., Budrahan, V. S., Lakin, N. D., Terrenghi, G., Wood, J. N., Polak, J. M., and Latchman, D. S. (1992). A novel POU family transcription factor is closely related to Brn-3 but has a distinct expression pattern in neuronal cells. Nucleic Acids Res. 20:5093–5096.

4. Budhram-Mahadeo, V., Lillycrop, K. A., and Latchman, D. S. (1995). The levels of the antagonistic POU family transcription factors Brn-3a and Brn-3b in neuronal cells are regulated in opposite directions by serum growth factors. Neurosci. Lett. 185:48–51.

5. Smith, M. D., Dawson, S. J., and Latchman, D. S. (1997). The Brn-3a transcription factor induces neuronal process outgrowth and the coordinate expression of genes encoding synaptic proteins. Mol. Cell. Biol. 17:345–354.

6. Smith, M. D., Morris, P. J., Dawson, S. J., Schwartz, M. L., Schlaepfer, W. W., and Latchman, D. S. (1997). Coordinate induction of the three neurofilament genes by the Brn-3a transcription factor. J. Biol. Chem. 272:21325–21333.

7. Lakin, N. D., Morris, P. J., Theil, T., Sato, T. N., Moroy, T., Wilson, M. C., and Latchman, D. S. (1995). Regulation of neurite outgrowth and SNAP-25 gene expression by the Brn-3a transcription factor. J. Biol. Chem. 270:15858–15863.

8. Smith, M. D., Dawson, S. J., and Latchman, D. S. (1997). Inhibition of neuronal process outgrowth and neuronal specific gene activation by the Brn-3b transcription factor. J. Biol. Chem. 272:1382–1388.

9. Lillycrop, K. A., Dent, C. L., Wheatley, S. C., Beech, M. N., Ninkina, N. N., Wood, J. N., and Latchman, D. S. (1991). The octamer-binding protein Oct-2 represses HSV immediate-early genes in cell lines derived from latently infectable sensory neurons. Neuron 7:381–390.

10. Howard, M. K., Mailhow, C., Dent, C. L., and Latchman D. S. (1993). Transactivation by the herpes simplex virus virion protein Vms65 and viral permissivity in a neuronal cell line with reduced levels of the cellular transcription factor Oct-1. Exp. Cell Res. 207:194–196.

11. Liu, Y.-Z., Lillycrop, K. A., and Latchman, D. S. (1995). Regulated splicing of the Oct-2 transcription factor RNA in neuronal cells. Neurosci. Lett. 183:8–12.

12. Evans, J., and Lillycrop, K. A. (1996). Serum growth factor regulation of the paired-box transcription factor Pax-3 in neuronal cells. Neurosci. Lett. 220:125–128.

13. Boland, L. M., and Dingledine, R. (1990). Expression of sensory neuron antigens by a dorsal root ganglion cell line, F-11. Dev. Brain Res. 51:259–266.

14. Dodd, J., and Jessell, T. M. (1985). Lactoseries carbohydrates specify subsets of dorsal root ganglion neurons projecting to the superficial dorsal horn of the rat spinal cord. J. Neurosci. 5:3278–3294.

15. Wheatley, S. C., Suburo, A. M., Horn, D. A., Vucicevic, V., Terenghi, G., Polak, J. M., and Latchman D. S. (1992). Redistribution of secretory granule components precedes that of synaptic vesicle proteins during differentiation of a neuronal cell line in serum-free medium. Neuroscience. 51:575–582.

16. Theveniau, M., Durbec, P., Gennarini, G., Wood, J. N., and Rougon, G. (1992). Expression and release of phosphatidylinositol anchored cell surface molecules by a cell line derived from sensory neurons. J. Cell. Biochem. 48:61–72.

17. Francel, P. C., Harris, K., Smith, M., Fishman, M. C., Dawson, G., and Miller, R. J. (1987). Neurochemical characteristics of a novel dorsal root ganglion X neuroblastoma hybrid cell line, F-11. J. Neurochem. 48:1624–1631.

18. Suburo, A. M., Wheatley, S. C., Horn, D. A., Gibson, S. J., Jahn, R., Fischer-Colbrie, R., Wood, J. N., Latchman, D. S., and Polak, J. M. (1992). Intracellular redistribution of neuropeptides and secretory proteins during differentiation of neuronal cell lines. Neuroscience 46:881–889.

19. Lundberg, J. M. , Terenius, L., Hokfelt, T., Martling, C. R., Tatemoto, K., Mutt, V., Polak, J., Bloom, S., and Goldstein, M. (1982). Neuropeptide Y (NPY)-like immunoreactivity in peripheral noradrenergic neurons and effects of NPY on sympathetic function. Acta Physiol. Scand. 116:477–480.

20. Hökfelt, T., Zhang, X., and Wiesenfeld-Hallin, Z. (1994). Messenger plasticity in primary sensory neurons following axotomy and its functional implications. Trends Neurosci. 17:22–30.

21. Kusano, K., and Gainer, H. (1993). Modulation of voltage-activated Ca currents by pain-inducing agents in a dorsal root ganglion neuronal line, F-11. J. Neurosci. Res. 34:158–169.

22. Boland, L. M., and Dingledine, R. (1990). Multiple components of both transient and sustained barium currents in a rat dorsal root ganglion cell line. J. Physiol. 420:223–245.

23. Kobrinsky, E. M., Pearson, H. A., and Dolphin, A. C. (1994). Low- and high-voltage–activated calcium channel currents and their modulation in the dorsal root ganglion cell line ND7-23. Neuroscience 58:539–552.

24. Naruse, K., McGehee, D. S., and Oxford, G. S. (1992). Differential responses of Ca-activated K channels to bradykinin in sensory neurons and F-11 cells. Am. J. Physiol. 262:C453–C460.

25. Faravelli, L., Arcangeli, A., Olivotto, M., and Wanke, E. (1996). A HERG-like K^+ channel in rat F-11 DRG cell line: pharmacological identification and biophysical characterization. J. Physiol. 496:13–23.

26. Francel, P. C., Miller, R. J., and Dawson, G. (1987). Modulation of bradykinin-induced inositol triphosphate release in a novel neuroblastoma × dorsal root ganglion sensory neuron cell line (F-11). J. Neurochem. 48:1632–1639.

27. Francel, P., and Dawson, G. (1988). Bradykinin induces the bi-phasic production of lysophosphatidyl inositol and diacylglycerol in a dorsal root ganglion × neurotumor hybrid cell line, F-11. Biochem. Biophys. Res. Commun. 152:724–731.

28. Francel, P. C., Keefer, J. F., and Dawson, G. (1989). Bradykinin analogs antagonize bradykinin-induced second messenger production in a sensory neuron cell line. Mol. Pharmacol. 35:34–38.

29. Cruciani, R. A., Dvorkin, B., Klinger, H. P., and Makman, M. H. (1994). Presence in neuroblastoma cells of a mu 3 receptor with selectivity for opiate alkaloids but without affinity for opioid peptides. Brain Res. 667:229–237.

30. Fan, S. F., Shen, K. F., and Crain, S. M. (1993). μ and δ opioid agonists at low concentrations decrease voltage-dependent K^+ currents in F11 neuroblastoma × DRG neuron hybrid cells via cholera toxin-sensitive receptors. Brain Res. 605:214–220.

31. Cruciani, R. A., Dvorkin, B., Morris, S. A., Crain, S. M., and Makman, M. H. (1993). Direct coupling of opioid receptors to both stimulatory and inhibitory guanine nucleotide-binding proteins in F-11 neuroblastoma-sensory neuron hybrid cells. Proc. Natl. Acad. Sci. USA 90:3019–3023.

32. Akopian, A. N., Sivilotti, L., and Wood, J. N. (1996). A tetrodotoxin-resistant voltage-gated sodium channel expressed by sensory neurons. Nature 379:257–262.

33. Sangameswaran, L., Delgado, S. G., Fish, L. M., Koch, B. D., Jakeman, L. B., Stewart, G. R., Sze, P., Hunter, J. C., Eglen, R. M., and Herman, R. C. (1996). Structure and function of a novel voltage-gated tetrodotoxin-resistant sodium channel specific to sensory neurons. J. Biol. Chem. 271:5953–5956.

34. Chen, C.-C., Akoplan, A. N., Sivilotti, L., Colquhoun, D., Burnstock, G., and Wood, J. N. (1995). A P2X purinoceptor expressed by a subset of sensory neurons. Nature 377:428–431.

35. Lewis, C., Neidhart, S., Holy, C., North, R. A., Buell, G., and Surprenant A. (1995). Coexpression of P2X2 and P2X3 receptor subunits can account for ATP-gated currents in sensory neurons. Nature 377:432–435.

36. Huettner, J. E. (1990). Glutamate receptor channels in rat DRG neurons: activation by kainate and quisqualate and blockade of desensitization by con A. Neuron 5:255–266.

37. Linnik, M. D., Hatfield, M. D., Swope, M. D., and Ahmed, N. K. (1993). Induction of programmed cell death in a dorsal root ganglia × neuroblastoma cell line. J. Neurobiol. 24:433–446.

38. Wiesner, D. A., and Dawson, G. (1996). Programmed cell death in neurotumour cells involves the generation of ceramide. Glycoconj. J. 13:327–333.

39. Mailhos, C., Howard, M. K., and Latchman, D. S. (1994). A common pathway mediates retinoic acid and PMA-dependent programmed cell death (apoptosis) of neuronal cells. Brain Res. 644:7–12.

40. Sah, D. W. Y., Ray, J., and Gage, F. (1997). Bipotent progenitor cell lines from the human CNS. Nature Biotechnol. 15:574–580.

41. Hoshimaru, M., Ray, J., Sah, D. W. Y., and Gage, F. (1996). Differentiation of the immortalized adult neuronal progenitor cell line HC2S2 into neurons by regulatable suppression of the v-myc oncogene. Proc. Natl. Acad. Sci. USA 93:1518–1523.

42. Raymon, H. K., Thode, S., Zhou, J., Friedman, G. L., Pardinas, J. R., Barrere, C., Johnson, R. M., and Sah, D. W. Y. (1999). Immortalized human DRG cells differentiate into neurons with nociceptive properties. J. Neurosci. 19:5420–5428.